Behavioural Distress

KT-486-608

COLLEGE

Please return this book

- if re

WITHDRAWN

3   JUN 2024

York St. John College

3 8025 00451467 8

For Baillière Tindall:

Senior Commissioning Editor: Jacqueline Curthoys
Project Development Manager: Karen Gilmour
Project Manager: Jane Shanks
Design Direction: George Ajayi

Behavioural Distress
Concepts and Strategies

Edited by

Bob Gates MSc BEd(Hons) DipNurs(Lond) CertEd RNT RNMH RMN
Senior Lecturer, School of Nursing, University of Hull, UK

Jane Gear MA PhD
Consultant in Learning, Development and Communication;
Hononary Fellow, Institute for Learning, University of Hull, UK

Jane Wray RGN BA(Hons) HETC
Research Associate, East Yorkshire Learning Disability Institute, University of Hull, UK

YORK ST. JOHN
COLLEGE LIBRARY

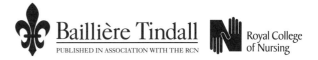

Baillière Tindall
PUBLISHED IN ASSOCIATION WITH THE RCN

Royal College of Nursing

EDINBURGH LONDON NEW YORK PHILADELPHIA ST LOUIS SYDNEY TORONTO 2000

BAILLIÈRE TINDALL
An imprint of Harcourt Publishers Limited

© Harcourt Publishers Limited 2000

is a registered trademark of Harcourt Publishers Limited

The right of Bob Gates, Jane Gear and Jane Wray to be identified as editors of this work has been asserted by them in accordance with the Copyright, Designs and Patents Act 1988.
All rights reserved. No part of this publication may be reproduced, stored in a retrieval system, or transmitted in any form or by any means, electronic, mechanical, photocopying, recording or otherwise, without either the prior permission of the publishers (Harcourt Publishers Limited, Harcourt Place, 32 Jamestown Road, London NW1 7BY), or a licence permitting restricted copying in the United Kingdom issued by the Copyright Licensing Agency, 90 Tottenham Court Road, London W1P 0LP.

First published 2000

ISBN 0 7020 2415 5

British Library Cataloguing in Publication Data
A catalogue record for this book is available from the British Library

Library of Congress Cataloging in Publication Data
A catalog record for this book is available from the Library of Congress

Note
Medical knowledge is constantly changing. As new information becomes available, changes in treatment, procedures, equipment and the use of drugs become necessary. The editors and contributors and the publishers have, as far as it is possible, taken care to ensure that the information given in this text is accurate and up-to-date. However, readers are strongly advised to confirm that the information, especially with regard to drug usage, complies with the latest legislation and standards of practice.

The
publisher's
policy is to use
**paper manufactured
from sustainable forests**

Printed in China

Contents

Contributors **vii**

Preface **ix**

SECTION 1 Understanding behavioural distress, terminology, and ethical and legal contexts 1

1. Towards understanding behaviour **3**
    Jane Gear, Bob Gates and Jane Wray
    Theoretical orientations towards understanding behaviour; Psychological explanations of behaviour; Sociological explanations of behaviour; Anthropological explanations of behaviour; APM-A (orientation) theory and 'psychological survival'.

2. Terminology **31**
    Peter Oakes
    Why words?; The language of disability; Image of disability; The language of behavioural distress; Expressions of behavioural distress; The language of intervention; The impact messages.

3. The ethical and legal context **49**
    Sam Ayer
    Ethical issues; Human rights; Ethical behaviour and professional practice; 'Special' rights of people with learning disabilities; Behavioural interventions and the client's rights; The 'pindown' experience; Use of medication: legal implications; Legal issues: background and relevant definitions; Legal issues and the manifestations of behaviour; Issues of consent; Risk assessment and risk management.

SECTION 2 Seven therapeutic interventions used in behavioural distress 77

4. Nonviolent (compassionate) Communication **79**
    Jane Gear
    What is Nonviolent Communication?; Personal growth and the development of NVC; Evidence base; The NVC process; The NVC model; Case illustrations of NVC in use; The interaction of APM-A (orientation) theory and NVC; The qualities and uses of NVC; Training.

5. The arts therapies   **107**
    Marian Liebmann
    History;The theoretical basis;The philosophical basis;The evidence base;
    Case illustrations of arts therapies in use; Limitations.

6. Chemotherapy and other physical treatments   **131**
    Ibrahim Y.A. Turkistani
    History; Chemotherapeutic treatment of some conditions with
    underlying behavioural distress; More general states of distress;
    Pharmacotherapy; Psychotropic drugs; Non-psychotropic drugs;
    Electroconvulsive therapy; Psychosurgery; Compliance with treatment.

7. Gentle Teaching   **159**
    Siobhan O'Rourke and Jane Wray
    Gentle teaching; The practical application of gentle teaching;
    Organisational principles of gentle teaching; Criticisms of gentle
    teaching.

8. Structured teaching   **185**
    Owen Barr, David Sines, Ken Moore and Gillian Boyd
    The nature of the spectrum of autistic disorders; History of structured
    teaching; The theoretical basis; The philosophical basis; The practical
    application of structured teaching; The empirical basis of structured
    teaching; Limitations of the structured teaching approach.

9. Behavioural interventions   **215**
    Michael McCue
    The behavioural approach; Theoretical bases for behavioural
    interventions; Practical applications; Planning interventions; Approaches
    to behavioural change; The limitations of behavioural approaches.

10. Cognitive behavioural interventions   **257**
    John Turnbull
    Historical overview; Theoretical development; The philosophical basis of
    cognitive behavioural approaches; Case illustrations of cognitive
    behavioural approaches in use; The strengths and limitations of the
    cognitive behavioural approach.

SECTION 3   Examining evidence   281

11. The problematic nature of evidence   **283**
    Jane Wray and Bob Gates
    Scientific evidence; What constitutes evidence and how is it obtained?;
    Comparing and contrasting the evidence and research base of
    interventions; Implications for organisations and settings.

A plate section can be found between pages 112 and 113.

Index   301

Contributors

Sam Ayer BSc(Hons) PhD RNT RNMH RMN FRSH
Senior Lecturer, School of Nursing, University of Hull, UK

Owen Barr RGN RMNH CertCNMH RNT BSc(Hons) MSc
Lecturer in Nursing, Learning Disabilities, School of Health Sciences, University of Ulster, Coleraine, UK

Gillian Boyd BPhil TCert
Principal, Foyle View School, Londonderry, UK

Bob Gates MSc BEd(Hons) DipNurs(Lond) CertEd RNT RNMH RMN
Senior Lecturer, School of Nursing, University of Hull, UK

Jane Gear MA PhD
Consultant in Learning, Development and Communication; Honorary Fellow, Institute for Learning, University of Hull, UK

Marian Liebmann BA MA CQSW RATh
Senior Art Therapist, Inner City Mental Health Service, Bristol, UK

Michael McCue RNMH BA
Additional Support Team Manager, Greater Glasgow Primary Care NHS Trust, Glasgow, UK

Ken Moore BSc(Hons) RNMH DipCouns UKRC
Residential Care Manager, Surrey, UK

Peter Oakes BA(Hons) DipClinPsychol CPsychol
Lecturer in Clinical Psychology, University of Hull, UK

Siobhan O'Rourke RNMH BA(Lond)
Consultant/Trainer, Highfields, Ceredigion, UK

David Sines PhD BSc(Hons) RMN RNMH PGCTHE RNT FRCN
Dean, Faculty of Health, South Bank University, London, UK

Ibrahim Y. A. Turkistani MB BS MSc MMedSc BCPsych DPM DipClPsych DDS
Psychiatrist, Hull and East Riding Community Health NHS Trust & Department of Psychiatry, University of Hull, UK

John Turnbull BA MSc RNMH
Director of Nursing, Oxfordshire Learning Disability NHS Trust, UK

Jane Wray RGN BA(Hons) HETC
Research Associate, East Yorkshire Learning Disability Institute, University of Hull, UK

Preface

Human behaviour has been described in many different ways by different academic disciplines over many centuries. The origins of this book lie in an interest in exploring the different therapeutic interventions used in learning disabilities. This initial conception, however, proved to be narrower than we wanted and risked giving the impression that behavioural distress was something peculiar to people with learning disabilities. Any of us may experience some kind of behavioural difficulty at some period in our lives. For most of us, even if we cannot bring about resolution, it may be possible to learn strategies for coping. This book identifies a range of strategies that can be used with people who may be unable to bring about changes for themselves.

Part of the difference in the ways in which behaviour is understood in different academic disciplines is attributable to different definitions. In the context of this book, 'behaviour' refers to the total response of a person to a situation that he or she faces, including both psychological and physiological elements. How we as individuals view behaviour, interpret it, understand it, and possibly respond to it depends on many factors, including our own attitudes and internal 'theories' about human nature. We use the term 'behavioural distress' to refer to expressions of psychological and physiological experience perceived by self and/or others as threatening, frightening, destructive, or self-destructive in direct or indirect ways.

The book is divided into three sections. The first section explores how we view behaviour and the impact of the language and terminology we use when referring to distressed and distressing behaviour; and introduces a discussion of ethical and legal contexts. The second, and most substantive section, provides a detailed overview of seven different kinds of intervention used by professional carers. The final section (Ch. 11) considers the problematic nature of evidence and refers again, briefly, to the interventions presented in Section 2.

Our rationale for the choice of interventions presented was to offer a sample of therapeutic approaches representative of the kind of continuum illustrated in Figure 1.1 (see Ch. 1). In Chapter 1 we touch on what can seem to be mutually exclusive ways of understanding the world: positivism versus anti-positivism (seeing the world as real, external to the individual and quantifiable in objective terms, versus seeing the world as more subjective, person created, and reflective of our interactions with the environment). This apparent dichotomy can also be seen as existing along continua ranging from objective to subjective; from seeing people as reactive to seeing them as proactive; and/or describing views of learning and behaviour from elemental (as a collection of parts) to holistic (taking the whole person into account).

As well as attempting to offer an overview of interventions rooted in a wide range of theoretical positions, we have also attempted to cover types of behavioural distress that can occur across an entire life-span; we have therefore chosen case illustrations, reader reflections and reader activities to represent a broad range of situations.

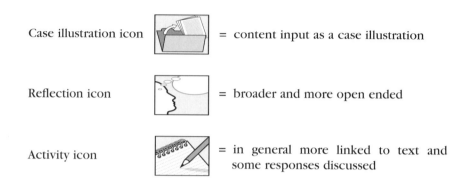

Case illustration icon   = content input as a case illustration

Reflection icon   = broader and more open ended

Activity icon   = in general more linked to text and some responses discussed

Some chapters have arisen specifically from work in the field of learning disabilities that also has wider applications, whereas other chapters are based on established interventions that are already generally acknowledged. We are nevertheless aware that this book covers only a sample of interventions that can be used in helping to change behaviours that either trigger, or result from, distress. Practical considerations have resulted in the need to draw boundaries.

The growth of interest and pace of development in the whole field of therapy during the last decade have heightened awareness of the short 'shelf-life' of some medical and non-medical approaches. Increased interest and rapid developments have also led to many tensions, controversies and ethical debates in the fields of counselling and therapy in general. Although we touch on some of these controversies (such as the debate about the efficacy of aversive and non-aversive therapies in Chs. 7 and 9), to address this and other issues fully would require a volume to itself. Our focus is primarily on interventions and understanding their use.

This book is aimed at both professional and lay readerships. It is intended both as an overview and as a source of information, but not as a means of developing competence in any of the approaches described. The authors hope that the book will inspire and encourage readers to pursue further knowledge and/or go on to develop specialist skills in the application of the interventions presented. The information may also be useful to people who have had direct experience of behavioural distress themselves, or to relatives or other carers who want to understand more fully the usefulness and boundaries of interventions that they have already come across. It is hoped that students will find it a resource that provides a comprehensive yet accessible body of knowledge concerning different therapeutic approaches. Finally, existing practitioners may wish to learn something of therapeutic approaches with which they have been thus far unfamiliar.

Hull 2000   BG, JG, JW

Understanding behavioural distress, terminology, and ethical and legal contexts

1 Towards understanding behaviour   **3**
Jane Gear, Bob Gates and Jane Wray

2 Terminology   **31**
Peter Oakes

3 The ethical and legal contexts   **49**
Sam Ayer

This first section comprises three chapters. The first chapter explores how we view behaviour and identifies how it has been described defined and accounted for in different ways by different academic disciplines over many centuries. The chapter focuses primarily on developments in the social sciences since the end of the 19th century. The chapter also touches on what can be seen to be mutually exclusive ways of understanding the world: positivism versus anti-positivism. Here these two positions are related to continua underlying different theoretical perspectives. Chapter 1 emphasises the complexity of behaviour and behavioural distress, and the need to acknowledge the validity of many different perspectives. The chapter also acknowledges the importance of being aware of the implications, theories and attitudes that inform our own approaches to behavioural distress. To this end, major psychological, sociological and anthropological approaches to understanding behaviour are briefly outlined, before introducing an alternative view that provides an inclusive and evolutionary framework.

Chapter 2 considers words used to describe people who experience behavioural distress and/or who trigger distress in others. The chapter explores how language can impact on people to whom it refers, and acknowledges the somewhat bitter irony that our thoughts and speech may indeed contribute to the distress we are aiming to resolve.

Chapter 3 explores the ethical and legal contexts of behavioural distress. In this chapter, the first two sections deal with broad ethical and human rights issues. The third section explores the implications of criminal and civil law arising from the treatment, care and control of people with learning disabilities who also present with severe challenging behaviour. The final section briefly explores the issue of risk and implications for the care, control and safety of people with learning disabilities.

1 Towards understanding behaviour

Jane Gear, Bob Gates, Jane Wray

Key issues
- Behaviour has been described, defined and accounted for from different perspectives in psychology and by different disciplines, including philosophy, sociology and anthropology
- Behaviour and behavioural distress are complex phenomena
- Our own theories and attitudes inform and influence our understanding of behaviour
- APM-A theory offers an alternative, inclusive and evolutionary framework for understanding behaviour

Overview
Chapter 1 considers ways of understanding human experience and behaviour. As touched on in the preface to this book, behaviour has been described, defined and accounted for in many different ways by various academic disciplines over many centuries. In this chapter we concentrate primarily on the latter half of the 19th century and on developments in the social sciences during the 20th century. In so doing, we describe what can seem to be mutually exclusive ways of understanding the world: positivism versus anti-positivism. Positivism refers to seeing the world as real, external to the individual, and quantifiable in objective terms, while anti-positivism sees the world as more subjective, person created, and reflective of our interactions with the environment. This apparent dichotomy can also be seen as being composed of various continua (Fig. 1.1). Views can range from objective to subjective; from seeing people as reactive to seeing them as proactive; and/or describing views of learning and behaviour from elemental (as a collection of parts) to holistic (taking the whole person into account). Whether we operate from formal theories or not, if we see people as reactive and behaviour as elemental, for example, we are likely to choose different interventions than if we adopt a holistic view or see people as proactive and autonomous.

This first chapter draws attention to how different ways of viewing the world have also pervaded views of behaviour. It emphasises the complexity of both behaviour and behavioural distress and the need to acknowledge the validity of many different perspectives. The chapter also acknowledges the importance of being aware of the implications of the theories and attitudes that inform our own approaches to behavioural distress. To this end,

3

Fig. 1.1
The seven interventions presented in Section 2.

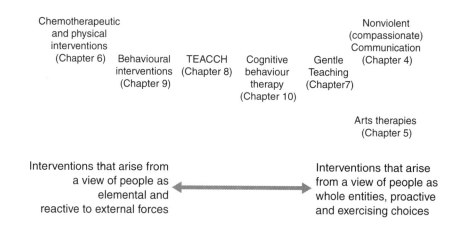

we briefly outline major psychological, sociological and anthropological approaches to understanding behaviour before introducing an alternative view that provides an inclusive and evolutionary framework.

We hope that this first chapter will demonstrate clearly that different theoretical positions are not necessarily mutually exclusive: more often they describe different facets of human nature. The intention is to offer awareness of the diversity of major theoretical positions that inform interventions and to increase awareness of our own concepts and attitudes to behavioural distress.

Theoretical orientations towards understanding behaviour

Whereas we might look towards psychology or sociology for an understanding of human behaviour, the contributions of both of these sciences are relatively new, and there is plentiful evidence from ancient history of academic communities attempting to understand the nature of the world and behaviour. The works of Plato and Aristotle are probably the most famous examples. Indeed, until the end of the 19th century the academic discipline of philosophy dominated ways in which knowledge, theories and 'laws' were constructed; and philosophy continued to dominate explanations of behaviour until the early decades of the 20th century. Plato argued that thought alone could furnish knowledge, and he dismissed the idea that observation was at all useful to the 'scientific method', because, he argued, observation was inherently unreliable. Plato disputed whether 'scientific testing' could, or ever would, assist us in the generation of knowledge. However, he did emphasise the importance of mental health and linked it to the development of a healthy body.

At a later stage, Aristotle (incidentally a student of Plato) argued for the scientific method. He rejected the idea that this approach was no more than the 'prying of man into the divine order of nature' as argued by Plato. Instead, Aristotle advocated a deductive approach that followed a linear progression: from theories that should influence what we choose to observe and then, dependent on the results of observations, to the modification of theory. Deduction remains one way of attempting to understand the world, and induction - starting with particular data in order to infer general conclusions - is another. A classic paper describing different approaches to science has been provided by Wallace (1971). Readers with an interest in this area might also refer to Papineau (1989) who discusses some of the complexities of different philosophical positions. Within the context of this book, awareness of some of the ways in which we attempt to construct knowledge is seen as important because of its influence on theories of behaviour and, in turn, on how we view and respond to behavioural distress.

In addition to these fundamentally different ways of construing behaviour and behavioural distress, geographical, cultural, social and historical factors also play a part in influencing our views. Some major theoretical positions that underpin current approaches are outlined (as far as possible in chronological order) below. There are also relatively new neurological and genetic findings, hypotheses and controversies beyond the scope of this book. However, some other views and explanations of more specific conditions and behaviours are offered in the chapters about interventions.

Psychological explanations of behaviour

Behaviourism

The earliest empirical research in psychology was concerned with observable behaviour only, and known as behaviourism. Mental experience was of no interest, and any phenomena occurring between speech or movement were seen simply as subliminal movements, and accounted for as implicit, or covert, stimulus–response connections (Watson 1907). Although Watson eventually became known as 'the father of behaviourism', by 1938 Thorndike's theory of connectionism (Thorndike 1898) was assessed as the starting point for all of the major developments in American psychology up to that time (Tolman 1938). Thorndike identified the most characteristic form of lower animal and human learning as 'trial and error': learning by 'selecting' and 'connecting'. The work of both Thorndike and Watson was based on mechanistic concepts that incidentally also reflected the language of the 19th-century industrial revolution. For example, responses to stimuli were 'stamped in' and 'stamped out', and were 'chained' in association with one another.

A more famous exponent of behaviourism was Pavlov (1902) who identified 'conditioning'. He described a relationship between what he called unconditioned responses and unconditioned stimuli. The original responses were referred to as 'unconditioned' because they were integral components of the repertoire of the behaviour of the animals he used in his experiments, most famously dogs. Pavlov found that if an unconditioned stimulus was paired with a conditioned stimulus then it would, through a process of association, be able to elicit a conditioned response. Box 1.1 illustrates this mechanism.

It can be seen that at Stage 1 the unconditioned stimulus of food causes the dog to salivate. If this unconditioned stimulus is paired for a sufficient period of time (Stage 2) with a conditioned stimulus (bell), eventually (Stage 3) the conditioned stimulus (bell) alone will elicit a now conditioned response (salivation). This definition of how behaviour was learned was called 'classical conditioning'. This early work was developed by other psychologists including Watson, and it is interesting to note the power of persuasive argument employed by behaviourists at that time. Consider the following statement by Watson (1924 cited by Stevanson 1974):

❝*Give me a dozen healthy infants, well-formed, and my own specified world to bring them up in and I'll guarantee to take any one at random and train him to become any kind of specialist I might select – lawyer, artist, merchant, chef and yes even a beggar man and thief, regardless of his talents, penchants, abilities, vocations, and race of his ancestors.* ❞

Box 1.1
Classical conditioning

Stage 1
Unconditioned stimulus   *Unconditioned response*
Food   →   →   →   →   →   Salivation

Stage 2
Unconditioned stimulus
Food paired with
Conditioned stimulus   *Unconditioned response*
Bell   →   →   →   →   →   Salivation

Stage 3
Conditioned stimulus   *Conditioned response*
Bell   →   →   →   →   →   Salivation

The significance of this is the underlying assumption of simplicity in how behaviour could be accounted for: shaped by external forces elementally and deterministically (in a quite different way from the determinism of Freud, see below).

It was B. F. Skinner, a leading exponent of behaviourism, who made the notion of 'shaping' behaviour famous, and the underlying assumptions of behaviourism explicit. For Skinner behaviour was not simply determined, it could be predicted and controlled by its consequences. Feelings were part of those consequences, and certainly not causal. In the 1950s, Skinner articulated the idea that if a specific behaviour were to be positively reinforced (i.e. satisfy a previously deprived drive), then the frequency of that behaviour was likely to be increased. Skinner's experimental rats and pigeons made associations between food rewards as reinforcement and responses made immediately prior to that reinforcement. Consequently, the animals replicated the behaviour in order to replicate the reinforcement. By way of contrast, if an organism were to be negatively reinforced (by the removal of aversive stimuli, such as loud noises, bright lights or extreme cold – as opposed to punishment), then the frequency of that behaviour would decrease.

One extraordinary example of the effectiveness of this was that Skinner was able to teach pigeons to play table tennis. He called this more complex form of conditioning 'operant conditioning'. The implications of Skinner's findings at the time were enormous; here was a way of accounting for the nature of behaviour, and behaviour could be modified by the use of reinforcement to either increase or decrease its frequency, according to its desirability. Skinner's work sparked many controversies, most of which are still being debated. However, behaviourism and operant conditioning, in the form of 'behaviour modification', has developed and provided an effective technology for helping people change behaviours distressing to themselves and others. A fuller account of the development of behaviourism, along with a contemporary account of the practical uses of behavioural interventions, is described by Mike McCue in Chapter 9. Readers who wish to explore behavioural approaches further are referred to Yule & Carr (1990), or can explore Skinner's own vision of behaviourism's potential for society in *Beyond Freedom and Dignity* (Skinner 1971).

Psychodynamic approaches

The origins of this perspective lie in the work of Sigmund Freud, whose papers 'Repression' and 'The Unconscious' (Freud 1925a, 1925b) were first published in 1915. The term 'psychodynamic' is a generic term that refers to a number of components concerned with at least two inter-related theories. The first is concerned with human emotional development and the second with the treatment of mental disorder by use of psychoanalysis. Freud suggested that 'abnormal' behaviour is a result of a dysfunctional mind, and therefore abnormal behaviour represents mental disorder. The earliest of his theories, object relations theory, identified the significance of instinctive drives in determining behaviour. The theory was concerned with relationships and the fundamental need for people to form relationships. Freud suggested that our earliest relationships become internalised and impact on the ways we behave towards others throughout our lives.

From birth, the impact of the relationships between child and mother, father and later 'significant others' lays the foundations for an individual's internal world. This internal world, depending on the quality of early relationships, may be full of doubt and anxiety, with a need to please, or, alternatively, secure and balanced. These early foundations of our psyche contribute to unconscious thought alongside powerful, instinctive drives. According to Freud, our personalities evolve through continual conflict between the unconscious selfish impulses driven by the desire for pleasure and the 'reality' encountered in conscious thought, as well as our infant experiences. The latter can impact in profound, unconscious ways, shaping and sometimes distorting experience and behaviour.

Freud called the part of the unconscious mind serving primitive drives the id. This was seen to contain the turbulence of socially unacceptable drives and sexual fantasies kept in place by the ego (housing learned skills of social and physical adjustment) and the superego (interpreting the moral beliefs of society as exemplified by parents) to protect the entire structure of personality. The unconscious mechanisms of control were called defence mechanisms, some of which are still referred to commonly as denial, rationalisation, sublimation, repression and projection.

However, psychodynamic approaches comprise a wide number of interrelated theories that collectively attempt to account for much of human behaviour. Readers wishing to explore psychodynamic approaches further are referred to Brown (1993).

Cognitive approaches

One of the earliest experiments offering insight into the interaction of behaviour and mental experience came from research by Tolman (1925) into maze learning in rats. Tolman's research was pivotal, especially so as an outcome of behavioural research. It also made a significant contribution to other developments from which cognitive psychology emerged.

At much the same time as the behavioural approach was gaining ground in the USA, another school of thought, Gestalt psychology, was emerging in Europe. In Germany, Max Wertheimer (1938), Kurt Koffka (1924) and Wolfgang Köhler (1925) were researching the structure of experience and thinking, how we 'see' problem situations, and other perceptual phenomena. The word 'Gestalt' translates as 'figure' or 'form', and in 1925 Wertheimer published a classic paper describing 'laws' of perceptual organisation. The

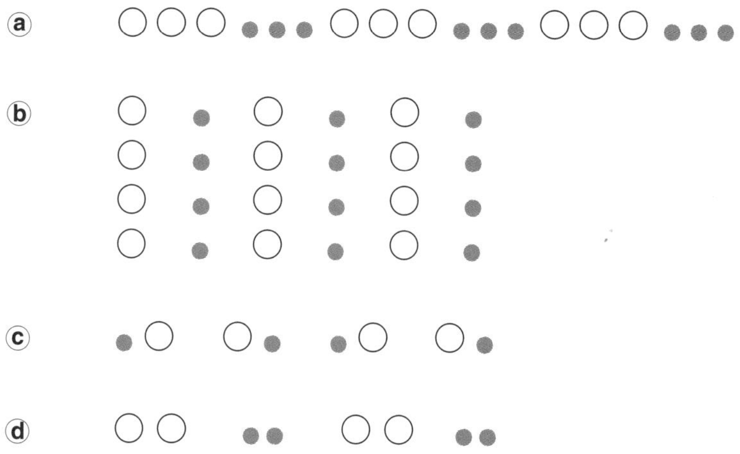

Fig. 1.2
Perceptual grouping by similarity, in this case of colour and size (Hilgard & Bower 1975, reproduced with kind permission from Prentice Hall International, London).

nearest to a general law of perception was later formulated as the 'law of Pragnanz' (meaning compact and significant). Part of our tendency to perceive 'good Gestalts' (i.e. complete forms and patterns) was seen to be a preference to group perceptions according to different attributes, such as similarity, proximity and simplicity. Figure 1.2 illustrates our tendency to perceive by grouping according to similarity.

Although these findings referred directly to visual perception, it can be argued that our tendency to perceive patterns and complete forms, and to fill in missing information, even when parts of figures are lacking, can affect the way we perceive patterns of behaviour and construe (or sometimes misconstrue) people and their motivations.

Köhler's major discovery was that chimpanzees could solve problems that required understanding of the relationship between a number of factors. Köhler's experiments exposed a quite different kind of learning from that discovered by the behaviourists: namely, problem-solving that depended on insight (see the accounting 'Sultan the chimpanzee'). Köhler's book *The Mentality of Apes* (1925) describes experimentation with a group of chimpanzees over a period of 6 years. His studies provided clear evidence that learning could not simply be explained in terms of connections and associations alone, and that mental activity and cognition were significant factors. Cognition includes thinking, valuing and judging as well as perceiving and other mental phenomena. None of these aspects of mind figured in behaviourism; they were rejected as internal constructs, invisible and non-observable.

The early work of Wertheimer, Koffka and Köhler formed the basis of Gestalt psychology, and paved the way for many more cognitive explanations of learning and behaviour which culminated in the 'cognitive approach' being formally adopted in 1956 (Matlin 1994). This branch of psychology is concerned with how individuals form cognitive structures within memory that enable information to be stored, retrieved, analysed and used in novel ways to resolve problems and situations. In Chapter 10, John Turnbull writing on cognitive behavioural interventions draws attention to the central work of other cognitivists; readers wanting to explore cognitive approaches further are referred to Matlin (1994).

Sultan the chimpanzee

A chimpanzee, Sultan, was placed in front of bars that led to a small enclosed area that contained fruit on the floor. Lying outside the bars was a small stick and inside the enclosed space were two further sticks; one medium sized, the other a long stick. On seeing the fruit in the enclosed space Sultan attempted to use the small stick outside of the bars to reach the fruit. He realised that this would not work and initially became frustrated and agitated. However, at some point Sultan appeared to develop insight. He realised that with the small stick, he could reach the medium stick, and with this he could reach the big stick, and finally with this he was able to reach the fruit. This was one of the earliest examples of insight learning and demonstrated an understanding of the relationships that were essential to solving a problem, and that this was not simply based upon trial and error learning.

Phenomenological approaches and humanistic psychology

During the 1950s, an approach to understanding experience and behaviour emerged that, instead of being based on the behaviour of rats, dogs, pigeons or chimpanzees, was based on the subjective experience of human beings. The ground for this new psychology had been laid by the influence of the German philosopher Edmund Husserl (1859–1938). Husserl's work had a deep influence across a range of disciplines that we now call human sciences (Husserl 1891 cited in Gregory 1987). He elaborated a radical philosophy of consciousness from which a general epistemological change took place, as well as the eventual development of a new kind of psychology. His fundamental theory of phenomena, including perception and creative thinking, allowed a reintegration of concepts and shifted psychology onto other levels. One of the philosophers who contributed to this shift was Maurice Merleau-Ponty with his analyses of the experienced body in 1942 and of perception in 1945 (cited in Gregory 1987).

An early exponent of the new approach that became known as humanistic psychology was Carl Rogers (1951). His theoretical approach was based on therapeutic practice in clinical psychology. Whilst behavioural explanations could adequately describe relatively unsophisticated kinds of behaviour, theories did not offer understanding of mental states, psychological needs or clinical conditions. Humanistic psychology articulated two underlying principles to understanding human behaviour. First, the person was seen as central to a subjective understanding of human behaviour, not simply as an object, responding passively and unknowingly to stimuli within the environment. People were viewed as dynamic, unique and interactive beings who are both subject and object, and therefore able to interact with their environments. Secondly, it was suggested that the ultimate purpose for human behaviour is simply 'being' and achieving self-actualisation (developing individual potential to its fullest). This was clearly articulated in an extract from a diary of a teacher with whom Rogers was working:

It is not the panacea, but it is a step forward. Each day is a new adventure; there are moments of stress, concern, pleasure – they are all stepping stones toward our goal of self actualisation.

[Rogers 1983, p. 52]

Abraham Maslow (1954), famous for his hierarchy of human needs, was the other major exponent in this field. Maslow described needs as ranging from basic physiological needs such as physical safety, food, water, and air to complex psychological needs such as the need to 'belong' and the need for self-esteem. According to Maslow, the motivation for all behaviour is simply being alive and moving towards self-actualisation, 'being whatever we can be'. Examples of how the approaches of Rogers and Maslow have influenced how we understand and respond to distressed behaviour are provided in Chapters 4 and 7. Both these chapters describe and promote interventions that are fundamentally phenomenological and humanistic in their approaches to working with distressed people.

Psychology has provided many different theories, explanations, and insights into human behaviour; and different schools of psychology promote different theories and models for our collective understanding. Some of these are located on the continuum in Figure 1.1. Table 1.1 (adapted from Ellis & Gates 1995) is based on the work of Pervin (1993), who provided a framework for identifying general differences that divide theorists.

Sociological explanations of behaviour

Sociology is concerned with the construction of social facts and ways of understanding the behaviour of groups within society, as opposed to a focus on the behaviour of individuals. When individual experience and behaviour are subjects of research and theory, phenomena are explained by reference to effects of belonging to groups, for example 'alienation' and 'social exclusion' and Bandura's social learning theory (Bandura 1962). As with psychology, sociology comprises many different theoretical stances (e.g. structural functionalism, symbolic interactionism, Marxist, neo-Marxist and feminist perspectives).

An example of how sociological theory assists in understanding human distress is offered by the work of French sociologist Émile Durkheim (1858-1917). His particular interest in suicide (Durkheim 1952) and its relationship to the well-being of society at large led him to address questions such as whether suicide was a barometer of a society's overall 'health', or level of distress. He concluded that, although suicide is a unique episode that culminates in the death of an individual, when studied as a phenomenon at the level of society there are a number of significant patterns. Firstly, suicide rates differ between countries. Secondly, within countries suicide rates appear remarkably stable when plotted against a temporal dimension. Finally, within single countries different rates exist for different social groupings and religions.

Despite methodological weaknesses in the collection of data, some of Durkheim's findings have stood up to continued scrutiny. Central to his work was a will to construct a social explanation for suicide, rather than an individual explanation that, in psychology, might be offered by a psychodynamic explanation, as one of many possibilities.

Another classic example of how sociological theory provides valuable insights into the nature of behavioural distress comes from the seminal work of Thomas Szasz (1961). In *The Myth of Mental Illness* he argued that people who were said to be mentally ill were inappropriately labelled. His theory was that many people so labelled were simply having problems with 'living'. At the heart of his preferred explanation lay scepticism concerning the centrality of the process of labelling itself, and its actual and potential outcomes. This sociological explanation suggested that mental

Table 1.1

Underlying assumptions and features of behavioural, psychodynamic, cognitive and humanistic models of human behaviour (adapted from Ellis & Gates 1995, with kind permission from Churchill Livingstone)

Issues	Behavioural	Psychodynamic	Cognitive	Humanistic
Philosophical view of the person	All behaviour learned in response to environment	Behaviour originates from our past experiences	Behaviour indicative of a problem-solving organism	Behaviour drives an individual to self-actualise
Internal versus external causes of behaviour	Emphasis placed on external world causing behaviour	Interactive relationship between inner and outer world	Reciprocal relationship between external and internal worlds	Balance is sought between two worlds to create harmony
Self-concept	Self is not central as it is unobservable and therefore unmeasureable	Concept of ego central to understanding self	Important in self-praise, self-criticism and self-regulation	Self a central concept combining thought, feeling and behaviour
States of awareness	Awareness and insight not relevant	Unconscious most important. Interplay between conscious and unconscious behaviour	Behaviour may not be unconscious but automatic and rehearsed	Mostly concerned with the here and now, and existentialism
Feeling, thought and behaviour	Behaviour central; thought and feeling not relevant (excluding cognitive behaviour therapy)	Feeling, thought and behaviour all important in understanding behaviour	Cognition central to understanding feeling and behaviour	Lived and unique experience central; feeling thought and behaviour should be in harmony
Role of past, present and future	Present and future important	The past is most important in understanding the present, and both interact	Cognitive maps and schemata enable expectation	Most importance placed upon present

health professionals constructed convenient diagnostic structures that would rid societies of their 'deviants' (Newell 1996). The issue of labelling is taken up in Chapter 2 which discusses the impact of terminology, and is referred to again in Chapter 4 with reference to Nonviolent Communication (NVC).

From Szasz's perspective, distressed behaviour is more adequately explained by reference to social structures than as a problem located within the individual. This point is especially relevant in the context of people labelled as having 'personality disorders' today, who in the main are treated within the National Health Service. Recent debate has focused on this very issue and on whether such individuals are amenable to treatment at all.

Sociology also offers insights into many other types of behavioural distress; for example, addictions to drugs and alcohol. Some sociologists view both of these types of behaviour as forms of 'retreatism'. This refers to the outcome of individuals' needs being unmet by the groups to which they belong, and their 'opting out' of society and engaging in self-destructive behaviour. Other, often-cited examples include explanations of violence taking account of levels of sex and violence shown in entertainment media, phenomena such as 'copy cat' crimes and linking crime rates to unemployment and social deprivation.

Anthropological explanations of behaviour

Haviland (1996 p.5) has explained the meaning of the term anthropology as follows:

> *Anthropology is the study of human kind everywhere, throughout time, and it seeks to produce meaningful generalisations about people and their behaviour and to arrive at the fullest possible understanding of human diversity.*

Pelto (1965) reminds us that a distinguishing feature of behaviour is that it is pervasively cultural. Culture is seen as the entirety of the expressed behaviour of communities and societies, and was first defined by Burnett Tylor in 1871 as:

> *That complex whole which includes knowledge, belief, art, law, morals, custom and any other capabilities and habits acquired by man as a member of society.*

The beliefs, laws, morals and customs representing 'rules' and standards (most of which may be tacit) are shared by a society, and accepted by members of that society as reasonable ways in which to behave. Those members who adopt or engage in behaviours that are unacceptable to others may be considered, and labelled as, 'deviant'. It is worth noting that smaller communities within a society may adopt sub-cultural ways that are also considered 'normal'. This is especially obvious in pluralistic societies that comprise many different religious, ethnic and other cultural groupings who have their own norms of behaviour.

How we behave towards infants, people with disabilities, disaffected youths or distressed others who exhibit behaviour we are unable to tolerate is likely to be affected in part, if not substantially, by cultural and sub-cultural standards. Since culture is learned, societies pass on its elements from one generation to the next, a process referred to as enculturation (an equivalent concept in sociology is socialisation).

It has been suggested that enculturation commences shortly after birth with the development of self-awareness, and enables us to construe ourselves as separate identities from those around us. It also enables us to modify our behaviour in response to others and to assume differing roles. For example, on a recent field visit to Jamaica one of the authors of this chapter was intrigued to learn that some people in Jamaica believe that a woman who has a handicapped child is being punished for something that she has done wrong in the past. As a result of this, some handicapped children are kept in their homes unknown to friends and neighbours. It is often the case that the local community does not realise that a child is being brought up in the home, because the mother does not want others to know that she has 'done something wrong in the past': a poignant example of the relevance of anthropology to the field of distressed behaviour. Similarly powerful examples of the influence of beliefs and norms can be found in the cultures of all institutions, peer groups and families worldwide.

As an exercise in considering the totality of culture on people's behaviour, and the possible effects of social conditioning, readers are directed to the reader activity below and invited to think about those parts of a culture that might account for the behaviour in question.

Cultural differences

Think of someone you know well who has behaved in ways that others have found unacceptable. Quite apart from the immediate factors that you may think offer explanation, identify aspects of the person's culture (or that of the group on whom the behaviour impacted) that might have influenced the behaviour or reactions in question. Consider, among other things, religion, ethnicity, exposure to ideas, books, art and music, other media, education, family background, place of birth and organisations and groups to which the person has belonged. This exercise might be undertaken with a colleague or as an anonymous case study with a student group, to share views and thoughts on the impact of culture on behaviour.

Finally, individual approaches, while having many applications, do not accommodate sufficient diversity to explain the complexity of human behaviour. This has led some to conclude that more eclectic and holistic approaches to understanding behaviour may be more useful than adherence to any single existing theoretical perspective.

The remainder of this chapter is devoted to a synopsis of an evolutionary and unifying way of looking at experience and behaviour known as APM-A (orientation) theory, the work of one of the authors, Jane Gear. Although this work is a theoretical perspective in its own right, rather than eclectic, it also provides a framework within which the theoretical approaches above can be related to one another and seen as describing different aspects of experience and behaviour. While other theories are not necessarily accepted in their entirety, major aspects (such as the power of the unconscious mind and psychological defences as aspects of psychodynamic theory) are accommodated and reinforced. Schools of psychology are also related to distinct stages of evolution of the brain and seen as referring to qualitatively different kinds of experience, learning and behaviour. Some detail of parts of the APM-A perspective is offered in order to help make connections between the different kinds of experience and behaviour identified by the approaches introduced so far.

The perspective offers a view that stands 'normal' and 'abnormal' experience and behaviour within the same theoretical context and explains dysfunctional behaviours and violence as expressions of unmet needs. Importantly, it also introduces the concept of vulnerability to ways of looking at behaviour, and draws attention to the arbitrariness of conventional categories and labels for behaviour we do not like. In addition, the theory draws attention to how stress alters the ways we perceive, think and act.

APM-A (orientation) theory and 'psychological survival'

In APM-A, or orientation theory (Gear 1985, 1989) APM-A stands for the interaction of attention (A), perception (P), memory (M) and arousal (-A), and 'orientation' relates to fundamental needs, defined as 'orientation needs', that are seen to affect both mind and body. The theory reinterprets established findings, mainly from the fields of psychology, anthropology, psychiatry and neuroscience.

APM-A theory accepts that we are subject to conditioning and habit formation, as well as problem solving and goal seeking; in part determined and in part autonomous; both homeostatic in seeking balance, and heterostatic, inevitably changing and growing. Primitive drives, the unconscious mind and defence mechanisms also play significant parts in this perspective, but in different ways from those formulated by Freud. Although we have evolved into rational beings, APM-A suggests that at the same time we have become more (not less) emotional; and although people are seen in terms of evolutionary development and personal history, moment by moment experience is also a key factor in understanding behaviour.

APM-A exposes greater human complexity than established schools of psychology. It offers a 'whole person' view of behavioural distress that links mind and body. All forms of behaviour categorised as dysfunctional or maladaptive are seen as 'stressed' (albeit in different ways), and as representing extremes on a variety of continua. The theory offers a general understanding that views violence, physical and psychological 'bullying' and other directly or indirectly destructive, self-destructive and abusive behaviours as expressions of emotional distress. They are seen as outcomes of unmet needs for orientation that affect us emotionally, and physiologically. APM-A suggests that feelings and needs expressed violently or in ways distressing to self or others could be expressed and fulfilled creatively and effectively, given appropriate skills and means (see reflection box below). This is not to deny the usefulness of some of the more invasive interventions (chemotherapeutic for example), but it is to suggest that the number of cases where these approaches are needed is minimal.

A brief summary of APM-A theory

APM-A theory can be briefly summarised as follows: as human beings we are emotionally as well as physically vulnerable beings in a potentially hostile environment. We interact consciously and unconsciously with stimuli that hold meaning and significance for us (as a species and as individuals) according to feelings and needs, in our efforts to meet mainly unconscious physical, social and other needs for orientation. Needs for orientation include needs for expression; and the ways in which we respond to other people and our surroundings depend on:

- The perceived threat or promise carried by stimuli
- Individual differences in levels and kinds of needs for orientation and expression
- Innate and learned skills and acces to means of expression.

Natural variability extends to our physiology and brain chemistry to affect adaptive styles: kinds of attention, experience and behaviour emotional vulnerability and dominance of kinds and levels of needs for orientation within our physical, social and cultural environments.

The emphasis is ultimately on feelings and (mostly unconscious) needs linked to variability in styles of perception and expression. As well as defining *kinds* of orientation need, the theory highlights individual differences in *levels* and *urgency* of needs for emotional expression that, for example, can result in either apparent coolness or impulsivity. While negative behaviours are seen as mostly unconscious expressions of distress in response to unmet needs, ironically, unmet needs are likely to include a need for conscious awareness of the very needs in question; as well as access to positive and effective means of expression.

Our physical environment – including everything that impinges on our senses – and our life experience – including social interactions and the changing worlds of ideas and culture – are seen to impact on us in a variety of unconscious as well as conscious ways, both moment by moment and in the longer term. Their impact affects our biochemistry, emotions and behaviour. All interact to affect needs and result in expressions of comfortable or uncomfortable feelings.

Factors in APM-A theory seen to be crucial to understanding and intervening in behavioural distress are:

- A wide range of individual differences not generally acknowledged or catered for in various institutions, particularly education
- Differences in kinds and intensities of dominant needs
- Differences in needs for, and styles of, expression (also not generally taken into account).

However, how we respond, internally and externally, and whether we respond in creative or destructive ways depends ultimately on the 'tools' for understanding and expression that we have available to us. As well as acknowledging minute and unconscious changes in biochemistry and emotion, moment by moment, APM-A theory identifies 'baseline' variability in patterns of release of transmitters and hormones. These personal norms are seen to be in part genetic and in part adaptations, 'tuned' by both pre- and postnatal experiences. Eventually these infinitesimal base-line differences show up as differences, alongside other factors, in what we call 'personality'.

APM-A also suggests that what are referred to as 'personality disorders' are expressions of unacknowledged and unmet needs, and that problems are more likely to be an outcome of inhospitable social contexts than located within individuals.

At this point it might be thought that what follows is reductionist and/or deterministic. However, the references to biochemistry, evolution and contexts are necessary to reveal greater complexity, variability, and human potential for choice, not to simplify or reduce in any way (see reflection box below).

One key implication of what follows is that so-called 'normal' ranges of human experience and behaviour are far wider than catered for by our social structures and institutions, so that fundamental needs of many people remain unmet. Another implication is that needs for understanding our emotions and for socially acceptable channels for expressing feelings are considerably higher than currently taken into account.

Orientation and disorientation

As well as APM-A standing for the interaction of attention, perception, memory and arousal, it also represents the core model of the theory. The model expresses the fact that mind and body and conscious and unconscious experience are all essentially interactive. Whereas it may be simpler to think of a linear process such as attention → perception → thought → feeling → memory, any constant order of these events or ultimate separability of one from another is seen to be conceptual only. Change in one leads to change in the others (Fig. 1.3).

The alternative name for the theory, orientation theory, refers to the function of APM-A as underlying the interplay of 'orientation' and 'disorientation' and, in turn, different kinds of behaviour as fundamental themes of the theory – and of life. While temporary and manageable experience of disorientation can have creative potential as we discover new ways of looking at things, disorientation perceived as unmanageable holds negative and destructive potentials. The theory suggests that we can help people move from disorientation and dysfunctional behaviours to 'reorientation', by moving through a process of identifying feelings and unmet needs, and facilitating socially acceptable ways of fulfilling those needs.

There are few concepts in psychology that evoke general agreement. The 'orientation response' and arousal observed by Pavlov as his experimental dogs reacted to novelty and change (see pp.5, 216), and basic impulses to either 'stop' or 'go' (act or not) are unusual in this respect: psychologists generally agree about their significance as findings. In humans, the orientation response is a state of alertness most obvious when we are surprised by a sudden noise or movement and are alerted to check out the source, and our own safety, before deciding whether to act or not.

All of these reactions and impulses are primitive responses governed by the autonomic (self-governing and involuntary) nervous system (ANS) composed of balancing sympathetic (SNS) and parasympathetic nervous system (PNS) activity. The SNS arouses us and spurs us into action while the PNS balances and counters this effect. The emphasis in the theory is on limbic arousal (the most primitive kind of arousal) associated with drives and emotion, and the effects of two specific hormones (adrenaline and noradrenaline) familiar via the ubiquitous 'stress response'.

APM-A is based on the notion that we orientate and reorientate ourselves from moment to moment, checking 'direction', focusing actions and identifying signals in order to survive. Every act of this checking our physical and psychological safety wherever we are, and whomever we are

Fig. 1.3
The core APM-A model (from Gear 1989, with kind permission from Routledge, London).

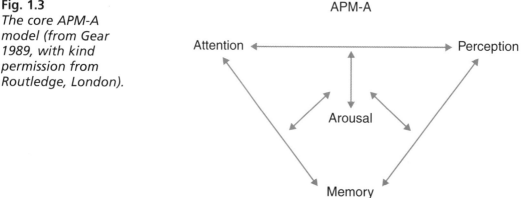

with, involves the interaction of attention, perception, memory and arousal. It is central to the theory that the balance of this process (and its biochemistry) is vulnerable; and that human beings display different kinds and levels of vulnerability to *dis*orientation (and needs *for* orientation) according to natural variability as well as the effects of life experience and adaptation.

Evolved complexity, imagination and vulnerability

APM-A theory views behavioural distress as involving the whole person. It accepts the significance of both biological and environmental influences on 'who' we are. Similarly, feeling and thinking, body and mind, conscious and unconscious functioning are all seen as highly interactive and dynamic. So-called 'normal' and 'abnormal' experience and behaviour, along with our personal styles that we call personality, exist along many continua with particularly vulnerable extremes lying at each end. The major theories referred to in the first half of this chapter can be seen as describing different aspects and stages of how we have evolved from being reactive to proactive beings (see Fig. 1.5) while retaining both possibilities. However, as our needs around physical survival became more complex, our psychological mechanisms for coping with challenges and defending against perceived threats are also seen to have become more complex. It is one of the arguments of the theory that this complexity, necessary growth in awareness and development of imagination, held its own threats to our survival. Our minds as well as our bodies became vulnerable to new kinds of threat in the form of what are now called, for example, anxiety, addictions, neuroses, psychoses and potential for both consciously and unconsciously driven infliction of pain and destruction. Hence an evolved need for 'psychological survival'.

Whether or not we maintain emotional balance and avoid disorientation and distress are seen to depend on fulfilling fundamental needs called 'orientation needs'. In turn, the kinds and levels of needs we experience as dominant are seen to depend on different levels and kinds of SNS-PNS activity, and different levels of vulnerability experienced consciously or unconsciously. On the one hand people are seen to vary as individuals; on the other hand these individual patterns of SNS-PNS activity and their effects (see Figs 1.4-1.9 below) change in reaction to the situations we find ourselves in, and as we become more or less aroused.

Arousal, awareness and needs for expression

SNS activity includes the secretion of adrenaline and noradrenaline. However, whereas the role of adrenaline in stress is fairly well known, if noradrenaline is mentioned at all its role in the 'fight-flight' response is rarely differentiated from that of adrenaline. APM-A suggests that both adrenaline and noradrenaline play key roles in perception and behaviour. Very early research by Ax (1953) and Funkenstein (1956) into the emotional effects of these hormones revealed marked differences highly relevant to behavioural distress. Their early findings related to fear and anger; since then others (Van Toller 1979, Campbell & Singer 1979, McGaugh 1980, Beatty 1982, Gale &

Edwards 1983) have drawn attention to differences in levels of mental and physical activity; tendencies to broaden and narrow attentional capacities; tendencies to scan and focus; and individual variability in secretions of the hormones in question.

In the detailed theory, another very significant finding by the Russian neuroscientist Luria (1976) is taken to suggest that when we are aroused it is necessary to move or act in some way to express that arousal. This is interpreted in ways highly relevant to understanding behavioural distress and the importance of helping to identify feelings and needs in order to reduce arousal (see Ch. 4 for one effective means of doing this).

Ultimately, APM-A suggests that people differ according to needs that arise *from* different patternings of autonomic nervous system activity, and that levels and kinds of more recently evolved needs associated with 'psychological survival' also differ. In turn, these differences are compounded by our perceptions, reactions, adaptations and learning from the situations we find ourselves in.

The four core areas of difference in experience and behaviour crucial to defining greater psychological variability than generally taken into account are defined in detail elsewhere (Gear 1989) as:

1. Individual biases and changes in physical and mental activity

2. Individual biases and changes in tendencies to scan or focus

3. Needs for orientation, including needs for understanding and expression

4. Potential for positive and negative outcomes of increases in energy and breadth of consciousness.

All of these factors are seen to interact and be of key importance to understanding different kinds of experience and behaviour; and, again, all relate to SNS and PNS activity (see below, Table 1.2 and Figs 1.6 and 1.7).

It is argued that under experience of threat, needs for orientation (which are ultimately needs for feelings of safety and security) dominate. At one pole the basic need for feelings of safety may be obvious and easily understandable, as in a need to withdraw from emotional involvement. At the other pole, the underlying need can be much less obvious, as is the case in needs for expression that may result in displays of anger or violence.

Although our responses to threat are now (superficially) more sophisticated than those of the Neanderthals or early hominids, APM-A argues that primitive needs related to physical survival are now compounded by needs for psychological and emotional survival. We all share needs for reassuring cognitive and sensory feedback from the whole of our perceived environments, particularly about the quality of connection with our fellow beings. However, as well as sharing needs, as individuals we are also seen to vary in our experience of intensity of needs. This variability includes relative dominance of needs for orientation and reassuring feedback of physical, social, cultural and spiritual kinds (Fig. 1.4). Table 1.2 (below) recognises differences between experiencing these needs as 'first-order', or as part of our natural variability, or more (or less) temporarily heightened through stress, as 'second-order' needs for orientation and 'psychological survival'. Needs for goals and 'purposes' and for 'mastery and growth' are all seen to become more important to maintaining balance (as offering focus and channels of expression) under the experience of heightened (second-order) needs.

Fig. 1.4
*APM-A orientation
needs (after Gear
1989, with kind
permission from
Routledge, London).*

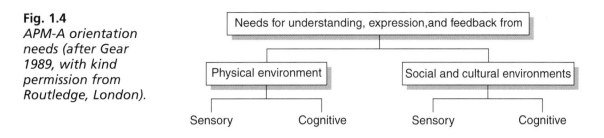

These needs are called 'orientation needs' because of their relationship to the orientation response and limbic arousal. Sensory needs include reassurance from unconsciously registering and identifying surfaces, sounds, smells, and sights as well as an optimal mix of familiarity and change. For example our need for contact with the natural world is borne out by research showing that even a view of nature through a window can aid healing (Ulrich 1984). Cognitive needs include those listed under the headings of autonomy, integrity and interdependence in Box 4.2 (see Ch. 4) and many, many more. Needs thought of as 'spiritual' needs are seen to encompass sensory and cognitive elements; for example, for some people aesthetic enjoyment via the senses may be the prime source of meeting spiritual needs, whereas for others cognitive elements, beliefs and rituals may play a very strong part.

*Imagination and
creativity, or
destruction and
self-destruction*

Under prolonged experience of threat, or as a result of highly stressful and disorientating events, the shifts to disorientation and back to reorientation can take us back to a different psychological, emotional and/or spiritual 'place'. A different patterning of biochemistry can also represent a noticeable shift in consciousness, and changes in needs and behaviour. For example Ed Mitchell, former pioneer astronaut, has spoken at length and made a film about his experiences of harmony, unity and insight as a result of his space flights; and fellow astronaut Charlie Duke has since been working and preaching to 'bring together' psychology and religion. In APM-A terms, negative kinds of disorientation, fear, tension or trauma can produce just as dramatic shifts in awareness. If people are then unable to understand why they feel as they do, and/or lack goals and purposes as channels of expression, they frequently need help to find reorientation. Remaining in a state of disorientation can hold danger for both self and others.

An APM-A explanation of a macro example of a species-wide shift in experience and behaviour may help to make the point. The first known unnecessary embellishment of a functional object, and its transformation into an object of beauty, is known as the Acheulian axe. Its creation coincided with the end of the harsh climatic conditions of the Pleistocene, the end of the last ice-age. This time was marked by a number of qualitative advances, including the production of beautiful decoration which bore no apparent relationship to functional demands. An APM-A explanation suggests that increased SNS activity, associated with stress, which is both self-perpetuating and wears off only slowly, happened as a result of harsh climatic conditions. The fact that the Acheulian culture coincided with the disappearance of the threat that had gradually raised SNS activity can be seen to be highly significant. A relatively sudden change in conditions and lessening of external demands is likely to have favoured those able to direct their new, excess (to survival needs) energies into other kinds of productive activity.

It would obviously have been counter-productive for individuals (and ultimately the species) for surplus energies to have been expressed randomly; perhaps in the form of gratuitous violence towards fellow tribesmen (or in more indirect threat to self, but to satisfy equally primitive urges) to direct energy towards the mates of fellow tribe members. The harmless (by comparison) hominid embellishers of axes are likely therefore to have been among those who survived long enough to procreate and exert influence over others.

There is of course more to creativity than the mere use of otherwise potentially self-destructive or socially disruptive energies. There is also enough evidence of current destructive and self-destructive behaviour to know that this was not selected against *per se*. However, just as creativity is about the expression of ideas as well as expression of energy in socially acceptable ways, and there are many repetitive activities that could have served the purpose of

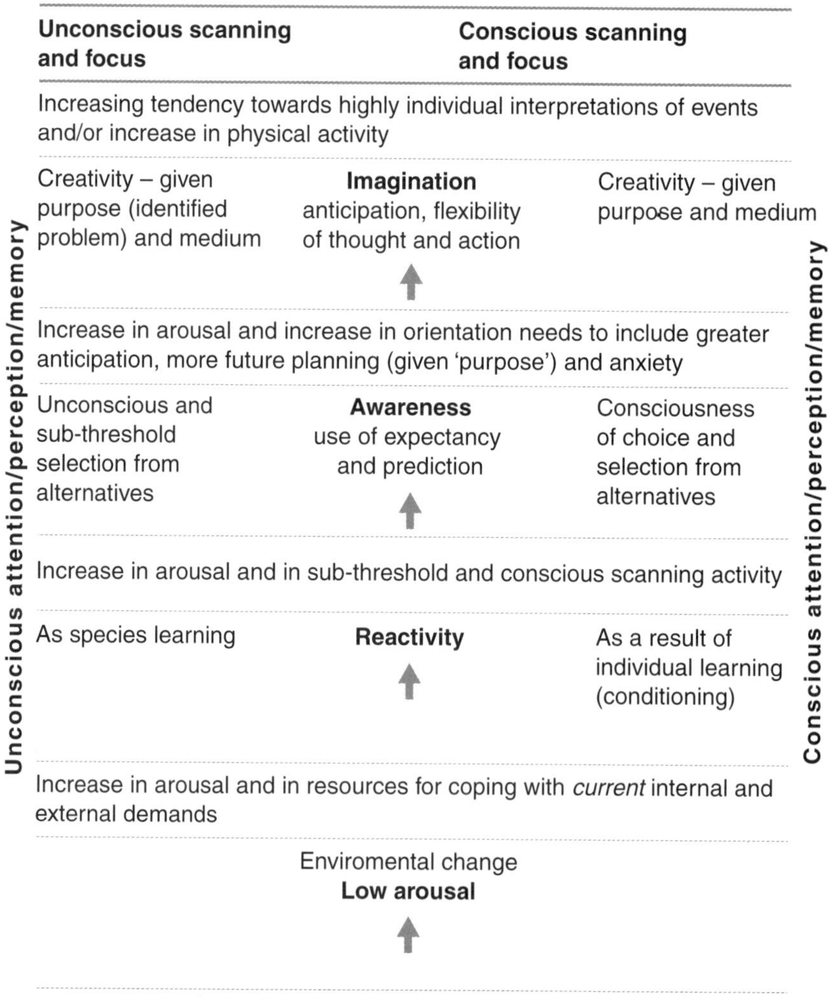

Fig. 1.5
Levels of conscious and unconscious 'awareness' (from Gear 1989, with kind permission from Routledge, London).

Unconscious scanning and focus		Conscious scanning and focus
Increasing tendency towards highly individual interpretations of events and/or increase in physical activity		
Creativity – given purpose (identified problem) and medium	**Imagination** anticipation, flexibility of thought and action ↑	Creativity – given purpose and medium
Increase in arousal and increase in orientation needs to include greater anticipation, more future planning (given 'purpose') and anxiety		
Unconscious and sub-threshold selection from alternatives	**Awareness** use of expectancy and prediction ↑	Consciousness of choice and selection from alternatives
Increase in arousal and in sub-threshold and conscious scanning activity		
As species learning	**Reactivity** ↑	As a result of individual learning (conditioning)
Increase in arousal and in resources for coping with *current* internal and external demands		
	Enviromental change **Low arousal** ↑	

(left vertical axis) Unconscious attention/perception/memory

(right vertical axis) Conscious attention/perception/memory

physical expression, so are current so-called 'clinical conditions' and criminal activities also about ideas as well as expressing energy; and repetitive activity is often a factor in self-injurious behaviour in particular.

The key point is about urgent needs for expression and understanding of disorientating and/or psychologically painful experiences that, when unmet, can result in distortions of thinking and expression, and behaviour that we have difficulty in handling.

Figure 1.5 describes shifts in consciousness, and the generally acknowledged shift to higher order needs that happened approximately half a million years ago. The diagram is just as relevant to dynamic and developmental changes within individuals as to species changes. Evolutionary changes in SNS activity and excitability inevitably imply changes in balancing PNS activity. The evolutionary change in question incidentally also compounded potential for human variability via increased adaptability and increased breadth of nervous system activity in general.

Figure 1.5 can also be seen to represent different kinds of learning and motivation recognised by the major schools of psychology (for more detail see Gear 1987). The 'reactive' level is consistent with behavioural findings about conditioning and habit formation; the next two levels are consistent with more recently evolved insight and problem-solving capacities identified by the Gestaltists; while autonomy and creativity, at the top of the diagram, are major areas of interest in humanistic psychology. The more recently developed views of memory and learning called information processing are represented by the core APM-A model representing interaction between attention, perception, memory and arousal (Fig. 1.3), and our dependency on identifying all messages conveyed by our senses, according to a hierarchy of priorities for physical and psychological survival (Gear 1987).

Different levels and kinds of vulnerability and a 'dynamic model of style'

Table 1.2 identifies relative dominance of needs for physical and psychological survival, as first- and second-order orientation needs. As explained above (pp. 17–18), second-order needs are higher level needs experienced as a result of more intense autonomic nervous system activity.

Table 1.2

First- and second-order needs (adapted from Gear 1989)

		Description of needs
Mastery and growth needs	Second-order orientation needs	Heightened orientation needs as a result of intensity of affect: need for more feedback/change; greater 'need to know', with reference to longer term, more complex and/or more abstract issues; increased communicative and expressive needs
Expectancy-value	First-order orientation needs	See Fig. 1.4 and pp. 18–19 for a summary of orientation needs
Drive reduction	Physical survival needs	Fulfilment of physiological demands: need for shelter, warmth, avoidance of danger, food drink, sleep, sexual expression

Note: Second-order orientation needs vary between and within individuals, as do the relative dominance of physical survival needs and kinds of orientation needs.

Figure 1.6 illustrates a model of styles based on differences in mental and physical activity as outcomes of variability in patterning of SNS and PNS activity. Differences in secretions of hormones and transmitters produce qualitatively different kinds of attention, perception, memory and awareness; differences in qualities of awareness in turn result in different levels and kinds of needs for orientation, including needs for understanding and expression. The whole forms a dynamic model of 'adaptive styles'. The term 'adaptive styles' refers to different ways of 'coping and defending' in the broadest sense: that is, identifying and classifying (mostly at an unconscious level) everything we experience, and defending against everything we perceive as either physically and/or emotionally threatening.

The dynamic model is based on the idea that, given a relative bias towards SNS activity, an individual may, or may not, display a further bias towards an increase in either mental or physical energy. This view acknowledges three key aspects of limbic arousal and autonomic nervous system activity:

1. Intensity of arousal

2. Predominantly adrenaline-biased arousal

3. Predominantly noradrenaline-biased arousal.

A further level of complication is variability in responsiveness, and relative dominance of SNS and PNS activity over each other. The interplay of all of

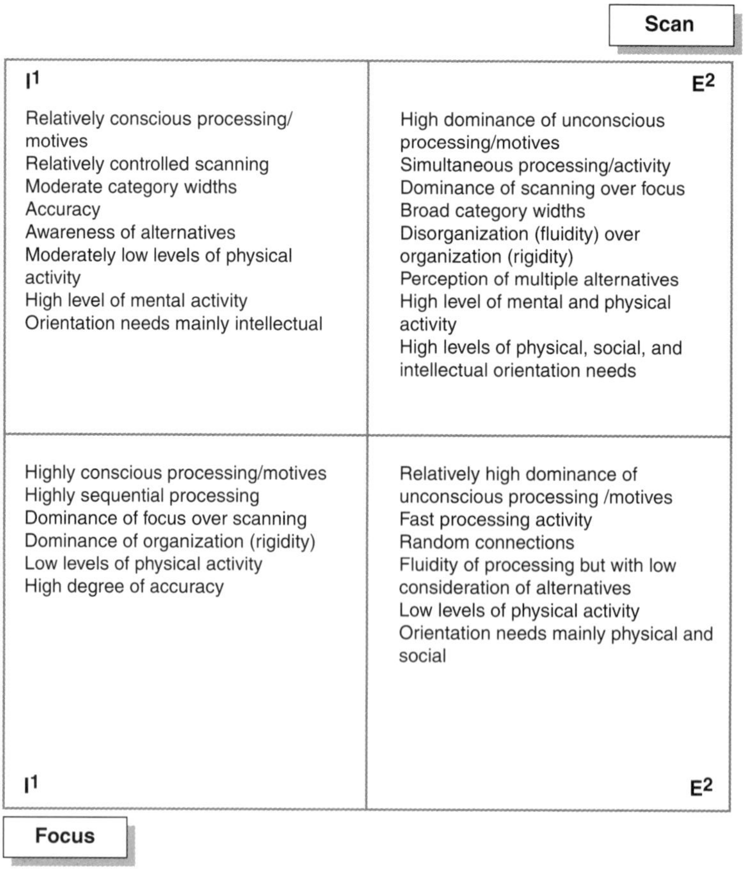

Fig. 1.6
Major APM-A styles: some fundamental differences within and between the major internal and external styles (adapted from Gear 1989, with kind permission from Routledge, London).

Scan

I1 / E2

Relatively conscious processing/motives; Relatively controlled scanning; Moderate category widths; Accuracy; Awareness of alternatives; Moderately low levels of physical activity; High level of mental activity; Orientation needs mainly intellectual

High dominance of unconscious processing/motives; Simultaneous processing/activity; Dominance of scanning over focus; Broad category widths; Disorganization (fluidity) over organization (rigidity); Perception of multiple alternatives; High level of mental and physical activity; High levels of physical, social, and intellectual orientation needs

Highly conscious processing/motives; Highly sequential processing; Dominance of focus over scanning; Dominance of organization (rigidity); Low levels of physical activity; High degree of accuracy

Relatively high dominance of unconscious processing /motives; Fast processing activity; Random connections; Fluidity of processing but with low consideration of alternatives; Low levels of physical activity; Orientation needs mainly physical and social

I1 / E2

Focus

these factors holds potential for a vast range of individuality. Expressed diagrammatically, this concept offers the framework of the 'dynamic model of style' (Fig.1.6).

In sum, the model in Figure 1.6 is of fundamental differences in ways in which we perceive and handle sensory and cognitive information: differences in how we are likely to think, feel and act in response to what happens around us. The extreme differences lie between the lower left quadrant (I^1) where behaviour is most passive and the upper right (E^2) representing the most active and expressive behaviours. The bottom left corner of the model (marked I^1) represents lowest arousal of any kind – in APM-A terms archetypal internalisers; the top right hand corner (marked E^2) represents highest levels of adrenaline and noradrenaline secretion – highest arousal, and archetypal externalisers. However, the model also allows variability within each of the four areas as well as a dynamic relationship between each area. It is not a static typology.

Although APM-A definitions of internalisers and externalisers are somewhat different from Eysenck's famous definition of introverts and extroverts (Eysenck 1981), the I^1–E^2 diagonal accommodates the Eysenckian polarity. This can be seen to represent the simplest possible bipolar way of defining differences in personality. The model also accommodates dimensions of neuroticism and psychoticism, represented by Eysenck as quite separate (Eysenck & Eysenck 1981), as well as other conventional categories of personality and perceptual disorders, but offers different explanations (Gear 1989). Some examples of positive and negative potentials of styles in each quadrant in Figure 1.6 are offered below.

Adaptive style, creativity, and behavioural distress

Conventionally defined neuroses and psychoses are located on the model (Gear 1989) in terms of characteristics of attention, perception, emotion and thinking. The strong links between creativity and schizophrenia, identified particularly by Laing (1971) and Arieti (1976, 1981), are accommodated in the quadrant E^2 (Fig. 1.6). It is important, however, to remember that there are many different kinds of creativity, and in translating the contents of the quadrants in Figure 1.6 into some everyday language and behaviours, examples from the arts are used to illustrate differences of 'style' (see below). It is stressed that each quadrant of the model itself contains variability and shading into other styles:

■ *First-order internalisers* (I^1) may be interpreted as having most 'stability' and control, displaying carefulness, orderliness, focus and liking for detail; or conversely, as being subject to rigidity of thought and actions and vulnerable to obsessive behaviours and withdrawal. Extreme fears are more likely to be relatively concrete, phobic rather than paranoid, with anger and other emotions less likely to be expressed directly than by externalisers.

Taking the example of artists, this group might be interested in realism, crafts and technical processes, or photography as an example that could also require least interaction with other people.

■ *Second-order internalisers* (I^2) are seen to have very similar characteristics to first-order internalisers, with more abstract interests and more flexible and sociable behaviours. Their vulnerabilities are again seen as similar to first order internalisers, but with any obsessions more abstract, and embracing ideas. Extreme fears would be more likely to be paranoid than phobic, and words more violent than actions.

As artists their work might include surrealism, writing or poetry, with ideas expressed in quite detailed ways.

- *First-order externalisers* (E^1) are seen as having particular likings for social and physical activity, and as having potential for impulsivity. If under stress and without socially acceptable means of expression, behaviour might spill into physical aggression.

  First-order externalisers are seen as more likely to be interested in sport than in art or craft. If they were artists, media might include physical activity such as stone- or rock-carving, to give scope for broad rather than precise forms of expression.

- *Second-order externalisers* (E^2) are seen as stereotypical opposites from first-order internalisers (I^1s), with behaviour showing more responsiveness, versatility, social awareness and abstract thinking than first-order internalisers. These characteristics might also be expressed as restlessness, instability, confusion or anxiety. Highly stressed conditions might include hallucinations, loss of touch with 'reality' and violence.

  Artistic styles could include abstract expressionism.

Potential for 'normal' variability is seen to be considerably wider, and emotional and expressive needs much higher than generally taken into account. For example, APM-A suggests that children currently referred to in mainstream schools as having 'special needs' may be unconsciously expressing their *unmet* needs and heightened vulnerability in their learning difficulties and behaviour. This seems especially likely when the proportions of special needs cases in some city schools can reach 60% and more of children (see, for example, the case illustration 'A teacher's use of NVC in the classroom' in Ch. 4, p. 91–93).

However, even at this stage the model is still based on the relatively simple notion of gradual dominance of SNS over PNS activity as arousal increases. To attempt to give as complete a picture as possible of real variability it would be necessary to place various overlays over the existing model to represent a variety of potential patterns and intensities of hormonal secretions.

These factors alone offer potential for an extraordinary range of variability in attention, perception, memory, excitability and kinds of response to everyday events, as well as variability in the kinds and levels of energy available to us. Add to this the habits of perception and behaviour we form, the mental maps we build, and social and cultural conditioning, and the possibilities for human individuality in psychological and emotional experience to affect behaviour becomes immense.

All styles are seen as having both strengths and vulnerabilities, and the model accommodates movement between quadrants as temporarily changed patterns of biochemistry, gradual adaptations, or highly stressed behaviours. The latter are detailed in the description of the whole theory where these stressed styles are related to well-documented conditions and 'psychopathologies'. In APM-A terms, the dividing line between so-called normality and abnormality and 'psychopathology' is seen to be extremely thin, very wavy and highly dependent on contexts. Figure 1.7 shows the

Fig. 1.7
Different kinds of potential for behavioural distress, with extreme passivity and potential for withdrawal located in the lower left side of the model, and attention deficit disorder (ADD), for example, on the right side of the model (from Gear 1989, with kind permission from Routledge, London).

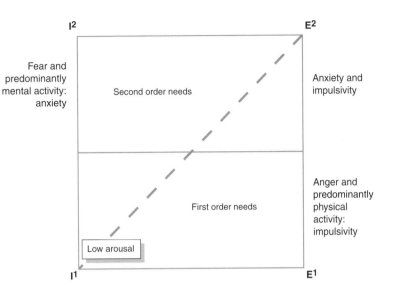

same model as Figure 1.6 with different kinds of potential for vulnerability and behavioural distress expressed in terms of fear and anger. These are the emotions most directly related to the hormones adrenaline and noradrenaline.

Some kinds of 'intelligence' and abilities have also been mapped onto the model to emphasise different kinds (rather than levels) of intelligence (Gear 1989). The model identifies different inborn potentials and vulnerabilities that we can become aware of, modify if necessary and, given opportunities, use in whatever ways are most rewarding.

In allowing for positive and negative potentials of personality traits, the model also accommodates socially acceptable and socially unacceptable ways of behaving. Which kinds of behaviour occur depends on environmental influences, including factors such as predominance of orientating or disorientating events and the availability or unavailability of means of understanding and expression. The same physiological type may achieve accolade or institutionalisation (or both), depending on whether energies are used creatively or destructively. The boundaries between behavioural difficulties – so-called 'abnormality' – and 'normality' are seen as tenuous and highly subject to social and political interpretation, adjustment and manipulation.

This view of people varying in terms of different kinds of vulnerability, and subject to different possible manifestations of individual styles (as either functional and adaptive or maladaptive to the circumstances they find themselves in) offers the possibility of what APM-A calls 'biological alternatives'. A well-known example of this phenomenon is the struggle to get needs met evident in the life of the reformed convicted murderer Jimmy Boyle, who now dedicates his life to helping other people.

Having passed through periods of his life unable to express feelings and needs orally, Boyle now talks movingly and eloquently about finding a creative outlet for his energies through sculpture in particular (Boyle 1977, 1984). He draws parallels between cutting away pieces of wood and 'finding things inside' at the same time as his own 'hard exterior' and defences were falling away, allowing him to experience a similar sense of

Fig. 1.8
A simple unitary model of regression that acknowledges changes in levels of engagement with physical and social environments and heightening of needs for both cognitive and sensory feedback as sympathetic nervous system (SNS) dominance increases. 'Threat' refers to perceptions of insecurity (from Gear 1989, with kind permission from Routledge, London).

Intensity of threat and increase in regressive behaviours ➡			
➡ Increase in mental and physical energy	➡ Increase in sensation-seeking behaviours	➡ Increase in attention to self/own needs	➡ Building up of defences that can include acquisition and ownership
➡ Dependency on available sources of gratification and increase in susceptibility to alternative rationales and belief systems	➡ Disengagement and polarization	➡ Self-neglect and/or abuse	➡ Withdrawal and/or disintegration

discovery about himself. All of this happened, he says, after he experienced trust for the first time. This happened in the special unit at Barlinnie prison where he was trusted with the sharp tools that enabled him to learn his craft.

The possibility of wholly different outcomes for individuals with high-level needs has also been highlighted by the recent controversial work of Bob Johnson, who video-recorded his own therapeutic work with murderers and other violent inmates of Parkhurst prison between 1993 and 1995. His videos show murderers eventually being able to show their own vulnerability as he helps them to revisit 'frozen terrors, buried fears, and toxic memories' from childhood. In each case he uncovered aggression rooted in deep emotional insecurity, and needs for 'respect' not experienced or witnessed in other ways than inspiring fear in others. Finding themselves in a new relationship of trust allowed prisoners to adjust to the reality that they were now 'safe', so that they could change attitudes and, apparently, 'personalities', as well as appearance (Johnson 1999).

Two further APM-A models that summarise very different uses of energy are a model of regression (Fig. 1.8) and a positive alternative, in which orientation needs are met from the experience of secure physical and social environments (Fig. 1.9). Figure 1.8 can be seen to be generally relevant to behavioural distress, and Figures 1.8 and 1.9 can both be seen as particularly relevant to 'Gentle Teaching' (described in Ch. 7), Nonviolent Communication (NVC) (Ch. 4) and all educational and therapeutic

Fig. 1.9
An alternative to the model of regression in Figure 1.8 when orientation needs are met. 'Promise' refers to perceptions of positive information and feedback (from Gear 1989, with permission from Routledge, London).

Increase in 'promise' ➡		
➡ Engagement	➡ Lowering of defences	➡ Interaction and learning
➡ Lowering of needs	➡ Growth in autonomy	➡ Attention to needs of others as well as self

interventions where creating emotionally safe environments, secure relationships and feelings of connection are important factors.

Conclusion

Some implications of APM-A theory

At its core, APM-A suggests that by helping people to identify feelings and unmet fundamental 'orientation needs' we can help them move from positions of disorientation to reorientation. It becomes possible to facilitate understanding and/or expression, and teach skills for needs to be met in alternative ways.

Broader understanding of the effects of changes in attention, perception, memory and arousal brings awareness of needs for optimal (to the individual) levels of arousal before some interventions (particularly those requiring focus) are likely to be effective. The same awareness and understanding of the relationship between high arousal and heightened needs offers understanding of the power of empathy in lowering arousal, and the deep value of helping people to get in touch with feelings and needs. Similarly, understanding of the huge potential for human emotional variability, and of different forms of vulnerability, can help us have more realistic expectations about differences in responses and behaviours, and again help us to maintain empathic connection.

APM-A offers an understanding of different kinds and levels of vulnerability and different styles of defence, as well as individuality in intensities of needs. For relationships in general as well as for counselling and other therapeutic interventions, deeper understanding of the significance of security, safety and trust, and of how they are created, is helpful in avoiding high defences and the barriers of withdrawal or attack. We can choose to connect with problems or symptoms, or we can choose to connect with people and their unmet needs. We can judge, blame or criticise, or identify feelings and needs (especially for understanding and expression) to help lower arousal, lower needs and aid concentration and focus.

Further kinds of understanding can help in choosing tools and interventions most likely to be helpful in particular cases. Examples include recognition of different biases and levels in needs for orientation, and recognition of different kinds of awareness and styles of thinking and learning in 'process' terms. Greater awareness of different kinds and levels of distressed communication and behaviour, and of the likely unmet needs behind them, may even avoid using other interventions. (Some specific implications of APM-A when linked to Nonviolent Communication (NVC) are discussed in Ch. 4.)

Consciousness of 'process' characteristics heightens understanding of flexibility and rigidity of thinking. At the same time it sharpens awareness of different kinds of so-called 'abnormal', 'deviant' , 'difficult' or 'challenging' behaviour (the last term at least acknowledges that the major difficulties might be our own) or diagnosed conditions and their relationships to 'normal' experience and behaviour. Awareness of individual differences in vulnerabilities as an integral part of human variability could help us to develop different kinds of diagnoses from the static labels currently in use. Instead, we may concentrate on identifying potentials linked to vulnerabilities.

There are many wider implications of APM-A, in terms of the range of needs perceived as not being taken into account in many fields such as health care, the law and in particular the education system. Education is seen to .have a crucial role to play in the avoidance of behavioural distress via curricula and other changes already identified (Gear 1989). More recently, moves towards encouraging emotional literacy and some aspects of the new 'citizenship' curriculum offer hope.

However, one direct implication of the theory is for the learning of interpersonal communication and relationship skills to be included in the school curriculum. If these were practised by both teachers and pupils from primary school level onwards it might eventually be possible for all members of society to have skills for reducing both 'inner' and 'outer' conflict. A specific tool for this purpose already being incorporated into some curricula outside the UK is Nonviolent Communication (see Ch. 4), for which APM-A provides a supporting theory.

Another implication is for the multiple roles of the arts (particularly in offering sensory experience, understanding and expression) and physical activities to be acknowledged as holding value in helping children and adults achieve optimal states for other kinds of learning.

General implications of theory

The established theories offered in the first half of this chapter are a mere sample from major disciplines in the human sciences, and from different schools of psychology, of volumes of theory that refer variously to all aspects of mind and behaviour.

Ultimately, as parents, other family members, informal helpers, educaters or other professionals, we construct knowledge ourselves, unconsciously if not consciously, and we will be operating from theory whether we realise it or not. The more conscious we become of the variety of theories available to us, the better position we are in to be conscious of the theories that inform our own actions. More importantly, we may then become more aware of their implications for the people we try to help.

We can choose to offer people tools, skills and choices or we can choose to intervene in more or less controlling ways. We can condition or 'shape' or we can enable development and change (or both) in differing degrees. How we have been taught, or choose, to view people and their behaviour will affect how we behave in return, the kinds of interventions (if any) we are likely to make and how successful some interventions are likely to be.

References

Arieti S 1976 The magic synthesis. Basic Books, New York

Arieti S 1981 Understanding and helping the schizophrenic. Pelican Books, Harmondsworth

Ax A F 1953 The physiological differentiation between fear and anger in humans. Psychosomatic Medicine 15: 433–442

Bandura A 1962 A social learning through imitation. In: Jones M R (ed) Nebraska symposium on motivation. University of Nebraska Press, Lincoln

Beatty J 1982 Task-evoked pupillary responses, processing load and the structure of processing resources. Psychological Bulletin 92 (2): 276–292

Boyle J 1977 A sense of freedom. Pan Books, London

Boyle J 1984 Art and personal development. Address to the conference: Support for the arts: recent evidence for the role of the arts in education. London

Brown J 1993 Freud and the post-Freudians. Penguin Books, Middlesex

Campbell F, Singer G 1979 Brain and behaviour. Pergamon Press, Australia

Durkheim E 1952 Suicide. Routledge and Kegan Paul, London

Ellis R, Gates B 1995 The person in communication. In: Ellis R, Gates R, Kenworthy N Interpersonal communication in nursing: theory and practice. Churchill Livingstone, Edinburgh

Eysenck H J 1981 A model for personality. Springer Verlag, Berlin

Eysenck H J, Eysenck S P G 1981 Psychoticism as a dimension of personality. Hodder and Stoughton, London

Freud S 1925a Repression. In: Collected papers. Hogarth Press, London, vol. 4, pp. 84–97

Freud S 1925b The unconscious. In: Collected papers. Hogarth Press, London, vol. 4, pp. 98–136

Funkenstein D H 1956 Norepinephrine-like and epinephrine-like substances in relation to human behaviour. Journal of Nervous and Mental Diseases 124: 58–66

Gale A, Edwards J A 1983 Physiological correlates of human behaviour. Academic Press, New York

Gear J 1985 Perception and the evolution of style: a unified view of human modes of behaviour and expression. PhD thesis, University of Hull

Gear J 1987 Attention, affect and learning. Newland Paper No 13, Department of Adult Education, University of Hull

Gear J 1989 Perception and the evolution of style: a new model of mind. Routledge, London

Gregory R 1987 The Oxford companion to the mind. Oxford University Press, Oxford

Haviland W 1996 Cultural anthropology, 8th edn. Harcourt Brace, Fort Worth

Hilgard E R, Bower G H 1975 Theories of learning. Prentice Hall International, London

Husserl E G A 1891 Philosophy of arithmetic.

Johnson B 1999 Is humanity born sociable, loveable and non violent? Address to the inaugural conference of the James Naylor Foundation: Building a violence free society. London

Koffka K 1924 The growth of the mind, trans. R M Ogden. Kegan Paul, Trench and Trubner, London

Köhler W 1925 The mentality of apes. Penguin Books, Middlesex

Laing A R 1971 The working brain. Penguin Books, Harmondsworth

Luria A R 1976 The nature of human conflicts. Liveright, New York (first published 1932)

McGaugh, J H 1980 Adrenalin a secret agency of memory. Psychology Today 14 (7): 132

Maslow A H 1954 Motivation and personality. Harper, New York

Matlin M 1994 Cognition, 3rd edn. Harcourt Brace, Fort Worth

Merleau-Ponty M 1942 Analyses of the experienced body.

Merleau-Ponty M 1945 Analyses of perception.

Newell R 1996 Mental health. In: Kenworthy N, Snowley G, Gilling C Common foundation studies in nursing. Churchill Livingstone, Edinburgh

Papineau D 1989 For science in the social sciences. McMillan, London

Pavlov I P 1902 The work of the digestive glands. Griffin, London

Pelto P 1965 The study of anthropology. Merrill, Ohio

Pervin L A 1993 Personality: theory and research, 6th edn. John Wiley, New York

Rogers C 1951 Client centered therapy: its current practice, implications and theory. Houghton Mifflin, Boston

Rogers C 1983 Freedom to learn for the 80s. Merrill, Columbus

Skinner B F 1971 Beyond freedom and dignity. Knopf, New York

Stevanson L 1974 Seven theories of human nature. Oxford University Press, Oxford

Szasz T 1961 The myth of mental illness. Harper, New York.

Thorndike E L 1898 Animal intelligence: an experimental study of the associative process in animals. Journal of Psychological Review Monographs suppl. 2 (no. 8): 28–31

Tolman E C 1925 Purpose and cognition: the determinants of animal learning. Psychological Review 32: 285–297

Tolman E C 1938 The determinates of behaviour at a choice point. Psychological Review 45 (1): 1–41

Tylor E B 1871 Primitive culture: research into the development of mythology, philosophy, religion, language, art and customs. Murray, London

Ulrich R S 1984 View through a window may influence recovery from surgery. Science 224: 420–421

Van Toller C 1979 The nervous body. Wiley, Chichester

Wallace W 1971 An overview of elements in the scientific process: the logic of science in sociology. Aldine, Atherton, Chicago

Watson J B 1907 Kinesthetic and organic sensations, the role of the reactions of the white rat to the maze. Journal of Psychological Monographs 8 (no. 33): 91–93

Watson J B 1924 Behaviourism. (Revised edn. 1930) Norton, New York

Wertheimer M 1938 Laws of organisation in perceptual forms. In: Ellis W D A source book of Gestalt psychology. Harcourt Brace, pp. 71–88 (translation and condensation of: Untersuchung zur Lehre von der Gesalt, II, Psychologische Forschung, 1925, 4: 301–350)

Yule W, Carr J 1990 Behaviour modification for people with mental handicaps. Chapman and Hall, London

2 Terminology

Peter Oakes

Key issues
- The words and language we choose to use to describe behavioural distress can have a profound impact upon the person to whom it refers
- Our understanding of distressed behaviour is best understood in terms of interpersonal relationships between the person experiencing the distress and others
- Behavioural distress can be explored and understood by examining the words, images and perceptions associated with the term disability

---

Overview
This chapter considers words which are used to describe people who experience behavioural distress, and who trigger distress in others. It explores how language may influence the person to whom it refers, and acknowledges the somewhat bitter irony that our thoughts and speech may indeed contribute to the distress we are aiming to resolve. Our understanding of behavioural distress will be illustrated by exploring the words, images and perceptions associated with the term 'disability' in particular. The aim of the chapter is to explore and develop a more positive approach to our thinking, and understand our perception of distressed behaviour in terms of interpersonal relationships between the person experiencing the distress and others. This chapter therefore suggests that we work alongside people to arrive at shared understanding of behavioural distress. The traditional categories of distressed behaviour are discussed and their meanings explained and related to the types of actions and characteristics to which they refer.

Why words?
To the author of this chapter, it would appear that we are moving away from taking care about the words that we use. Think for a moment; people appear more comfortable using phrases like 'the disabled' and 'behaviour problems' and it has become more acceptable to make the odd joke at the expense of someone who is vulnerable. There is a range of reasons for this relaxation and many people may confess to a sense of relief. It is possible that we grew tired of minding our p's and q's and the 'political correctness police' telling

us what to say; and perhaps the attempt to change attitudes by changing words was doomed to failure – did anyone really believe they were 'challenged' by 'challenging behaviour'?

There have also been some new demands made upon the attention of people working in this area, such as the ever growing call for evidence based practice. This drive for evidence is to be supported; however, it can lead to a culture of technique, where we are solely concerned with the impact a particular way of working has upon the person. Is the undesirable behaviour reduced by our actions? If it is, good. If not, then we talk in somewhat vague terms about maintaining current levels and standards of behaviour and how bad things would have been if we had not acted in the way we did.

So a series of new demands might mean that we have been unable to give much thought to the meaning of our language and the models of distress that we promote. Yet what of the person who experiences this distress, their family and carers, the services that support them and the wider community? They may have seen and heard a number of labels come and go, yet continue to feel hurt and rejected by the harshness and sense of blame which are carried by the words we choose to use. They may continue to tolerate the actions of family members, carers, members of staff and professionals who simply do not understand the meaning of their behaviour and the distress that they feel. Unfortunately, it would appear that the life experiences of people who exhibit behavioural distress are largely unchanged over the years (Williams 1994). People continue to be excluded from the discussions which attempt to understand and respond to their distress. They continue to live in a world which sees distress in terms of personal tragedy, firmly located inside the person, as essentially medical in nature, and needing to be controlled or changed by the actions of formal professionals and paid supporters.

In writing about the importance of language, Slee (1996) noted that words bring assumptions, represent history and define practice. These elements of assumption, history and practice could be seen as the *message* carried by the words. This can best be explored and illustrated by discussing the application of the medical model to the notion of disability. The impact of such messages can then also be understood in terms of distress. Firstly, the medical approach assumes that the disabled person is biologically or physiologically inferior to the ordinary person. Here, the disability is quite definitely inside the person. Secondly, the approach has a history of medical interventions which have involved institutional care, segregation and control of all aspects of a person's life. The third element involves practice which seeks to predict and control behaviour and to restore functional loss (Slee 1996).

An alternative approach would be to see disability in terms of the relationship a person has with others in their community. Disability in this sense arises from the failure of society to adjust to the wide variety of needs among the individuals who make up a community. The assumption within this alternative approach is that a person with a disability is different in the same way that all people are different from each other. The focal point of this model is the need to analyse and reverse the prejudice found in the wider community. The implications for practice of this model are that families, communities and services aim to support and empower a person, wherever that may lead, within accepted legal and social frameworks. These issues will be explored throughout this chapter. (Before moving on, look at the activity 'How was it for you?')

How was it for you?

Think for a while about a situation in which you have been misunderstood. It might have been at home, school or work. It might have involved people you spend other time with. What were the words which showed you that the other people did not understand you? What actions followed from the wrong words and the wrong conclusion? What would you like to say to those people now?

The language of disability

An apology

In writing this account, it has been necessary to use a number of terms in the text which are highly offensive to most people – with and without learning disabilities and/or in behavioural distress. These words are therefore set in inverted commas and the intention is to demonstrate the destructive influence of such words upon the experience of the people concerned. However, there is a sense in which using these words within these pages keeps them alive. The author keen to apologise to anyone who may be upset by their presence and assure you that their use has not been taken lightly. It is hoped that past mistakes can be avoided by modern practitioners who seek to understand and move on.

First words

Charting the history of the definition and legal terms relating to learning disability provides a helpful starting point for exploring the use of language and labels. This approach has been used by Gates (1996) and will be repeated here.

Until the beginning of the 20th century there was just one separate legal reference to people with learning disabilities. This was contained in an obscure law of 1325 called De Praerogative Regis. It concerned the disposal of land and referred to people with learning disabilities as 'born fools'. This distinguished them from people with mental health needs for the purpose of the act (Potter 1993), and represented the last clear distinction between learning disability and mental health until the Mental Deficiency Act of 1913.

More recent legal and professional definitions can be used to track the thinking of the 20th century. The Mental Deficiency Acts of 1913 and 1927 referred to people as 'defectives' and sought to categorise the extent of disability by reference to four sub-categories. Three of these relate specifically to the extent of disability and use language which can still be heard on the streets and in the playgrounds of today. These are 'idiot', 'imbecile' and 'feeble minded'. The fourth category is one of the earliest descriptions of a person who is distressed: the term 'moral defective'.

The *message* of these words is that the person is incomplete, that the person is summed up by a difficulty and that the difficulty lies within the person. The words also serve to separate and distance the person from the ordinary population. This naturally places a person with others who share similar problems, rather than with others who share interests, humour, family and so on.

In the new Mental Health Act (1959) the words were changed for legal purposes and the sub-categories were reduced from four to two. The new offering was 'subnormality'; a person was defined as either 'subnormal' or 'severely subnormal', depending on the extent of her or his learning disability. The four-way categorisation of 'mild, moderate, severe and profound' has lived on in professional circles where these terms have tended to suggest the extent of difficulties experienced by an individual.

The message contained within these categories was much the same as that of the first part of the century. If anything, the idea of 'subnormality' was a little more sinister, possibly because the use of this term can be placed within the historical context which included the eugenics movement. The eugenics movement sought to distinguish those people in society who, classed as genetically subhuman, were considered a threat to the wider community. This movement found its ultimate and terrifying expression in extreme fascism which involved the systematic destruction of people who were considered to be, in some sense, inadequate or incomplete, including people with learning disabilities.

The current parlance

The 1983 Mental Health Act could be said to have moved matters forward. The images of people as incomplete and subhuman were left behind and the term 'mental impairment' was introduced. In addition to this, services moved from referring to 'the mentally handicapped', through 'people with mental handicap', to 'people with learning disabilities'. These could be said to be the mainstream terms. Other terms have been less frequently used and have included 'people with learning difficulties'. This last term has been the consistent preference of groups representing people who receive services, and 'people with intellectual impairments' has been the term favoured by some members of the academic community.

In considering the *message* carried by these more recent descriptions, there remains an assumption of damage and weakness. However, there is also a clear concern to establish the person as a person, before identifying the disability. The conflict between the need in formal services for an accurate, shared set of terms and the views of people themselves is of interest. This will become even more apparent as we search for appropriate ways of defining and describing distressed behaviour. Clearly, there are demands for the use of common language and terms to help plan services, establish eligibility and research the issues concerning people with learning disabilities and people who exhibit behavioural distress. This is especially the case for formal and organised services. However, shared perceptions, images and assumptions are framed by language and guide behaviour (see the activity 'Messages').

Messages

Think about the terms you yourself have used to describe people with learning disabilities. Some of these terms may be professional descriptions (such as 'people with learning disabilities') and others may be the language used on a day-to-day basis ('them' or 'the lads' or 'the girls'). What is the message carried by these terms, and which ones would you like to be called if you were disabled in some way?

Images of disability

Allied to the professional and legal terms which have been used are the ideas and images which are held by wider society. These are described by a number of authors (Wolfensberger 1972, Gates 1996). Some of these perceptions can be found in the language used by people as they talk to, or about, people with disabilities. Wolfensberger (1972) gives the following eight headings:

1. Subhuman

2. Object of ridicule

3. Object of dread

4. Menace

5. Holy innocent

6. Eternal child

7. Object of pity

8. Sick.

Each of these perceptions seems to have been dominant for a period of time before being replaced by one of the other perceptions. Each, however, continues to have some influence on the way people think today. A brief review of modern media images of people with learning disabilities would reveal evidence of many of these ideas. This is especially the case given a continuing difficulty in the wider community when seeking to distinguish between people with learning disabilities who exhibit behavioural distress and people with mental health needs. It follows that many people will bring these perceptions along with them when they work with, and care for, people who receive their support.

It also seems probable that the message from our overall models of disability and the continuing presence of the ideas from the wider community will have an influence on the thinking and language which are used to described distressed behaviour. The more specific use of terms to describe distressed behaviour can now be considered.

The language of behavioural distress

There has been little consistency in the use of language to describe behavioural distress in people (both with and without learning disabilities), apart from a period between the late 1980s and the mid-1990s when the term 'challenging behaviour' was used very widely in the UK. Prior to this there was a tendency to use such terms as 'problem behaviour' or 'behaviour problems', 'disturbed behaviour', 'maladaptive behaviour' or 'difficult behaviour'. The new term 'challenging behaviour' was introduced by Blunden & Allen (1987), who had a clear message for those involved in this field. The message was that behaviour should be seen as a challenge to the services and individuals involved with a person, rather than the challenge being located within the person.

In considering the language of behavioural distress, there is no common agreement regarding a definition of the phenomenon. It is necessary, therefore, to present issues which surround the *definition* of distressed behaviour, and to describe the things which people do to attract the label 'challenging'. This will lead to an exploration of the *perceptions* of behavioural distress which, as before, are framed by words and influence our behaviour.

In recent years, much reference has been made to the important work of Emerson (Emerson et al 1988) about what was termed as challenging behaviour. Emerson's definition (p. 16) was as follows:

> *Severe challenging behaviour refers to behaviour of such an intensity, frequency or duration that the physical safety of the person or others is likely to be placed in serious jeopardy, or behaviour that is likely to seriously limit or deny access to and the use of ordinary community facilities.*

It seems here that a person's behaviour can be described as 'challenging' if it raises issues of safety and/or access to the community. Wray (1999) has identified two main difficulties with this approach. The first is that some people express their distress in passive ways, such as stereotyped movements or withdrawal. Although these behaviours are still 'challenging' they might not be included in the definition above. Also, the second part of the definition which relates to community access seems to assume that access would normally be straightforward. This is patently not the case.

In rejecting the term 'challenging behaviour', Slevin (1995) reverts to the notion of problematic behaviour, suggesting that such behaviour needs to be reduced because of the difficulties it causes to the person and to those around the person. Whilst this carries a certain honesty, there remains the difficulty of locating the behaviour with the person and assuming that it is negative.

Perhaps the most promising way forward has been produced by the Mental Health Foundation in its document *Don't Forget Us: Children with Learning Disabilities and Severe Challenging Behaviour* (Mental Health Foundation 1997). Emerson's definition (Emerson et al 1988, p. 12) is expanded as follows:

> *Severe challenging behaviour refers to behaviour of such an intensity, frequency or duration that the physical safety of the person or others is likely to be placed in serious jeopardy, or behaviour that is likely to seriously limit or deny access to and the use of community facilities, or behaviour which is likely to impair the child's personal growth, development and family and which represents a challenge to services, to families and to the children themselves however caused.*

This definition of distressed behaviour seems to deal with some of the difficulties which have impeded progress up to this point. It certainly widens the definition to include personal growth and family. It also locates responsibility for a response with services, families and the individual concerned whilst not seeking to place blame for the causes of behaviour. However, there remains a range of difficulties which simply cannot be addressed by a single definition. These difficulties include questions such as:

- Is it the behaviour which limits community access and personal growth or something else?
- At what point can a way of behaving be said to become challenging?

To include all possible forms of distress, both active and passive, the definition seems to cover an enormous range of possible behaviour. There is no means of distinguishing distress that needs a response from a range of behaviours which would satisfy this definition but not require a response of any kind.

These definitions have been so important to the provision of services for people who are distressed, they still have the effect of summing up the person in terms of the label of distress. Distress may have to be at a certain level to trigger eligibility for special services, and consequently the person becomes defined by the distress which they experience and its attendant label. This is the classic problem of labelling and stigma. A small part of a person's behaviour is taken and used to sum up the whole person. How often have we heard phrases such as:

'He's a "runner"' (of someone who seeks to leave a building without support to do so).

'She's a "pincher"' (of a woman who attempts to pinch people).

'This is Gary, be careful he "nips"' (of a man who attempts to pinch people).

Such descriptions give a most unhelpful first impression. They deny the massive range of other characteristics which will distinguish this person from others, many of which will be positive. They send an immediate *message* – to beware – and so break any positive expectations which someone might have when meeting the person. They act as a constant reminder to the person of a part of his or her life which is negative and which, no doubt, everyone is trying to change.

A key reason why this book takes the title of 'distress' rather than 'problem', 'challenge' or 'difficulty', is that this seems as far as we can go without detailed reference to the person and his or her current behaviour and experience. We are talking simply about people who manifest behaviour that is distressing for themselves and for others. As this chapter develops, it is becoming increasingly evident that the next step in understanding such distress is to seek to understand the experience of the person and those who are in contact with the person. If that presents difficulties for research and eligibility criteria for special services, then these problems are our problems, not the individual's. However, before moving to an exploration of an alternative and perhaps more appropriate model, it is important to describe the kinds of actions which tend to attract the labels discussed here and to give some idea of their prevalence.

Expressions of behavioural distress

How many people are distressed?

One of the fundamental difficulties in determining prevalence and incidence of behavioural distress is that it is likely that everyone will experience some significant distress at some point in their lives. This may, or may not, lead them to do things which cause concern amongst other people. This in turn may, or may not, lead to the involvement of specialised staff employed to help support people when they are distressed. (See also the activity 'Who decides?'.) Consequently, reliable estimates of prevalence in total populations cannot be calculated. However, it is possible to look at one group of people (such as people with learning disabilities who present with behavioural distress) and obtain approximate estimates. Mansell (Department of Health 1992) has suggested that 20 people per 100 000 total population will express significant distress at any one time where there is a defined learning disability. Murphy (1994) goes on to suggest that this figure is increased as the level of disability increases. These are helpful guide figures, yet the issue of definition remains and can be explored in more detail at this point.

' Who decides? '

Consider anyone you know who is not learning disabled, and who is (or has been) distressed. At what point did they seek help? Where did they seek help? How did they decide to seek professional help? If they did not seek help, what happened?

Now consider a person with a learning disability in distress. How can that person seek help from someone who is not paid to help them and who is not involved in all other aspects of their lives? Who decides to seek additional support from an outside professional? Why are the two experiences so different?

What do people actually do?

There have been various approaches to understanding the ways in which people might express their distress. Some of those methods involve simply describing what people do – these are known as descriptions of topography. The best examples of this approach are found in the development of the Adaptive Behaviour Scale (Nihira et al 1993). This gives the following sub-categories of behaviour:

- Social behaviour
- Conformity
- Trustworthiness
- Stereotyped and hyperactive behaviour
- Sexual behaviour
- Social engagement
- Disturbing interpersonal behaviour
- Self abusive behaviour.

An alternative to this approach is that adopted by Pyles & Bailey (1990), who explain the expression of distress in terms of the function or purpose of that behaviour. This is clearly influenced by behavioural approaches to the management of distress in which functional analysis forms the core means of assessment and formulation. Seven categories have been identified under the terms of this approach:

- Self-stimulation
- Escape from demands, people or settings
- Attention seeking/attempting to communicate
- Reinforcement of behaviour or history of reinforcement
- Medication side-effects
- Illness, pain, discomfort or deprivation
- Physiological.

A third approach has been to combine the topographical and the functional. McBrien & Felce (1992) give five categories which describe both action and proposed function:

- Aggressive approaches to others (e.g. hitting, pulling hair)
- Self-injurious behaviours
- Destructive behaviours
- Disruptive, nuisance, antisocial, dangerous behaviours
- Stereotypic/self-stimulatory behaviours.

What is of interest in considering these different categories is that each of them carries a message in much the same way as the models of disability carried messages. Inherent in each of the approaches are some assumptions about the meaning of the behaviour, the system of support and the theoretical approach of the people who have developed these measures. This is particularly so for the functional approach where it is assumed that the person is doing something to gain attention or to provide stimulation. The basis for such an interpretation is unclear and the theoretical approach denies the possible importance of such things as early childhood or emotional trauma, the need to belong or to be close to other people.

However, the topographical elements also carry value judgements in regard to what is inappropriate, antisocial or rebellious. There is a sense here of an order or a regime which needs to be complied with. If a person objects to that regime or is so distressed about something that the order has no meaning, then their behaviour is seen as 'inappropriate'. Is it not possible that the circumstances which are imposed on a person are inappropriate and antisocial, and that the response is reasonable and appropriate?

These difficulties are largely ignored because the professional community needs a system of description in order to gather evidence about prevalence and the effectiveness of various interventions. Once again, however, the meaning of an action to an individual is lost and the words used to describe that action are almost entirely negative, value laden and focusing on the person rather than the relationships which he or she may have with other people.

The language of intervention

Up to this point we have considered the words used to describe disability as a whole and the words used to describe distress. It has been clear at every stage that the words carry a wider message and that this message is imposed on the person by the practitioner rather than the other way around. Before moving to consider the possible impact of this process on the people who exhibit distress, it is important to contemplate the words which are used to describe the services and support which people receive. Again it is a question of exploring the words to uncover the message which they carry. For example, people with learning disabilities can be in receipt of services ranging from the occasional visit by a support worker through to full-time detention in a special hospital. It is likely that people who become distressed will gradually attract the attention of a wider group of support services as their distress increases. This has been shown to lead to the planning and implementation of intervention strategies and moves to more intensively supported settings (Emerson et al 1994).

Some of the theoretical background underpinning the different models of intervention has been outlined in Chapter 1. However, it remains important to determine both the message of specific approaches which are used and also how these messages relate both to the general provision of care and to responses to distress.

Baldwin (1985) takes us through five separate models of service delivery which apply to both general services and interventions. These are as follows:

- Child development model
- Medical model
- Social–ecological model
- Behavioural model
- Psycho-educational model.

In a similar vein, Sumarah (1989) gives an excellent account of three metaphors which tend to govern the relationship between people who receive a service and people who work in a service. These are:

- Organic (animal)
- Mechanical
- Personal.

Here, in both words and actions, the person is seen either as an animal who is cared for, patted and stroked, but who is essentially not human; a machine which is essentially technical in nature and needs to be predicted and controlled; or as a person with agency and the ability to relate to others.

These ideas can be synthesised to give the following models and messages:

Child development model

Within this model there is an assumption that people with learning disabilities have been delayed in their social, cognitive, emotional and psychological development and this has involved missing key developmental milestones. Thus, in understanding behavioural distress, theories of child development are brought into play and the person is helped to move through the appropriate period and so resolve the distress.

What, then is the message of a 'child-centred service' and a 'child-centred approach' to distress? There can be some positive answers here. There is certainly likely to be more of a sense of compassion towards children who are behaviourally distressed and also a reluctance, at least occasionally, to blame children for the circumstances of their difficulties. However, there are four clear dangers inherent in this approach and its message to the people involved with someone who is distressed:

1. Baldwin (1985) notes a lowering of expectations when dealing with a child and to this can be added a tendency to divert the child from the reasons for his or her distress and behaviour. This can amount to a belittling of the difficulties, because a child will cry so much more frequently than an adult. Such an approach can be particularly dangerous should the person be in an abusive situation.

2. When considering a child-centred approach, the need to involve the person in understanding behavioural distress and in making plans to respond is paramount. Whilst the approach for older children may be an involving or empowering one, the issues with younger children can legitimately be those related to boundaries where a child needs to learn to comply with adult instructions as a matter of obedience and good behaviour. However, this is not a helpful message for any adult experiencing or manifesting behavioural difficulties or distress.

3. The third issue is one of applying child-centred ideas to other parts of a person's life because their distress has been understood in these terms. If an episode of extreme anger is referred to as a tantrum much like that of a 2-year-old child, it is possible that issues of sexuality or a need to work will be ignored because they can be seen to be wholly inappropriate to the world of a 2-year-old.

4. At its extreme, these approaches become akin to the organic approach detailed by Sumarah (1989). Here people are trained to behave in particular ways without concern for their own personal thoughts, meanings and feelings.

Medical model

This model has already been mentioned because it remains dominant, especially where there are possible overlaps between the field of learning disability and mental health. Within this model, behavioural distress is seen as an illness with some form of physical cause and consequently the response is found in the use of medication. Without exploring the model in depth, it is important to understand the message of the medical model. Again there are some positive aspects to this. Medicine is clear in its understanding of the person as a person with physical integrity. Good practice within this model means that the person is to be respected and listened to. However, there are two main difficulties with the message of this model:

1. The medical model involves locating the need to get better inside the person, and the form of distress is explained in terms of the person's physiological make-up. Thus, the reduction of distress may deny the other elements of a person's life and experience such as his or her history, relationships or spiritual situation. Resolution of the distress is through the administration of drugs or other medically approved interventions to achieve change.

2. The other difficulty with a medical approach lies in the idea of diagnosis. Here is a process which seeks to exclude various possibilities (differential diagnoses) and so conclude that the person's behavioural distress falls into a particular category alongside that of a number of other people who experience similar 'symptoms'. This can lead to false assumptions and to a loss of the individual experience of the person. Once again the person 'is' the disease. Thus, if it is concluded that someone is depressed, it may be assumed that all of that person's behaviour can be understood in terms of the depression. There may be a whole range of different reasons why someone refuses to eat or does not sleep well. Instead, these are seen as symptoms of depression and consequently, it is assumed, should respond to antidepressants.

Technical model

The growth of evidence based practice and the continuing dominance of functional analysis (see Ch. 9) has made many improvements in people's lives. This technical approach incorporates a range of interventions in addition to the behavioural approach. These include psychotherapeutic and 'Gentle Teaching' methods (see Chs 1 and 7 respectively). People have received painstaking and thorough assessments of their behaviour and its context. Each intervention is a mini experiment which ensures that only the responses which bring results are pursued. Technical interventions are now almost entirely positive, offering the person the opportunity to learn alternative means of expressing distress or meeting needs. This is in many ways a human approach with the message that the person is fully an individual with a complex history and current environment. The message is also one of structure, accuracy and effectiveness.

The difficulties of this model of intervention are seen in some of the other approaches:

- There remains a sense that a person can be predicted and controlled as long as the technician has sufficient information. This is simply not the case. Moreover, we can be clear that however good a technician the worker may be, success is likely to depend on the relationship with the person.

- It seems clear that people are more than the sum of their parts, and it may not be possible to build up evidence to a point where the whole person can be understood.

Social–ecological model

In this model, people are understood within the context of their environment – in its broadest sense. The model has been gaining ground in both the thinking and practice of recent years. The advantages are clear. This model sees the person as an individual who interacts with other people and their contexts and as an equal partner in an environment which either enhances ability or which further disables the person. Behavioural distress is understood to communicate that relationships and environments are not meeting needs. The response involves working alongside the person to establish what it is that needs to change, and to work with the system of care to achieve that change. The message of the model is that the person is fully human and in relationship with others. The meaning of distress is to be understood from the individual's point of view, and everyone involved is therefore responsible for achieving change. This chapter proposes that this is the model of choice, in conjunction with elements of the technical model.

However, there is a key problem which still needs to be addressed. When applied to the distress of an individual, the social–ecological model in its purest form can be interpreted as somewhat pessimistic, as it sees the person as a rather passive victim of the behaviour of those around him or her. As a small boat tossed upon a mighty sea, the person is powerless and must grasp onto a single hope: that the professional can change the system. Also, the impact of personal factors and/or any disability which a person carries must not be denied. If someone has additional sensory disabilities or has suffered a lifetime of abuse, this will have an influence on that person's behaviour. Any approach based on this model will need to be honest about experience and disability and ensure that the message is one of empowered individuals who can withstand and influence the context in which they find themselves.

The work of Sumarah (1989) required an approach which was *personal*. This meant that the person was to be seen as a human being, responsible for action whilst in relationship with others. This represents a synthesis of the technical as it has now become and the social–ecological. It addresses the social perspective in that the person is seen as being in relationships with others. It also maintains a systematic and evidence based practice which nevertheless recognises the individual as a unique and valuable human being with the full range of complex histories, motivations and inspirations, hidden or otherwise. (Look now at the activity 'What's the difference?')

'What's the difference?

Using the metaphors of organic (animal), mechanical and personal outlined by Sumarah (1989) on p. 40, think about how we reflect those differences in our relationships and responses to people who are in behavioural distress.

The impact of messages

When thinking about the words we use and the message which they carry, there is a temptation to return to the position stated at the beginning of this chapter. Does it really matter if we send each other the wrong message when we discuss approaches, or plan a response, to people who are distressed? What are the implications for the people who are so labelled, and how does this affect our own relationships and behaviour towards them?

There are a number of ways to assess the impact of the message on the individual. Two are highlighted here. The first is to widen the search for information about individuals to other client groups and the experiences of other people who come across the messages, and the expectations of professionals and service personnel. The second is to consider research into the impact of words and labels on people who exhibit distress. This twin approach helps to use the articulate impressions of people who are not distressed and to enrich the direct information from those who are.

The field of education was one of the first to understand the impact of the message of words on the growing self-concept of the child. In 1974, Chet Bowers, an American educator, used the accounts of people about their experience to examine the impact of expectations within a particular school on the individual (Bowers 1974). In particular, he notes the impact of the school's belief system on a young black boy. Various terms of abuse were seen to alienate and isolate the child, and in addition a more subtle form of discrimination occurred. The school was very clear in its message to the child: a young black person from a rural community would never be a lawyer. Consequently the child's self-esteem was damaged by the school's low expectation of him.

In such cases children lose certain opportunities because they are not expected to achieve them. Having established a process whereby a school can work to alter the self-concept of a child, it was demonstrated that self-concept and academic achievement are linked. That is to say, a child's belief about academic ability will influence actual level of academic achievement. The failure to achieve then provides evidence for, and so confirms, the school's original belief about the child (Byrne 1984).

For an adult perspective, Scott (1969) gives an early and fascinating account of the process whereby a person becomes 'socialised' as a client of a special service. His book, brilliantly titled *The Making Of Blind Men*, describes the ways in which the loss of sight leads a person to become 'blind'. Two stages are noted. In the first instance, Scott describes the recruitment process. This is where the person identifies a sight loss and seeks help. There follows an increasing involvement in services which become more and more specialised. The response of these services forces the individual to redefine him or herself. Whilst initially the person was treated as an ordinary person who had trouble seeing, the service response treats the person as a blind person who has some residual vision (Scott 1969). Indeed any attempt to resist the pressure to be blind is interpreted as denial by services and becomes the object of some kind of intervention. This seems familiar as we remember the issue of who decides whether a person exhibits a behaviour requiring specialist attention.

Having given up an ordinary identity, the blind person now moves into the service agencies. The first stage involves a complete assessment of the person's situation. This tends to follow an established format and sees the individual's ideas of the problem somewhat patronisingly as 'the presenting problem' (Scott 1969). In considering this process, much of its power lies, rather ironically, in good practice as defined by modern professionals. The assessment no longer concerns itself with the practical problems accompanying failing eyesight. The services are concerned with carrying out holistic assessments of everything from sexual to spiritual needs. Consequently, part of a person becomes all of a person. From this point onwards the organisation and delivery of services are the responsibility of the professionals, and the person who arrived needing help with failing sight can say goodbye to his or her identity along with the sharp visual images of the past.

Clearly, this is presented as an extreme position as we seek to apply it to modern services. However, the parallels are striking. There has been a move to involve people who receive services in the organisation and delivery of those services, yet to what extent is this a reality for people who receive services because they have expressed their distress? Seeing the person as a whole person has been essential to many positive developments in recent years, yet it would appear that we may not have taken sufficient notice of the person's own perspective, and we may, on occasion, be exploring other areas of a person's life with neither cause nor permission.

Having considered some instances of the impact of words on the individual, the small number of accounts of this type of work among people with learning disabilities provide more striking examples. Heyman (1990) examined the self-concept of children with learning disabilities and related self-concept to their academic achievement. This included a measure of how the children understood their learning disability. This measure asked children about their learning disability across three dimensions:

- Delimited or global
- Modifiable or permanent
- Stigmatising.

It was found that the children with the most positive view of their disability were the children with the most positive self-esteem and academic self-concept. It seems that the message received about disability has an impact on a range of other ways in which children see themselves.

The importance of the impact of the message of disability upon the individual has since been documented in a number of papers (Nunkoosing 1995, Dodd & Webb 1998), although Dodd & Webb (1998) remain concerned that the professional community needs to develop accurate categories which can be used to define both behaviour and disability. The categories are needed to predict behaviour and share research, even if there may be some cost to the individuals being studied.

Hastings et al (1993) conducted a piece of work that suggests that such a position may not be tenable. He carried out an analysis of labels which have been applied to people with learning disabilities. College students were asked to rate a series of general labels such as 'mental handicap' and 'learning disability' along with some specific descriptors such as 'autism' and 'exceptional'. All terms were viewed equally negatively with the exception of 'exceptional'. This certainly leaves us with a long way to go with these issues. It is now possible to suggest some places to start and some directions to choose.

Throughout this chapter, it has been suggested that the message carried by our words may not be particularly helpful to the people who receive services or other kinds of support. There are a number of reasons for this.

Broadly, these relate to the ways in which our words, and the messages that they contain, take control away from the people to whom they refer. This has a serious impact on the person's sense of identity, and can in turn influence the person's behaviour. This leads to the unfortunate situation in which the work of professional and academic communities assist people in distress may itself be contributing to that same sense of distress.

There are two possible sources of a solution to this dilemma. First, we can turn to the sociological literature, where work to understand the effect of words and labels began. Slee (1996) draws upon studies conducted across marginalised groups. The problem as understood by Slee (1996) is that the language we use has always been conceived by people other than those to whom it refers. It is extremely rare for people who receive help or support from services to develop the language for themselves. A shift in power may allow people to find their own messages and leave some of the destructive responses behind. Slee (1996) calls for a move to shared language and definitions, with others stressing the need for more creative forms of expression such as multimedia and artistic presentation (Fulcher 1996).

In a similar piece of work, Oliver (1996) notes how passive people who receive help from services can be involved in developing the language and understanding of their distress or condition. Once again the impact of this is rehearsed and leads to four criteria for the development of helpful and possibly more appropriate language:

- *Emancipation*: language should lead to growth and release from oppression
- *Inclusion*: developing language should involve the people to whom it relates
- *Collection*: language should enable people to come together to define their experience
- *Working*: language should always be open to change and to development.

What is stressed in each of these social approaches is the need for professionals to come together with other groups of people such as clients and families to develop a shared language of distress. This may be seen as a little 'soft' for the current era of clinical governance, eligibility criteria and evidence based practice. However, if considered carefully it is fully consistent, for example, with the most up-to-date models of disability from clinical and professional practice.

The second possible source of a solution to our dilemma is the field of learning disabilities which provides us with a simple but powerful model to understand the concept of behavioural distress. In seeking to take forward the definition and classification of learning disability, the American Association for Mental Retardation (AAMR) developed a new model (AAMR 1992). This represented a series of shifts in thinking from previous ideas. The model can equally be applied to behavioural distress.

These shifts were analysed by Luckasson & Spitalnik (1994) in a later paper. The AAMR definition understands learning disability as a relationship or interaction between the person, their environment and the support they receive. This is given as a triangle (see Fig. 2.1). In this way a person who is learning disabled or distressed is seen in relationship with other people, communities and physical environments. The model stresses the need for

Fig. 2.1
Model of learning disability (AAMR 1992 with kind permission from American Association on Mental Retardation, Washington).

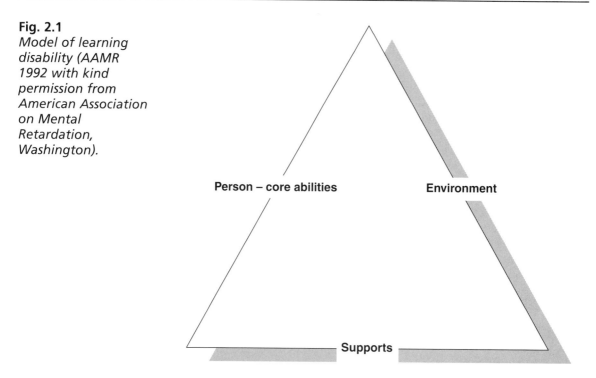

Person – core abilities   Environment

Supports

people to be understood as adults, and to be involved in the services they receive. The person is not seen as belonging to a set classification but as requiring a unique set of supports and relationships in order to cope with the challenges of everyday life.

Clearly, this model meets many of the difficulties expressed by social theorists and by people who have come into contact with services. It relates to general issues of disability, yet seems to apply equally strongly to people who exhibit behavioural distress. The implication would be that we work with people both individually and collectively to develop shared understanding. The words used would be shared by the people to whom they apply, involving independent advocates in those instances where people cannot express their distress for themselves. Likewise, in considering the range of interventions and models which are described in a book such as this, it would be necessary to involve the person concerned and others who know him or her well. Words would stress the positive and unique elements of a person's experience, and evidence would be gathered on an individual basis to test assumptions which may come from professional ideas and models.

Conclusion   More recently, services have begun to involve clients and significant others and ensure that they are at the centre of planning and decision making (Ramcharan 1997). Sadly, this seems to be left behind once someone becomes distressed and challenges the system in some way. The impact of this can further disempower the person by imposing models of assessment and intervention which are not shared. Applying the AAMR model of disability to distressed behaviour in general seems to be a means by which professional practice could make sense to those who are on its receiving end. (Now look at the reflection below.)

Issues for reflection

1. First, return to the activities which run through the chapter and consider them in the light of the chapter as a whole. Then consider your involvement with individuals who exhibit behavioural distress. How can you work as a partner in understanding this distress? Would this approach change any of your current assumptions?

2. Consider the words that are used in your service to describe the people who receive care and support. What message do they carry and what alternatives might there be? Move on to reflect on the words used to talk about distressed behaviour. Once again, what is the message and could there be more helpful alternatives? Finally, are you always comfortable with the jokes which may be made at the expense of people who receive services?

Further reading

Lovett H 1996 Learning to listen: positive approaches to people with difficult behaviour. Jessica Kingsley, London
This book explores the politics of labelling before giving some very practical insights into its impact on clinical practice. The traditional technical approaches to people who are distressed are challenged and more positive alternatives are proposed.

Cocks E, Fox C, Brogan M, Lee M (eds) 1996 Under blue skies: the social construction of intellectual disability in Western Australia. Centre For Disability Research, Edith Cowan University
The social model of disability is explored in great depth here. A historical analysis of services for people in Australia leads to a demand for an ethical approach to modern service delivery.

American Association on Mental Retardation 1992 Mental retardation: definition, classification and systems of supports, 9th edn. American Association on Mental Retardation, Washington

Cincotta K 1995 Doug's story: the struggle for a fair go. Deakin University, Australia
Take a look at the book which describes the AAMR model (AAMR 1992). Then, read 'Doug's Story' (Cincotta 1995) which gives a personal account of life in the system and then draws out some of the theories which have been helpful in understanding the system.

References

American Association on Mental Retardation 1992 Mental retardation: definition, classification and systems of supports, 9th edn. American Association on Mental Retardation, Washington

Baldwin S 1985 Models of service delivery: an assessment of some applications and implications for people who are mentally retarded. Mental Retardation 23 (1): 6–12

Blunden R, Allen D 1987 Facing the challenge: an ordinary life for people with learning disabilities and challenging behaviours. King's Fund, London

Bowers C 1974 Cultural literacy for freedom. Elan, Eugene, Oregon

Byrne B 1984 The general/academic self concept nomological framework: a review of construct validation research. Review of Educational Research 54: 427–456

Cincotta K 1995 Doug's story: the struggle for a fair go. Deakin University, Australia

Department of Health 1992 Mansell report on services for people with learning disabilities and challenging behaviour or mental health needs. HMSO, London

Dodd K, Webb Z 1998 Defining and classifying learning disabilities in practice. Clinical Psychology Forum 111(Jan): 12–15

Emerson E, Cummings R, Barrett S, Hughes H, McCool C, Toogood S 1988 Challenging behaviour and community services: who are the people who challenge services? Mental Handicap 16: 11–19

Emerson E, McGill P, Mansell J 1994 Severe learning disabilities and challenging behaviour: designing high quality services. Chapman and Hall, London

Fulcher G 1996 Beyond normalisation but not Utopia. In: Barton L (ed) Disability and society: emerging issues and insights. Longman, London

Gates B 1996 Understanding learning disability. In: Gates B (ed) Learning disabilities. Churchill Livingstone, Edinburgh

Hastings R, Sonuga-Barke E, Remington B 1993 An analysis of labels for people with learning disabilities. British Journal of Clinical Psychology 32(4): 403-405

Heyman W 1990 The self perception of a learning disability and its relationship to academic self concept and self-esteem. Journal Of Learning Disabilities 23(8): 472-475

Luckasson R, Spitalnik D 1994 Political and programmatic shifts in the 1992 AAMR definition of mental retardation. In: Bradley V, Ashbaugh J, Blaney B (eds) Creating individual supports for people with developmental disabilities: a mandate for change at many levels. Paul H Brookes, Baltimore

McBrien J, Felce D 1992 Working with people who have severe learning difficulty and challenging behaviour. A practical handbook on the behavioural approach. British Institute of Mental Health, Kidderminster

Mental Deficiency Act 1913 HMSO, London

Mental Deficiency Act 1927 HMSO, London

Mental Health Act 1983 HMSO, London

Mental Health Foundation 1997 Don't forget us: children with learning disabilities and severe challenging behaviour. Mental Health Foundation, London

Murphy G 1994 Understanding challenging behaviour. In: Emerson E, McGill P, Mansell J (eds) Severe learning disabilities and challenging behaviour: designing high quality services. Chapman and Hall, London

Nihira K, Leland H, Lambert N 1993 AAMR adaptive behaviour scale: residential and community. Examiners manual, 2nd edn. Pro Ed, Texas

Nunkoosing K 1995 Learning disability: psychology's contribution to diagnosis, assessment and treatment. In: Bull R, Carson D (eds) Handbook of psychology in legal contexts. Wiley, Chichester

Oliver M 1996 A sociology of disability or a disablist sociology? In: Barton L (ed) Disability and society: emerging issues and insights. Longman, London

Potter D 1993 Mental handicap: is anything wrong? Kingsway, Eastbourne

Pyles D, Bailey J 1990 Diagnosing severe behaviour problems. In: Repp A, Singh N Perspectives on the use of non aversive and aversive interventions for persons with developmental disabilities. Sycamore Publishing Company, Illinois, Ch 25

Ramcharan P, Roberts G, Grant G, Borland J 1997 Empowerment in everyday life. Jessica Kingsley, London

Scott R 1969 The making of blind men. Russell Sage Foundation, New York

Slee R 1996 Clauses of conditionality: the reasonable accommodation of language. In: Barton L (ed) Disability and society: emerging issues and insights. Longman, London

Slevin E 1995 A concept analysis of, and proposed new term for, challenging behaviour. Journal of Advanced Nursing 21: 928-934

Sumarah J 1989 Metaphors as a means of understanding staff–resident relationships. Mental Retardation 27(1): 19-23

Williams D 1994 Somebody somewhere. Corgi, London

Wolfensberger W 1972 The principle of normalisation in human management services. National Institute of Mental Retardation, Toronto

Wray J 1999 Children with learning disabilities and behavioural difficulties: a comparison of two therapeutic approaches used in the management of behavioural difficulties. MPhil dissertation, University of Hull

3

The ethical and legal context

Sam Ayer

Key issues
- The management and treatment of people experiencing behavioural distress raise serious ethical and human rights issues for practitioners and carers
- Some interventions in particular (such as 'pindown' and medication) expose specific ethical and legal issues
- There are considerable implications for criminal and civil law arising from the care, treatment, control and safety of people who exhibit behavioural distress

Overview

This chapter is divided into four main sections. The first two deal with broad ethical and human rights issues. In these sections, a management strategy (behaviour intervention) is used to explore specific ethical and human rights issues on the one hand and issues relating to ethical behaviour in professional practice on the other. The experience of young people who underwent the intensive training regime called pindown (Levy & Kahan 1991) is also profiled. Section three explores the implications of criminal and civil law arising from the treatment, care, control and safety of people with learning disabilities who also present with severe challenging behaviour. The use of medication as a management strategy is explored and some of the specific legal issues relating to drug intervention are examined. The final section briefly explores the issue of risk and its implications for the care, control and safety of people with learning disabilities.

Ethical issues

Philosophy ('love of wisdom'), of which ethics is a branch, comprised all forms of knowledge. In the 1400s 'natural philosophy' or science began to be studied as a separate discipline from 'moral philosophy'. The humanities (subjects such as history, art and literature) were still included in philosophy, as were ethics, law and religion.

Some knowledge rests on belief and cannot be measured; examples include philosophy, religion and ethics. These kinds of knowledge are called metaphysics (from Greek 'after or beyond the physical things which are nature' (Partridge 1983)). Anything that is not physical (that is, not measurable or perceivable by the senses) is metaphysical. Reber (1985) defines metaphysics as a branch of philosophy that seeks out first principles and, of necessity, must go beyond what can be learned by mechanical or physical analysis. Often, because of its intellectual heritage, it is used as a label for any philosophy that is obscure. American psychologist and philosopher William James (1842–1910), characterised metaphysics as 'nothing more than an unusually obstinate effort to think clearly'.

The word 'ethics' is derived from the Greek word *ethike tekne*, meaning 'the moral art'. The word 'ethics' was commonly used in place of the word 'custom' until a few decades ago (Cutter 1893).

'Ethics' and 'morals' are words whose significance and meaning enter into all areas of human thought and actions. This chapter makes no distinction between 'ethics' and 'morality'. For our present purposes we can follow the convention of regarding the terms 'ethics' and 'morality' as synonyms (see for example Singer 1979, 1991; Thompson et al 1988; Seedhouse 1989; Reber 1985; Michaels & Kelly 1991), and use all variations of the words interchangeably. Ethics is concerned with views of how men and women 'ought' to live their lives (Seedhouse 1989, Edwards 1996). It is clear that the majority of people hold ethical views, and that our moral intuitions have been internalised and developed as part of our upbringing and socialisation.

Edwards (1996) points out that it is possible to make a distinction between personal ethics, group ethics and philosophical ethics. Ethics in the personal sense refers to the beliefs which individuals hold about ethical issues. Such beliefs stem from various sources such as parents, schoolteachers, religious figures and the media. These sources influence our views with regard to moral matters and it is standard for such views to inform the intuitive judgements we make in relation to ethical issues (Singer 1993, Edwards 1996).

Edwards's second use of the term involves reference to the ethics of a group. These may be formal statements of standards of behaviour which members are expected to act in accordance with. Such groups might be professionals (e.g. nurses, doctors, and psychologists) or organisations (such as, for example, a religious group). Nurses and psychologists are useful examples of professional groups which have proposed various codes of ethics. The United Kingdom Central Council for Nursing, Midwifery and Health Visiting (UKCC) has set out a *Code of Conduct* for nurses (UKCC 1992). The American Nurses Association in 1976 and 1985 has also set out a *Code of Ethics* which identifies the standards of behaviour expected of its members (Benjamin & Curtis 1986). Likewise, the American Psychological Association has a code of ethics for psychologists (American Psychological Association 1977).

The third sense of the term 'ethics' refers to ethics as a more informal and academic enterprise. This can be described as 'philosophical ethics'. Philosophical ethics is concerned with a branch of philosophy normally termed moral philosophy. This form of philosophical enquiry is concerned with study of human conduct with respect to the 'rightness' and 'wrongness' of actions and the 'goodness' and 'badness' of the motives and ends of such actions. The focus is on concepts such as 'good', 'bad', 'right', 'wrong', 'should', 'ought', 'obligations', 'duty' and other similar terms (Hare 1952, Hanfeing 1972, Bloch & Chodoff 1991). When these words are used in sentences it is likely that some kind of ethical claim is being made (see Box 3.1).

A fundamental premise of the moral philosopher is that human conduct occurs within a context of values. The moral philosopher attempts to address such questions as: 'Is it right to prescribe contraceptives to a 12-year-old girl

Box 3.1
Examples of sentences that are making ethical claims

- That was a *good* (or *bad*) thing to do.
- It is not *right* that children are subjected to physical punishment.
- Clients have a *right* to be told the truth about their condition.
- Nurses have an *obligation* to protect patients.
- You *ought* to act in the best interests of your clients.
- You *should* protect your neighbour from being assaulted.
- It is the *duty* of care professionals to protect their clients from harm.
- It is *wrong* to provide treatment against the will of your client.

against parental wishes?', 'Should life support machines ever be switched off?', 'Should parents with learning disabilities be allowed to bring up their children?', 'Should all girls with learning disabilities be sterilised?' When people have a choice of one or more courses of action and their activities are not completely prescribed, the inevitable question presents itself as to whether the particular action chosen is right or wrong, good or bad (Ketefian 1981, 1989; Rest 1979; Bloch & Chadoff 1991). As Seedhouse (1989, p. 18) observes:

> *We have all experienced discussions on moral issues. Debates about right and wrong [and] about what is moral behaviour and what is immoral behaviour are very common. These distinctions happen daily, at work, over shop counters, in public houses, on trains, at bus stops – everywhere people are interested and are concerned enough to discuss issues affecting human life and relationships.*

There is also the growing awareness that some patients or clients are particularly vulnerable. When patients or clients cannot act for themselves, conflicts can arise between professionals' personal values and the need for surrogate actions taken on behalf of patients or clients by professionals. This requires insight, empathy, courage, self-control and self-respect.

Human rights   Internationally, the Geneva Convention on Human Rights provides a code which governments and nations should observe in order to guarantee people's rights. Nationally, governments and nations have created written constitutions, such as that in the USA, designed to guarantee citizens rights and identify their responsibilities. Even when there are no written constitutions, as in the UK, laws and legislation contain many rights and entitlements which are designed to safeguard and protect the citizen. International conventions and national constitutions, legislation and laws, all seek to uphold people's basic rights. It is also the case that professional groups may be expected to observe and protect human rights (RCN 1986, Department of Health 1990, Department of Health and the Welsh Office 1990).

In this context, the decisions and judgements which carers, professional practitioners and service providers make in their everyday work with vulnerable people have important implications for freedom and human rights.

The UK signed the United Nations Declaration of Human Rights in 1948. Broadly speaking, these rights relate to individual freedoms and the responsibilities accorded to them. The idea of associated responsibility is important, as it constrains the right of personal freedom which should be exercised in such a way that it does not impede the freedom of others. Osmanczk (1985) has outlined some of the basic rights of individuals in the following way:

1. All human beings are born free and equal.
2. The rights and freedoms apply to everyone without discrimination on any grounds.
3. Everyone has the right to life.
4. Everyone has the right to own property.
5. Everyone has the right to freedom of thought, opinion and expression of these opinions.

Ethical behaviour and professional practice

There are two main theories of ethics which govern professional behaviour about judgements in caring situations. These are the deontological perspective and the utilitarian perspective. There is the view that the essence of morality depends upon people acting according to certain given principles, which is their duty (deontology means 'the science of duty'). The other view (utilitarian) holds that the essence of morality rests upon a calculation of the benefits and disadvantages of the consequences of actions (see, for example, Seedhouse 1989, Bloch & Chodoff 1991).

Principles that are traditionally cited for ethical behaviour in caring situations are:

1. Autonomy, or respect for personal choice and self-rule. This is derived from a respect for the rights of the individual in society. Personal choice should be made intentionally with understanding and without external controlling influences (Beauchamp & Childress 1994, Merrell & Williams 1995).

2. Non-maleficence, or causing no harm to the client or patient: practitioners do not kill, cause pain or disability or detract from quality of life, summed up in the Latin motto: 'Primum, non nocere' ('Above all, do no harm').

3. Beneficence, or the moral duty to promote goodness or benefit to the patient or client and family. This is not merely equivalent to non-maleficence or not doing bad, but implies preventing evils from occurring (Gert et al 1989). Indeed, this is the source of the phrase 'acting in good faith', which is identified as the pertinent motivator within professional practice (Jones 1988, Department of Health and Social Services 1976, UKCC 1992).

4. Justice refers to respect for society's value system of fairness in the distribution of health care resources. The practitioner should respect fairness for individuals as well as resources, including the costs and availability of therapeutic resources (Seedhouse 1989).

Comment

The clauses in the UKCC *Code of Conduct* (UKCC 1992) attempt to set out the professional duties of the nurse. Clause 1 of the code states that registered nurses must:

Act always in such a manner as to promote and safeguard the interests and the well-being of patients and clients.

The similarity between this clause and the principle of beneficence is significant. The clause makes clear that it is a major part of a nurses' professional duty to promote the well-being of patients and clients. As Edwards (1996) has pointed out, the principle of beneficence generates moral obligation to act in ways which promote the well-being of others.

Clause 2 states that a nurse must:

ensure that no action or omission on his, or her part ... is detrimental to the ... safety of patients and clients.

According to this clause, nurses must ensure that none of their actions or omissions expose clients to risk of harm. It is significant that this sounds very similar to the principle of non-maleficence which, again as described above, generates obligations not to act in ways which result in harm to others.

Just as the principles of beneficence and non-maleficence underpin Clauses 1 and 2 of the nurses' code of conduct, the principle of respect for autonomy provides the moral foundation for Clauses 5, 7 and 10. Clause 5 obliges nurses to foster independence of clients, Clause 7 states that nurses must recognise and respect the uniqueness and dignity of each client, and Clause 10 is concerned with an obligation to respect confidential information. The principle of justice might reasonably be said to underpin all the clauses since it generates obligations to treat others fairly (Beauchamp & Childress 1994, UKCC 1992, Edwards 1996).

Summary

The principles of beneficence, non-maleficence, autonomy and justice clearly underpin the codes of conduct of professional groups. Nevertheless, these principles are broad concepts, and have considerable scope for individual interpretation in their application. They serve as a useful basis from which practitioners and other carers can consider appropriate respect for, and protection of, vulnerable people. They also provide helpful starting points for any discussion of management strategies and the obligations of practitioners and carers.

'Special' rights of people with learning disabilities

Historically there have been two dominant public perceptions of people who have learning disabilities. They have been perceived either as sick people with medically diagnosable conditions or as individuals who have suffered from a slowing down in their intellectual and personal development. There is also a perception of the person with learning disability as a subhuman organism, who may be denied the full range of social and legal resources that are implied by the term 'citizen' (see, for example, Seeley 1964, Friedman 1974, Wolfensberger 1975, William 1978).

In order to emphasise their essential humanness as valued citizens (Wolfensberger 1977), there is a need to address ethical, moral and legal issues which should underpin the relationship between people with learning disabilities and those who manage or care for them.

The 'special' rights for people with learning disabilities have their origin in the Congress of the International League of Societies for the Mentally Handicapped which was held in Jerusalem in 1968. These rights were endorsed by the United Nations in December 1971. There is a brief summary of the seven articles which constitute the special rights of people with learning disabilities in Box 3.2.

Box 3.2
The special rights of people with learning disabilities (United Nations 1971)

Article One says: 'The mentally retarded person has, to the maximum degree of feasibility, the same rights as other human beings.'
Article Two refers to the right to medical care 'and educational training as will enable the retarded to develop his [sic] ability to the maximum potential.'
Article Three refers to the retarded person's right to economic security: they have the right to productive work or meaningful occupation.
Article Four states: 'Whenever possible the mentally retarded person should live with his [sic] own family or in surroundings as close as possible to those in normal life.'
Article Five states: 'The retarded person has a right to a qualified guardian.'
Article Six says: 'The mentally handicapped should have the right to protection from exploitation, abuse and degrading treatment . . . if prosecuted for any offence the right to the due process of law should be recognised.'
Article Seven says: 'Whenever the mentally retarded are unable to execute all their rights, procedure used for the restriction or denial of rights must contain proper legal safeguards.'

In marked contrast to countries like the USA, the UK does not have a written constitution. Thus a problem arises because the rights enshrined in the declaration have no legal status. Minority groups such as people with learning disabilities may find that the exercise of their rights is subordinated to the exercise of the rights of the majority. In addition to these basic rights, the government has afforded individuals other rights, in particular those that relate to health and social care and public services. These rights are outlined in the Patient's Charter (DoH 1976a), the National Health Service and Community Care Act (1990) (DoH 1991) and the Citizen's Charter (DoH 1976b). However, some of these rights do not have the force of statute and therefore the person with learning disability does not have the right to legal redress if these are denied.

Behavioural interventions and the client's rights

Professionals and therapists engage in all types of therapeutic interventions. Many criticisms and objections have been raised about therapeutic interventions which have the potential to be used as tools by which those in charge can manage and manipulate those in their care. Brown et al (1975) argue that although concerns and criticisms are raised about all types of interventions, behaviour modification seems to have acted like a 'lightning rod' in the midst of the current stormy ethical and legal controversies, drawing to it highly charged issues (see Ch. 9).

In particular, the explicit use of aversive control in behaviour modification practice has attracted much critical attention as a consequence of specific abuses attributed to the programmes. The use of the drug suxamethonium chloride to punish prisoners has also been described as behaviour modification (Reimringer et al 1970). 'Time out' – which is only effective when used for short periods of time (that is, a few minutes), in settings where behaviour is also positively reinforced – has in some settings involved extraordinarily long periods of isolation in small quarters (Opton 1974). People are afraid of being controlled, and they are increasingly concerned with how society deals with deviance, and sensitive to the potential consequences of the power imbalance between therapist and client. People may well also be reacting to extravagant claims made by some intervention analysts regarding the effectiveness of behavioural intervention (see, for example, Stolze 1976, 1978).

Thus, there are those concerned about any systematic attempt to change behaviour through the use of such techniques as 'therapeutic holding' (Wong et al 1998, Barlow 1989), 'physical restraint' (Favell et al, 1978, 1981) 'seclusion and time out' (Lieberman & Wong 1984, Tyler & Brown 1976, Solnick et al 1977, Bostow & Bailey 1969) and 'behavioural modification' (Wong et al 1988, Friedman 1975). Several authors have argued that therapists using behavioural methods should seriously question whether the behaviour they are being asked to change should in fact be changed, on the grounds that the clients' goals may be too far removed from the therapists' own values (Begelman 1975, Davison 1976, O'Leary 1972, Serber & Keith 1974).

When the therapist's 'client' is the employer, and not the vulnerable person whose behaviour is to be changed or modified, there are ethical issues to consider. Therapists who find that their services are being used by employers in a way that is not beneficial to the vulnerable person have an obligation to make their observations known to their employers and to propose necessary modification or termination of the intervention. Adequate guidelines should be provided to deal with the much more complex issues that may arise during the use of such behaviour interventions as those listed above (see, for example, Mental Health Foundation 1997).

The American Psychological Association points out that the primary purpose of safeguarding clients' rights is not to provide therapeutic benefit, but to ensure that power over individuals is not abused. The exploration of ethical and legal issues in the management of people with learning disabilities who display challenging behaviour serves to emphasise the vital point that an individual's rights may take precedence over the need for treatment.

The 'pindown' experience

The nature of pindown

The intensive training unit known as 'pindown' was in existence between November 1983 and October 1989 (Levy & Kahan 1991). The Staffordshire pindown inquiry in 1991 (Levy & Kahan 1991) revealed unacceptable practices in the management of young persons with challenging behaviour. They found that the regime was designed to exercise control over the young people by depriving them of their liberty and subjecting them to social isolation.

The pindown regime was designed to make children 'do as they are told'. The philosophy behind the approach considered that the regime was being undermined if the 'rules of the establishment' were not strictly adhered to. The rules made it clear that 'privileges are to be earned through co-operation with staff'. A list of the apparent reactions of the people who experienced pindown were taken from log books (see Box 3.3); the list crystallises the impact of pindown on those subjected to it.

The view of the inquiry team pointed to the likely negative effects of the use of a regime that was intrinsically dependant on elements of isolation, force, humiliation, confrontation, denial of basic human rights and an affront to human dignity. Clearly, the pindown regime demonstrates the ethical and

Box 3.3
Reported reactions to pindown (Levy & Kahan 1991)

> Clients reported the following reactions:
> Anger, depression, weeping, sobbing, anxiety, talking in sleep, talking to self, staring into space, lost confidence in people, frustration, boredom, banging on walls, loneliness and despair, inability to eat, frantic attempts to get out, temper tantrums and absconding. In addition, there were incidents of wrist slashing and the taking of overdoses (para 12.33).

legal difficulties inherent in the management of people with severe challenging behaviour. The inquiry was firmly of the view that pindown, in all its many manifestations, was intrinsically illegal, unethical, unprofessional and unacceptable. The inquiry documented seven profiles (see Levy & Kahan 1991, pp. 107–116) of the young people who underwent the 'Pindown Experience' in an attempt to encapsulate the reality of the experience in human terms (précis of two cases are given in the case studies 'Pindown profile: Jane (13 years old)' and 'Pindown profile: Simon (9 years old)').

**Pindown profile:
Jane (13 years old)**

Manifestations of Jane's behaviour
Jane had serious difficulties in her relationship with her foster parents, and a tendency to self-harm, self-abuse and suicidal behaviour. She had attempted to cut her wrists, and regularly absconded from the care of her foster parents.

Description of Jane's pindown experience
Jane was given a nightdress to wear and her clothes and shoes were taken away in a black plastic bag. She was placed in the back pindown room which had in it a bed, a table and a wardrobe. She was told not to go out of the room and if she wanted anything she had to knock on the door (this included wanting to go to the toilet).

Jane said: 'I was informed that I had done wrong by running away from my foster parents and that I had lost all my privileges. To regain these privileges I had to prove that I could be good by doing what the staff told me. I had to sign a "contract" to say that I would keep it. If I disobeyed anyone on this contract a privilege would be taken away.' The programme written by staff for Jane at the intensive training unit (pindown), included the following: 'foster breakdown – very loose programme. She was to attend school and allowed visitors/phone calls/letters. She was to rise at 7.15 a.m. and have a bath. Her bedtime after a bath was 9.00 p.m.'

Jane's comments about her experience
Jane's view of what happened to her was that: 'It was a degrading experience ... I ran away a lot because I got so frustrated at not being allowed to see anyone and not being allowed to talk to anyone ... I remember being really upset one night and going out of the pindown room because I needed to talk and I got dragged back in.' She felt frightened when she was in pindown. She had no exercise and the only conversation she had with anyone was when her meal was brought. She had no books or magazines and no television or radio. The door was not locked. A chair was put next to the outside of the door, or pots and pans hung on the handle: 'It made you feel everyone was against you, you were always in the wrong, no one would listen, it made me very depressed. It made you hard, a loner. I don't trust people anymore, it makes you distrust all sorts of authority.'
　　Jane spent a total of 4 weeks in 1985 in pindown.

Pindown profile: Simon (9 years old)

Manifestations of Simon's behaviour
Simon was described as 'a difficult child to control, fighting and swearing at teachers, being extremely active, mischievous and accident prone . . . He also displayed very aggressive behaviour towards other children . . . regularly bullied other children . . . was accused of assaults of a sexual nature against both boys and girls, indecently exposing himself on a number of occasions.'

Description of Simon's pindown experience
Simon's log book outlines his programme of training: 'a totally negative approach to be adopted . . . plenty of stern looks and telling off to make him glad to go home. He will be based in the back pindown room and will eat in there . . . under no circumstances is he to communicate with other children . . . he is to perform tasks . . . of a negative kind . . . if it appears that he is enjoying a task, stop him and make him do another one.' On arrival he was put into a room which he thought was then locked and his slippers and pyjamas and trousers were taken away. The room contained a chair, a desk and a bed with a mattress, a sheet and a blanket. There were no books or writing materials in the room. He was told that he had to stay in the room because he had been 'pratting around' at school. After knocking on the door he was allowed out only to go to the toilet and to have a bath.

Simon's comments about his experience
Meals were brought to his room . . . was not allowed to contact other children . . . soon after being put in the pindown room he was allowed to go to the toilet and he opened a window in the bathroom, climbed out onto the roof and down a drain pipe and ran off in his underpants and pyjama jacket. He was not wearing any footwear. While in pindown he had been very frightened after seeing another boy from the adjoining room who had just slashed his wrists.

Social work records contained comments that the use of pindown produced no positive results and that, if anything, his behaviour became worse. Simon went into the unit on two separate occasions in 1986 for a total period of not less than 8 days and probably much longer.

The accounts of clients, staff, practitioners and independent observers (officials of the inquiry) give vivid insights illustrating the ethical, legal and human rights issues that the previous sections of this chapter have attempted to highlight and explore.

Use of medication: legal implications

In dealing with the management of clients who display severe challenging behaviour, including some people with learning disabilities, practitioners are known to use medication (Schaal & Hackenburg 1994). Drugs should be administered in good faith and their use should be the least restrictive and detrimental alternative to help the client. Certain relationships are deemed to be so proximate as to entail a duty of care not to endanger others by exposing them to an unreasonable risk of harm. It is well established that parents owe such a duty to their children; so do practitioners such as doctors, nurses, social workers and paramedics to their clients/patients.

The legal issues concerning the use of medication relate to:

- Negligence
- Issues of consent.

Negligence in relation to the long-term use of medication

Prosecution of doctors for criminal negligence is rare. In the case of *R.* v. *Bateman* (1925, p. 48, A11 ER Rep 45), Lord Hewart LCJ stated:

> *In order to establish criminal liability, the facts must be such that … the negligence of the accused went beyond a mere matter of compensation between subjects and showed such disregard for the life and safety of others as to amount to a crime against the State and conduct deserving punishment.*

Smith & McCalls (1990, pp.225–226) state:

> *Clearly, there must be some extra dimension to medical negligence before it can be regarded as criminal … In short, there must be a deviation from or a reckless disregard of normal practice or instruction that it represents a danger to the public.*

Essentially, the criminal law is reserved for those cases in which death results from a doctor's reckless disregard for life. For example, an anaesthetist left the operating theatre for a drink of milk, and during his absence the patient became disconnected from the oxygen supply and died. The anaesthetist was found guilty of manslaughter (Tribe & Korgaonkar 1991). Thus, it is the case that the doctor who fails to obtain consent to treatment or to inform the patient of the risks of treatment will not be liable in criminal negligence unless his failure represents a reckless disregard for human life and a danger to the public.

Negligence is a pertinent issue in relation to the long-term use of medication in that drug treatment may be prescribed without the doctor explaining his actions. The consequences of using the drugs so prescribed is commonly referred to as the Bolam test. The case of *Bolam* v. *Friern, Hospital Management Committee* ([1957] 1 WLR 582) concerned the administration of electroconvulsive therapy (ECT) to a patient who was suffering from depression. During the therapy the doctor failed to give muscle relaxants and the patient suffered physical injury. Judge McNair held that the treatment would be lawful if administered in accordance with a responsible body of skilled medical opinion. He added that a doctor will not be liable merely because there is a body of medical opinion which adopts the opposite view.

In the case of *Sidaway* v. *Board of Governors of Bethlem Royal Hospital* ([1985] AC 871) a patient's spinal cord was damaged during an operation and this led to severe disability. The patient attempted to sue the hospital for negligence for failure to inform him of the risks involved in surgery. In evidence, it was shown that there was a 1–2% risk of spinal cord damage and medical witnesses stated that they would have warned the patient of unfavourable results but not of the specific risk of paralysis. Adopting the Bolam test, Lord Diplock stated that as a reasonable body of medical opinion would have warned the patient, and since the doctor did so, he was not negligent.

Before any consideration is given to the long-term use of drugs, the prescriber must identify a diagnosis, syndrome or symptom which the treatment is aimed at, and both the prescriber and carer should be aware of this 'target symptom' and should monitor the patient. Any drug used should be identified as one which will be effective in the treatment of the given symptoms. The prescriber, carer and patient should be aware of the possible side-effects. As with the use of medication in an emergency, the decision to prescribe must be an act of good faith, in the person's best interests, and should be the least detrimental and restrictive alternative. The prescriber has a responsibility to find out what other treatments (not necessarily drug treatments) have been tried, and what might be available.

Enfield (1990) gives guidance to practitioners who use psychotropic medication as part of a long-term treatment programme. Enfield identifies procedures which should occur before the drugs are prescribed, as they are prescribed, and the steps to be taken whilst the treatment is occurring.

Before drugs are prescribed

Before a long-term drug treatment is embarked upon there must be a comprehensive assessment of the efficacy of previous drug and non-drug treatments; an elucidation of the biological, psychological, environmental and social contributions to presenting problems; and the formulation of precipitating, perpetuating and palliating factors in the presentation. Proper consideration must be given to receiving informed consent from the client or others, generally a parent, who may lawfully give it. It has to be agreed that the drug treatment will be an integrated part of concurrent treatments and there must be interdisciplinary liaison on the role of the drug in relation to established treatment programmes – for example it must be decided whether the drug treatment and a behaviour modification programme should be altered concurrently or sequentially; the latter might have the advantage of making it easier to determine which intervention is responsible for the observed change in behaviour or emotion.

As drugs are prescribed

The precise symptoms for which the psychotropic medication is being prescribed must be stated. In other words what exactly is it hoped that the psychotropic medication will treat? It should be used in order to achieve therapeutic specificity. As Werry (1988, p.92) has said:

> *generalised suppression of behaviour can be acquainted with clinical depression and is only one small advance on physical restraint.*

It must be expected that the drugs will be effective in alleviating the stated target symptom. Conclusions as to effectiveness may be derived from published literature and from clinical experience of psycho-pharmacological principles. The temptation to prescribe because 'something must be done' should be avoided, and a means of validly and reliably assessing changes in target symptoms should be created – for example a specially formulated questionnaire such as the Developmentally Delayed Children's Behaviour Checklist (Enfield & Tonge 1989) could be used to facilitate the assessment. It is best to have at least two persons making ratings independently and have the behavioural record completed at predetermined regular intervals, and not only when the client presents troublesome behaviour.

During the use of drug treatment

Records must be maintained and any positive responses recorded. If initial doses do not produce the desired effect, then dosages can be increased, but they must not go above a predetermined maximum level. If this level is reached and those concerned are in agreement that the treatment is unsuccessful, the treatment is withdrawn.

Withdrawing treatment

When target symptoms are reduced or absent for a reasonable period, then reduction in dosage should be considered; however, a proper withdrawal regime must be established. Sudden cessation of psychotropic medications, especially when they have been used for lengthy periods, is usually undesirable.

If the above guidelines are adhered to, then there should be no cause for any legal proceedings to occur (Lyon 1994). (See Ch. 6 for a detailed account of the use of medication in the management of behavioural distress.)

Legal issues: background and relevant definitions

Following the introduction of the Children Act 1989 (Department of Health 1989b), the Crown Prosecution Service (the government department responsible for prosecuting an offence through the courts) sought to consider the implications of the criminal and civil law arising from the treatment, care, control and safety of children and young people with learning disabilities who also present with severe challenging behaviour. Both criminal and civil law provide some guidance about the legal issues involved in this area of care.

Criminal law

A developed and civilised society will generally ensure that certain types of conduct will not be considered acceptable, and will legislate for that conduct to be unlawful through its criminal law. The criminal law of England and Wales is made up of offences to be found either in statutes passed by parliament or in judge-made or customary law referred to as the 'common law'. When a person engages in any sort of conduct which has been designated a 'criminal offence', if the police are notified then they will investigate and consider charging the individual concerned with the particular criminal offence. If the circumstances surrounding the commission of the alleged offence cause the police (perhaps in consultation with social services) difficulties – as, for example, in the case of suspected false imprisonment of, or assault and battery against, a person with learning difficulties presenting severe challenging behaviour – they may pass the matter on to the Crown Prosecution Service, for its advice. The Crown Prosecution Service will then consider all the circumstances of the case and decide whether to prosecute. In practice, it would appear that very few cases that relate to people with learning disabilities are actually reported to the police. This might suggest that as a nation we are either extremely tolerant of what might in other circumstances be deemed to be criminal behaviour, or that as a society we are reluctant to appear to be meddling in other people's private family situations (see for example the Mencap (1997) study *Barriers to Justice*, which illustrates how the criminal justice system treats people with learning disabilities).

Civil law

Whilst the criminal law provides for conduct to be treated as unlawful by breaching a general standard of conduct deemed to be acceptable in a civilised society, the civil law in England and Wales is concerned with the regulation of conduct between individuals on a one-to-one basis. This law requires that if any person is aggrieved or injured by the conduct of another, then they must individually take action against that other person in respect of the civil wrong, sometimes referred to as a 'tort', which the conduct discloses. The same circumstances which give rise to the possible prosecution of an individual under the criminal law may also, in addition, amount to the commission of a civil wrong. If both a criminal and a civil wrong arise out of the same conduct (for example in the case of assault and battery), the individual will find that in addition to criminal prosecution by the police, the victim may take some action in the civil courts and claim damages, a sum of money by way of compensation for the injury received. It should be pointed out, however, that even though the police or the Crown Prosecution Service may decide not to proceed with a criminal prosecution, nevertheless an action may still be taken by the victim (or by the victim's parents on his or her behalf) in the civil courts. Indeed, in many situations the conduct being complained of may not be serious enough to constitute the commission of a criminal offence, though it may still give rise to an allegation of a civil wrong or tort and result in a damages claim for the consequences of the wrong which has been perpetrated.

Legal issues and the manifestations of behaviour

In discussing legal issues, the term 'severe challenging behaviour' is adopted for descriptive rather than diagnostic purposes, since there is no universally accepted definition of what constitutes a challenge (Blunden & Allen 1987; Barrett et al 1989a, 1989b; McCue 1993). Empirical studies highlight certain behaviours that are regarded as challenging by those who live and work closely with clients who have learning disabilities and with other vulnerable people who also present severe challenging behaviour (Jacobsen 1982, Lund 1989). (The manifestations of challenging behaviour are documented in Ch. 2.)

One approach to identifying those behaviours that constituted a 'challenge', involves asking staff to identify the sorts of behaviour that they have found challenging; this information is then used as a checklist for other staff to assess the presence or absence of a particular behaviour. However, as Turnbull (1994, p. 68) points out (see also Royal College of Psychiatrists 1986, Hofkens & Allen 1990, Groeman et al 1992):

> *This approach to assessment has often been criticised for taking a unidimentional view of challenging behaviour. Although there may be broad agreement about what constitutes a challenge, this approach reveals little about the additional dimensions, such as the origin of the behaviour, how severe it is considered to be, or even whether the agreed constituents of challenging behaviour are valid.*

In considering the legal issues to treatment, care, control and safety of people with learning disabilities who also present with severe challenging behaviour, knowledge of the manifestations of the problem behaviour provides valid sources for consideration by the criminal and civil law of the land. The next section of the chapter discusses in detail criminal and civil law in relation to challenging behaviour. (In addition to these legalistic definitions, the reader is referred to Ch. 2 where the social implications associated with labelling are more fully explored.)

Criminal law

A number of criminal offences need to be considered in relation to the potential responses which may be adopted by institutions and individuals to problems posed by persons with learning disabilities who also present severe challenging behaviour. The areas in which criminal liability may apply in common law are false imprisonment, assault and battery. Under statute, an individual may also be liable if they act contrary to the Children and Young Person's Act 1933 (s.1) (Department of Health and Social Security

1933), or the Mental Health Act 1983 (s.127). There is no need for damage to the person to be established in these offences. If a person is harmed in any way, then the perpetrator will be liable, in criminal law, for additional offences.

The restriction of liberty

The liberty of a person is restricted when he or she is:

- Secluded. (Seclusion is the confinement of a person in a room, which may be locked.)
- Prevented from leaving a particular place in a building. This would include:
  — physical restraint such as holding
  — blocking exits
  — using: gates, high handles, buxton chairs, chair nets, cot sides, medication, arm splints
  — sewing the sleeves etc. of clothes
  — tying a person to any part of a building or furniture.

False imprisonment

An individual who so restrains a person may be liable for false imprisonment, which is defined as the unlawful and intentional or reckless restraint of a victim's freedom of movement from a particular place. Such restraint may also amount to an assault, as in the case of *Hunter* v. *Johnson* ([1884] 13 QBD 225), where a schoolmaster was held to have assaulted a child whom he kept after school without lawful authority.

False imprisonment would thus include the situation where a person was prevented from leaving a room, building, chair, bed or the grounds of a hospital, residential home, school or home. It is sufficient to constitute false imprisonment if a person is ordered to go to another place and the person goes because he or she feels compelled to do so. The restraint need only be momentary. In the case of *Simpson* v. *Hill* ([1795] 1 Esp 431, per Eyre CJ), it was held that a tap on the shoulder accompanied by the words 'you are my prisoner' was sufficient to constitute imprisonment.

Assault

The actual definition of the criminal law offence of assault is not to be found in any criminal law statute, although the offences themselves are statutory and are principally to be found in the Offences Against the Person Act 1861 (see the decision of the Divisional Court in *DPP* v. *Little* [1992] 1 All ER 299). The definition of assault and of battery is then to be found in the common law, that is, the law to be found in decided cases. Thus in *Fagan* v. *Metropolitan Police Commissioner* ([1969] 1QB) it was held that:

> *an assault occurs when a person intentionally or recklessly does an act which causes another to apprehend immediate and unlawful personal violence.*

Apprehension of any unwanted touching is sufficient.

Unlawful imprisonment may also be an assault (*Hunter* v. *Johnson* (1884) 13 QBD). Recklessness in common assault consists of foresight of the possibility that the person will apprehend immediate and unlawful violence (*R.* v. *Spratt* [1990] 1 WLR 1073). An assault usually requires some action on the part of the defendant intended to cause the person to apprehend immediate unwanted touching or recklessness. This would include such acts as: shaking a fist, throwing an object, drawing up an injection, or presenting a device intended to restrict the liberty of the person which in order to implement would involve some form of touching (such as a buxton chair, arm splint, or rope).

There is conflicting authority over whether words alone can constitute an assault, for example if a teacher threatened to put arm splints on a child or remove a child from a room. In the case of *Meads* v. *Belt* ([1823] 1 Lew CC 184), Holroyd J stated that, 'no words or singing are equivalent to an assault'. However, in the case of *Wilson* v. *Wilson R.*, Lord Goddard stated obiter dicta: 'He called out "get out the knives" which would itself be an assault ...' ([1955] 1 All ER 744 745).

Some legal authorities consider words alone as being capable of amounting to an assault. Smith & Hogan (1991) and Allen (1993) adopt this position. Words may negate what would otherwise amount to an assault. In the case of *Tuberville* v. *Savage* ([1669] 1 Mod Rep 3), the defendant placed his hand on his sword and said, 'If it wcrc not assize-time, I would not take such language from you'. Assize time was a period during which the judges were in town. If an individual said, 'If it was legal I would tie you to a chair', this would not amount to an assault. This situation is to be differentiated from that where an individual says, 'Behave or I will tie you in a chair'. This is conditional upon the person behaving and could amount technically to an assault, although it must be considered in the light of the circumstances of the case and the practicalities of the situation. This example shows that in case law issues are judged within a particular context and in the light of the individual circumstances of the case.

Battery   The rationale behind the criminal offence of battery is the inviolability of every person's body. Battery occurs when an individual either intentionally or recklessly inflicts unlawful personal violence on another.

Personal violence includes unlawful touching or holding, touching a person's clothes whilst he or she is wearing them (*R.* v. *Thomas* (1985) 81 Cr App Rep 331), thrusting or pushing (*Cole* v. *Turner* [1705] 6 Mod 149), or throwing an object which touches a person (*Scott* v. *Shepherd* [1773] 2 W B1 892).

Thus, any action which involves the touching of a person, if unlawful, would amount to battery. Blocking exits, either physically or with objects such as 'baby' gates, secluding or getting a child to take oral medication, if they involve no physical contact, will not amount to a battery. Recklessness in battery involves foresight that the person will be exposed to unlawful force (R. v. Spratt, ibid.). Clearly, contact which occurs during the course of ordinary life needs to be distinguished. In the case of Collins v. Wilcock, Goff L J ([1984] 3 All ER 374, 378) stated that:

> *most of the physical contacts of ordinary life are not actionable because they are impliedly consented to by all who move in society and so expose themselves to the risk of bodily contact. So nobody can complain of the jostling which is inevitable from his or her presence in, for example, a supermarket, an underground station or a busy street; nor can a person who attends a party complain if his or her hand is seized in friendship, or even his or her back is (within reason) slapped . . . among such forms of conduct, long held to be acceptable, is touching a person for the purpose of engaging his or her attention, though of course using no greater degree of physical contact than is reasonably necessary in the circumstances for that purpose.*

It is submitted that the following should be seen to be outside generally acceptable conduct within ordinary daily life:

- Restraining a person physically
- Tying a person to part of a building or furniture
- Putting on clothing with the arms stitched up
- Putting a person in a chair, bed or room
- Putting arm splints on a person
- Injecting a person with medication.

Thus, if unlawful touching is involved, a battery will have been committed in criminal law. Any of the actions described above must, of course, be considered in context and in the light of any reasons put forward to justify the taking of such action.

Civil law

In seeking to provide for the treatment, care, control and safety of children with learning disabilities who also present severe challenging behaviour, professionals, parents and carers may be compelled in extreme circumstances to use methods of restraint which may give rise to an action in civil law in the law of tort. An action may arise under the general tort or trespass to the person, which encompasses the specific torts of false imprisonment, assault and battery. The tort of trespass to the person is actionable *per se* which means that there would be no need for the person to have suffered any damage. Given the rather hostile nature of making allegations of trespass to the person, and the acknowledged difficulties in caring for persons with learning disabilities who also present severe challenging behaviour, it is unlikely that parents, professionals, carers or others with parental responsibility for the person would generally consider lodging a claim in the courts. It is suggested that generally such an action would only be brought where there was evidence of bad faith or malice on the part of the carer concerned.

The four specific torts of false imprisonment, assault, battery and negligence are very relevant in legal issues relating to treatment, care, control and safety of persons who have learning disabilities who also present with severe challenging behaviour. This is because each of these specific torts are relevant to legal proceedings in cases where a person experiencing challenging behaviour has been subjected to an intervention (for example pindown) which may have violated their rights. These specific torts are now briefly considered:

The restriction of liberty leading to the tort of false imprisonment.

Definition of false imprisonment

The definition of the tort of false imprisonment is:

> ❝ *an act of the defendant which directly and intentionally or negligently causes the confinement of the plaintiff within an area delimited by the defendant.* ❞

[Brazier et al 1989, p. 28]

What constitutes the tort of false imprisonment

The tort of false imprisonment would include the situation where a person was prevented from leaving a room, building, chair, bed or the grounds of a hospital residential unit, school or home. The restraint must be total. This includes the situation where a person can only escape if he or she risks injury or it would be unreasonable to expect him or her to escape.

A person may be restrained even if, in the absence of restraint, he or she would be incapable of moving due to handicap or illness. This was established in the case of *Grainger* v. *Hill* ([1838] 4 Bing NC 212). It should be noted that the restraint need only be momentary. It is sufficient if a person is told to go to another place and the person goes because he or she feels compelled to do so. In the case of *Harnett* v. *Bond* ([1925] AC 669), a commissioner erroneously used his authority to persuade the plaintiff to stay in his office. He was held liable for false imprisonment. False imprisonment is actionable per se so there is no need for the person to have suffered any damage. Also, it is not necessary that the person be aware of the fact that he or she is imprisoned (*Meering* v. *Graham-White Aviation Co.*, ibid.).

Comment   Most people who are involved with looking after children of even 'normal' capacities, reading this account of the tort of false imprisonment, may be wondering how this is compatible with many aspects of ordinary parenting and care. This is, of course, where the balance has to be struck between the necessity to practice restraint which is necessary and in the person's interests, with the corresponding responsibility to take all reasonable care, where failure to do so could equally render the parent or carer liable in negligence. Thus, all would acknowledge that children are often compelled to do things which they may not want to do but which demonstrate that their parents are acting responsibly. Examples of this include: attending school, accompanying parents out shopping because there is no one else at home to look after them, being kept in at home when traffic on the road outside the house is exceptionally heavy, or if it is dark and a child is considered by the parent to be too young to be allowed out.

No one would sensibly seek to maintain that this could constitute false imprisonment because in truth it represents the 'responsible' exercise of parental or professional responsibility. Similarly, in seeking to provide for the care, control and safety of people with learning disabilities who also present severe challenging behaviour, responsible carers might take action which might otherwise be construed as false imprisonment such as the use of locks, double-handled doors, or other restraints to prevent such vulnerable people from being at risk. Thus, parents and carers often lock external house or school doors to prevent any person from possibly wandering off, but equally also to prevent risk from possible intruders who could put anyone in the house at risk.

Assault   An assault in civil law is:

> ❛ *any act of the defendant which directly and either intentionally or negligently causes the plaintiff immediately to apprehend a contact with his person.* ❜

[Brazier et al 1989, p. 28]

Some act on the part of the defendant is needed (examples of what would constitute such an 'act' are given in the previous section on criminal assault (p. 62–63).

The use of surveillance devices to observe children should not amount to an assault. In the case of *Murray* v. *Minister of Defence* ([1985] 12 NIJB 12), a photographic picture was taken of an individual against his wishes, and it was held that this did not amount to an assault in tort.

Battery   Battery is:

> *any act of the defendant which directly and either intentionally or negligently causes some physical contact with the plaintiff without the plaintiff's consent.*

[Brazier et al 1989, p. 28]

Where the contact occurred due to the carelessness of the defendant, the action will usually lie in negligence. The case of *Cole* v. *Turner* ([1704] 6 Mod 149), suggests that the 'least touching of another' will suffice to amount to battery. Battery is actionable without proof of damage or injury to the child. The defendant need not have intended the child any harm. The contact must be direct. In the case of *Pursell* v. *Horn* ([1838] 8 Add & El 602), water was thrown onto the clothes of the plaintiff, and it was held that such contact did not necessarily amount to a battery. Thus, touching a child's clothes while the child is wearing them may not amount to a battery in tort unless force is communicated to the person's body. Undoubtedly, tying a child's clothes to a bed while the child is wearing them would involve the application of force, particularly if the child was struggling to free him or herself. Such force would merely represent the continuation of the act of so tying the child (*Scott* v. *Shepherd* [1773] 2 W B1 892). Throwing an object which then hit a child would also be considered direct application of force.

As in the crime of assault, the contact must have been beyond that which occurs in the ordinary course of daily life.

Comment   It is clearly the case that personal violence towards children who present with severe challenging behaviour is unacceptable. It should be emphasised that these are behaviours which are generally, but not always, considered unacceptable. Thus, where a child is seriously self-abusive, then the use of stitched sleeves or cotton mittens may be appropriate where the family or agency have used their best endeavours to stop the child's injuries from being infected. If self-injurious behaviour occurs at particular times of the day, the planned use of special clothing may avoid serious self-injury pending more effective behavioural approaches to the problem. Many parents use such clothing for young children with eczema, for example, and could not be described as acting in any other way than a responsible manner.

Similarly, in the set of circumstances in the case illustration below, the mother without further tangible assistance from her local authority would not be seen as guilty of the tort of battery. In view of the home environment and the lack of support, this mother can only be described as acting responsibly and as not being guilty of battery or false imprisonment. If she was unable to control her child physically by putting him into the harness, she would probably cease to be able to care for him and this would not be in his best interests or in accordance with the terms of s.17(1) Children Act 1989.

Restraint

The family lives in a fifth floor run-down council flat with no lift and poorly fitting windows. The family has four children, one of whom, a boy with severe learning disabilities and severe challenging behaviour (due to meningitis as a baby), is very active and has already fallen out of a window. He survived with a broken leg but in consequence the mother is terrified of another accident and now fastens him to a chair with a car harness attachment when she has to bathe or give time to the other children. She considers that even if she were to be re-housed without any further form of care support she could not survive without some periods when the child is restrained.

Negligence

The tort of negligence in civil law is defined as:

> *a breach by the defendant of a legal duty to take reasonable care which results in damage being caused to the plaintiff.*

[Brazier et al 1989, p. 28]

The four major components of negligence are that:

- The defendant owes a legal duty of care to the plaintiff
- The defendant has breached this duty by falling below the required standard of care demanded of him
- The plaintiff has suffered damage as a result of the breach of duty
- The damage suffered by the plaintiff was not too remote.

As was pointed out above, certain relationships are deemed to be so proximate as to entail a duty of care not to endanger others by exposing them to an unreasonable risk of harm (see for example the section on the 'pindown' experience). It was also pointed out that parents owe such a duty to their children, as do any other persons placed in positions of responsibility with respect to children subject to their care, such as carers, teachers, child-minders, doctors and nurses.

Brazier et al (1989, para 10.61) point out that the reasonable performance of one's duty of care:

> *depends on the balance between on the one hand, the degree of likelihood that harm will occur, and on the other hand, the cost and practicability of measures needed to avoid it, the seriousness of the consequences, the end to be achieved, including the importance and social utility of the activity in question, and the exigencies of an emergency, dilemma or sport.*

Brazier et al (1989, para 10.62) also point out that:

> *the pattern of a reasonable person's behaviour is determined with reference to the likelihood of harm before and irrespective of its occurrence.*

More importantly, in relation to children, they further comment that:

> *the likelihood of harm will also depend on any abnormality of the plaintiff of which the defendant knew, or should have known.*

Parents can certainly be held liable to their children; so for example in *Jauffur* v. *Akhbar* (*Times*, 10 February 1984) the parent was held to be negligent when he knew there were candles in his house and he had failed to instruct and supervise his children with regard to their use and injury had occurred. Thus parents, carers and practitioners must take all reasonable steps to ensure that their children are not put at risk. This would tend to suggest that to fail to provide proper and appropriate measures for the treatment, safety, care and control of vulnerable people presenting with severe challenging would amount to negligence. Such liability in negligence would extend also to all those who are expected to act responsibly in providing for the safety of the persons in their care.

Issues of consent

A patient's rights in accepting treatment

Under common law a person has a right to give or withhold consent before being subjected to a medical examination or treatment. This is one of the basic principles of health care, and the failure to obtain consent may result in action for damages occurring. Patients are entitled to receive sufficient information, in a manner they can comprehend, about the proposed treatment, the possible alternatives and any substantial risks.

Such an approach enables any person to make an *informed* decision as to whether to consent to treatment or not. A patient may refuse treatment or withdraw consent at any time. The Law Commission consultation paper no. 129 (Law Commission 1993), gives advice on current 'basic information' which is relevant to the patient being able to take a decision about medical treatment (para 2.9).

Consent can be given by the patient, or the patient's parent or someone with parental responsibility if the patient is a child; differential tests will be applied to determine whether a child can consent or refuse to consent to treatment. In *Gillick* v. *West Norfolk and Wisbech Area Health Authority* in 1986 (IAC 112, HL) it was stated that:

> *Where a child has reached sufficient understanding and intelligence they may validly give consent to treatment.*

The issue of consent is central to the charges of battery and negligence. In battery, only where there is no consent will the touching be rendered unlawful. In negligence, the doctor may be liable for failing to obtain consent to treatment or to obtaining consent without informing patients of the risks involved.

Problems which may occur in obtaining consent

Although it can be assumed that most people will wish to be well informed about the risks of certain treatments, account should be taken by the doctor of those who may find it distressing. Furthermore, the patient's ability to appreciate the significance of the information should be assessed. This is particularly pertinent to the case of people with learning disabilities, or mental health difficulties, who also present with challenging behaviour, as their capacity to give consent to treatment can be problematic. In these instances, it may be that another party – a parent or someone with parental responsibility, that is, an advocate – will need to be present to help the patient make an informed decision in relation to consent to treatment. The issue of consent is of particular relevance since the introduction by the Law Commission of the consultation Green Paper on mental incapacity (Law Commission 1995).

Doctors will use their professional skill and judgement in deciding what risks the patient should be warned of, and in what terms the warning should be given. Guidance on the amount of information and warnings of risks to be given to patients can be found in the judgement of the House of Lords in the case of *Sidaway* v. *Board of Governors of Bethlem Royal Hospital* ([1985] AC 871). Lord Bridge (ibid. p. 879) indicated that the amount of (ibid. p. 879) information given must primarily be a matter of clinical judgement, and that, further:

> *a judge might in certain circumstances come to the conclusion that the disclosure of a particular risk was so obviously necessary to an informed choice that no reasonably prudent medical man would fail to make it.*

If a doctor is to avoid liability in battery, he will be need to provide proof that he had a legal justification for treatment without consent. Treatment which does not require the sanction of the court can be administered under the doctrine of necessity. In his speech in *Re F (mental patient: sterilisation)* (1990 p. 55) 2AC, Lord Brandon stated that:

> *In my opinion, the principle is that, when persons lack the capacity, for whatever reason, to take a decision about the performance of operations on them, it is necessary that some other person or persons, with appropriate qualification, should take such decisions for them. Otherwise they would be deprived of medical care which they need and to which they are entitled.*

It was further established in the case of *Re F* that the defence of necessity will be available to a doctor if his decision to treat the patient without consent was in the best interests of the patient and is in line with a responsible body of medical opinion skilled in that particular field (i.e. the Bolam test).

Risk assessment and risk management

Risk is an important word in current English language usage, and especially so as it features prominently in debates about health and welfare. The Chambers English Dictionary (Schwartz 1993) defines 'risk' as:

> *hazard, danger, chance of loss or injury, the degree of probability of loss, a person, thing or factor likely to cause loss or danger. Vb. to expose to risk, danger; incur the chance of unfortunate consequence by some action.*

Risk assessment and risk taking are linked to the concept of hazard. Risk assessment is concerned with identifying the hazards which can cause an accident or disaster, whereas risk analysis is concerned with the factors that may result in accident or disaster. Risk taking and risk management focus on responses to risk; the former is concerned with individual decisions, whereas the latter is concerned with collective or group responses. For a detailed discussion of the concept of risk and its implications, see Douglas (1990), Wharton (1992), and Alaszewski et al (1998). It is only recently that notions of risk assessment and risk management have explicitly entered the vocabulary of the literature on learning disability (see for example Parton et al 1997, Alaszewski et al 1997). Even though the development of state intervention during the 19th and 20th centuries reveals the changing political perceptions of adults with learning disability as 'vulnerable' and 'dangerous', the language of risk assessment and risk management is not explicitly used (Tindall & Alaszewski 1996, Tindall 1997).

Official identities: vulnerability and dangerousness

Legislation at the beginning of the last century perceived adults with learning disability in terms of a risk to society, and this official identity was reinforced in the 1929 report of the Mental Deficiency Committee (Mental Deficiency Committee 1929). In this report (part 1, para 20) the committee identified a distinct group of 'feeble-minded' (moral defectives) who posed a special threat to society, where:

> *defects are less prominent, but they are accompanied by such a marked lack of sense of right and wrong, or responsibility and social obligation, together with such strongly marked anti-social propensities as to cause the individual to be a great danger.*

Thus, a sub-group, the 'moral defectives', were identified as 'dangerous to society'.

Despite the acknowledgement of vulnerability, and the tension between the liberty of the individual and the protection of the community (Mental Deficiency Committee 1929, part 1, para 10), the main concern was the potential for danger. The primary official identity of adults with a learning disability remained entrenched as being the source of risk. In the case of children and young persons, the concern and emphasis was on vulnerability, the need for protection and the welfare of the child, even when risk arose as a direct consequence of the child's antisocial behaviour. This emphasis was endorsed in the Children and Young Persons Act 1933 (Department of Health and Social Security 1933, part 3, para 44[1]) by the principle that:

> *every court in dealing with a child or young person who is brought before it either as being in need of care and protection or as an offender or otherwise, shall have regard to the welfare of the child or young person and shall in a proper case take steps for removing him from undesirable surroundings and for securing that proper provision is made for his education and training.*

The need to *further the best interests* of the child and young person 'at risk' was enshrined in subsequent child-centred legislation, (see for example Children Acts: Department of Health 1963, 1969, 1975, 1989b).

The perception of the adult with learning disability as a danger to society was abandoned by the 1959 Mental Health Act [Department of Health and Social Security 1960]. The definition of 'severe subnormality' adopted within the Act [4(2)] emphasised vulnerability with no reference to dangerousness:

> *In this Act "severe subnormality" means a state of arrested or incomplete development of mind which includes subnormality of intelligence and is of such a nature or degree that the patient is incapable of living an independent life or guarding himself against serious exploitation, or will be so incapable when of an age to do so.*

The Mental Health Act 1959 sought to prevent unnecessary institutionalisation, but it was less concerned with the right to autonomy and self-determination of the vulnerable adult. The emphasis was on protection rather than empowerment.

The dual emphasis upon vulnerability and dangerousness is clearly expressed in respect to sexuality, where the 'socially inappropriate behaviour of a minority' is contrasted with the 'vulnerability of some mentally handicapped people to sexual abuse by other people' (Department of Health and Social Security 1985, para 30). Whilst previously these risks would have been managed by segregation and institutionalisation, community integration policies have decreed that the overall aim of control and protection be achieved by professionals providing training in socially acceptable behaviour (Department of Health and Social Security 1985, para 30).

National policy, professional/carer accountability and client choice

User participation and empowerment has been a developing policy theme in respect of adults with a learning disability following official endorsement of the normalisation principle (Wolfensberger 1980). It has been consolidated in Caring for People (Department of Health 1989a) which specifically puts a premium on the participation of vulnerable adults in the assessment process, thus asserting the general rule that service users should be enabled to achieve control over their own lives (para 2.2). In other words, service users should be enabled to exercise choice. It is by successfully making choices and thereby taking risks that people demonstrate competence and so become socially valued (Wright et al 1994). Thus, participation is a key feature of the normalisation principle in practice.

Once a formal responsibility for care is established through a contractual relationship, unqualified care givers are subject to mechanisms of accountability should a service user experience harm. For example, the Health and Safety at Work Act (1974, para 7a) (DoH 1976c) imposes a duty upon employees:

> *to take reasonable care for the health and safety of himself and of other persons who may be affected by his acts or omission at work.*

Failure to carry out these requirements can constitute an offence punishable by a fine (para 33(1)).

Direct care is also given to patients and clients by professionals, such as nurses, who are not only accountable through the general legal framework, but are also subject to the rigours of a professional code of conduct. For example the introductory paragraph of the code of conduct for nurses (UKCC 1992) states that:

> *Each registered nurse, midwife and health visitor shall act, at all times, in such a manner as to: safeguard and promote the interests of individual patients and clients.*

In paragraph 5 the code also requires nurses to:

> *work in an open and co-operative manner with patients, clients and their families, foster their independence and recognise and respect their involvement in the planning and delivery of care.*

Thus the code of conduct also endorses the participation, empowerment and choice of service users. Through the wording of the code and the accompanying document *Exercising Accountability* (UKCC 1989), registered nurses are left in no doubt as to the expectations of their regulatory body or the extent of their personal accountability for practice. Registered nurses therefore work in an environment of care which promotes patient participation and empowerment, but which also profiles professional responsibility and accountability. The registered nurse is directly responsible for ensuring the safety of patients and clients and thus open to a charge of negligence should a service user experience harm as a consequence of his or her practice. Look now at the activity opposite.

Conclusion

Through the law, social policy and professional accountability the scope of the state's interest in risk assessment and risk management has been extended from the narrow focus upon concerns about dangers from vulnerable people to encompass wider forms of risk, in particular the vulnerability of some groups of people to exploitation and abuse.

The Department of Health (1989a) document *Caring for People* puts a premium on the participation of vulnerable people in the needs assessment process, thus asserting the important principle that service users should be enabled to achieve control over their own lives. This policy puts great emphasis on issues such as care accountability and responsibility, user advocacy, autonomy, confidentiality and empowerment. These issues have to be considered in order to ensure that the objective to control, ameliorate or manage unacceptable behaviour in people does not lead to the infringement of their dignity and basic human rights. Look now at the activity below.

Issues for reflection

1. Write down your own brief definition of the following terms: ethics, morals. In a group discussion, reflect on the extent to which there is agreement in the perceptions of these terms between the members of the group.
2. List all the things you consider to be your rights (for example: free speech, clean air, education, choice). Discuss under what circumstances you would be prepared to allow a professional decision to override one of your basic rights.
3. Assuming that clients have a *right to know*, what duties and obligations do these imply for practitioners and carers?
4. Consider the following question: Why should the law interfere with professional decision making?

Further reading

Neuberger J 1992 Ethics and health care. King's Fund, London
Discusses the role of research ethics committees in the UK.
Clark E 1994 Ethics in nursing and midwifery research. Research Awareness Module No. 6. Southbank University, London
Discusses some of the vocabulary and concepts relating to ethics and some of the particular ethical dilemmas that arise in health and social care research.

Faulder C 1985 Whose body is it? The troubling issue of informal consent. Virago, London
Discusses the right of clients to be involved as equal partners in decisions about their bodies and their lives.
Fletcher N, Holt J 1995 Ethics, law and nursing. University of Manchester Press, Manchester
Offers students and practitioners a provocative and lively introduction to ethical and legal dilemmas. It is designed to provoke the practitioner's reflection on the nature of professional obligation and practice.

References

Alaszewski H, Alaszewski A, Ayer S 1997 Teaching and learning about risk working paper. Institute of Health Studies, University of Hull

Alaszewski H, Ayer S, Manthorpe. J 1998 Researching professional education. Assessing and managing risk in nursing educational practice: supporting vulnerable people in the community. ENB, London

Allen M J 1993 Textbook on criminal law. Blackstone Press, London

American Psychological Association 1977 Ethical standards of psychologists: revision. APA, Washington DC

Barlow D J 1989 Therapeutic holding: effective intervention with the aggressive child. Journal of Psychosocial Nurse Mental Health Services 27(1): 10-14

Barrett S, Cummings R, Emerson E, Hughes H, McCool C, Toogood A 1989a Challenging behaviour and community services 6: evaluation and overview. Mental Handicap 17(3): 104-107

Barrett S, Cummings R, Emerson E, Hughes H, McCool C, Toogood A 1989b Challenging behaviour and community services 4: establishing services. Mental Handicap 17(1): 13-17

Beauchamp T L, Childress J F 1994 Principles of biomedical ethics, 3rd edn. Oxford University Press, New York

Begelman D A 1975 Ethical and legal issues of behaviour modification. In: Hersen M, Eisler R M, Miller P H (eds) Progress in behaviour modification, vol 1. Academic Press, New York.

Benjamin M, Curtis J 1986 Ethics in nursing, 2nd edn. Oxford University Press, Oxford

Bloch G, Chodoff P 1991 Psychiatric ethics. Oxford University Press, Oxford

Blunden R, Allen D (eds) 1987 Facing the challenge: an ordinary life for people with learning difficulties and challenging behaviour. King's Fund Paper No 74. King's Fund, London

Bostow D E, Bailey J 1969 Modification of severe disruptive and aggressive behaviour using brief timeout and reinforcement procedures. Journal of Applied Behaviour Analysis 2: 31-37

Brazier M, Sweet N, Maxwell K 1989 The law of torts, 16th edn. Oxford University Press, London

Brown B S, Wienckowski L A, Stolz S B 1975 Behaviour modification: perspective on a current issue. DHEW Publications No ADM 75-202. US Government Printing Office, Washington DC

Cutter E 1893 Address on dietetics: medical food ethics now and to come. Journal of the American Medical Association 20: 239-244

Davison G C 1976 Homosexuality: the ethical challenge. Journal of Consulting and Clinical Psychology 44: 157-162

Department of Health 1963 Children's Act. HMSO, London

Department of Health 1969 Children's Act. HMSO, London

Department of Health 1975 Children's Act. HMSO, London

Department of Health 1976a Patient's Charter. DoH, London

Department of Health 1976b Citizen's Charter. DoH, London

Department of Health 1976c Health and Safety at Work Act 1974 HMSO, London

Department of Health 1989a Caring for people: community care in the next decade and beyond. Cm 849. HMSO, London

Department of Health 1989b Children's Act. HMSO, London

Department of Health 1990 Guidelines on standard for residential homes for elderly people. HMSO, London

Department of Health 1991 National Health and Community Care Act 1990. HMSO, London

Department of Health and Social Security 1933 Children and Young Persons' Act. HMSO, London

Department of Health and Social Security 1960 Mental Health Act 1959. HMSO, London

Department of Health and Social Security 1985a Government response to the second report from the Social Services Committee 1984/85 session: community care with special reference to adult mentally ill and mentally handicapped people. Cm 9674. HMSO, London

Department of Health and Social Security 1985b Mental Health Act 1983. HMSO, London

Department of Health and Social Services 1976 Management of the violent or potentially violent individual. HMSO, London

Department of Health and The Welsh Office 1990 Code of Practice. Mental Health Act, 1983. HMSO, London

Douglas M 1990 Risk as a forensic resource. Dadalus, Journal of the American Arts and Science 119: 1-16

Edwards S 1996 Nursing ethics: a principles based approach. MacMillan, London

Enfield S L 1990 Guidelines for the use of psychotropic medication in individuals with developmental disabilities. Australia and New Zealand Journal of Developmental Disabilities 16 (1): 71-73

Enfield S L, Tonge B J 1989 Development of an instrument to measure psychopathology in intellectually handicapped children and adolescents. Longman, London

Favell J E, McGimsey J F, Jones M L 1978 The use of physical restraint in the treatment of self-injury and as positive reinforcement. Journal of Applied Behaviour Analysis 11: 225-241

Favell J E, McGimsey J F, Jones M L, Cannon P R 1981 Physical restraint as positive reinforcement. American Journal of Mental Deficiency 85: 425-432

Friedman P R 1974 Mental retardation and the law: a report on status of current court cases. Mental Health Law Project, January. Office of Mental Retardation Co-ordination, Washington DC

Friedman P R 1975 Legal regulations of applied behaviour analysis in mental institutions and prisons. Arizona Law Review 17: 39-104

Gert B, Nelson W A, Culver C M 1989 Moral theory and neurology. Neurological Clinics 7: 681-696

Groeman N H, Slevin O D A, Buckenham M A 1992 Social and behavioural sciences for nurses. Campion Press, Edinburgh

Hanfeing O 1972 Kant's Copernican revolution. Open University Press, Milton Keynes

Hare R H 1952 The language of morals. Oxford University Press, Oxford

Hofkens A, Allen D 1990 Evaluation of a special behaviour unit for people with mental handicaps and challenging behaviour. Journal of Mental Deficiency Research 34: 213-228

Jacobsen J W 1982 Problem behaviour and psychiatric impairment with a developmentally disabled population: behaviour frequency. Applied Research in Mental Retardation 3: 121-139

Jones R 1988 Mental Health Act manual, 2nd edn. Sweet and Maxwell, London

Ketefian S 1981 Moral reasoning and moral behaviour among selected groups of practising nurses. Nursing Research 30: 171-176

Ketefian S 1989 Moral reasoning and ethical practice in nursing. Nursing Clinics of North America 24: 509-521

Law Commission 1993 Working Paper No 129. Mentally handicapped adults and decision making. Medical treatment and research. HMSO, London

Law Commission 1995 Green Paper on mental incapacity. Paper No 231. HMSO, London

Levy A, Kahan B 1991 The pindown experience and the protection of children: the report of the Staffordshire childcare inquiry 1990. Staffordshire County Council, Bambury

Lieberman R P, Wong S E 1984 Behaviour analysis and therapy procedures related to seclusion and restraint. In: Tardiff K (ed) The psychiatric uses of seclusion and restraint. American Psychiatric Press, Washington DC

Lund J 1989 Measuring behaviour disorder in mental handicap. British Journal of Psychiatry 155: 379-383

Lyon C 1994 Legal issues arising from the care, control and safety of children with learning disabilities who also present severe challenging behaviour. Mental Health Foundation, London

McCue M 1993 Helping with behaviour problems. In: Shanley E, Starrs T A (eds) Learning disabilities: a handbook of care, 2nd edn. Churchill Livingstone, Edinburgh, pp. 149-203

Mencap 1997 Barriers to justice: a Mencap study into how the criminal justice system treats people with learning disabilities. Royal Society for Mentally Handicapped Children and Adults, London

Mental Deficiency Committee 1929 Report of the Mental Deficiency Committee, being a Joint Committee of the Board of Education and Board of Control. HMSO, London

Mental Health Foundation 1997 Don't forget us: children with learning disabilities and severe challenging behaviour. Mental Health Foundation, London

Merrell J, Williams A 1995 Beneficence, respect for authority and justice: principles in practice. Oxford University Press, Oxford

Michaels R, Kelly K 1991 Training in psychiatric ethics. In: Block S, Chodoff P (eds) Psychiatric ethics. Oxford University Press, Oxford

O'Leary K D 1972 Behaviour modification in the classroom: a rejoinder to Winett and Winkler. Journal of Applied Behaviour Analysis 5: 592-601

Opton E M J R 1974 Psychiatric violence against prisoners: when therapy is punishment. Mississippi Law Journal 45: 605-644

Osmanczk E 1985 Encyclopaedia of the United Nations. Taylor and Francis, London

Parton N, Thorpe D, Wattam C 1997 Child protection, risk and the moral order. MacMillan, London

Partridge E 1983 A short etymological dictionary of modern English. Greenwich House, New York

Reber A S 1985 The Penguin dictionary of psychology. Penguin Books, Harmondsworth

Reimringer M J, Morgan S W, Bramwell P F 1970 Succingcholine as a modifier of acting-out behaviour. Cultural Medicine 77(7): 28-29

Rest J 1979 Developments in judging moral issues. University of Minnesota Press, Minneapolis

Royal College of Nursing 1986 What the RCN stands for, 2nd edn. Royal College of Nursing, London

Royal College of Psychiatrists 1986 Psychiatric services for mentally handicapped adults and young people. Bulletin of the Royal College of Psychiatrists 10: 321-322

Schaal D W, Hackenburg T 1994 Toward a functional analysis of drug treatment for behaviour problems of people with developmental disabilities. American Journal on Mental Retardation 99 (2): 123-140

Schwartz C 1993 Chambers English dictionary. Chambers, Edinburgh

Seedhouse D 1989 Ethics: the heart of health care. Wiley, Chichester

Seeley J R 1964 The law of the retardate and the retardation of the law. Mental Retardation 14: 6-9

Serber M, Keith C G 1974 The Atascadero project: model of sexual retraining programmes for incarcerated homosexual paedophiles. Journal of Homosexuality 1: 87-97

Singer P 1979 Practical ethics. Cambridge University Press, Cambridge

Singer P 1991 A companion of ethics. Oxford University Press, Oxford

Singer P 1993 Practical ethics, 2nd edn. Cambridge University Press, Cambridge

Smith J C, Hogan B 1991 Criminal law, 6th edn. Blackstone Press, London, pp 377-378

Smith M, McCalls A M 1990 Law and medical ethics, 3rd edn. Oxford University Press, London, pp 225-226

Solnick J V, Rincover A, Peterson C R 1977 Some determinants of the reinforcing and punishing effects of timeout. Journal of Applied Behaviour Analysis 10: 415-424

Stolze S B 1976 Why no guidelines for behaviour modification? Journal of Applied Behaviour Analysis 10: 541-547

Stolze S B 1978 Ethical issues in behaviour modification. Report of the American Psychological Association Commission. Jossey-Bass, London

Thompson I E, Melia K M, Boyd K M 1988 Nursing ethics. Churchill Livingstone, Edinburgh

Tindall B 1997 People with learning disabilities, citizenship, personal development and the management of risk. In: Kenshall H, Pritchard J (eds) Good practice in risk assessment and risk management 2: protection, rights and responsibilities. Jessica Kingsley, London

Tindall L, Alaszewski A 1996 National policies and the care of adults with learning disabilities: a brief historical review. Working Paper 11. Risk and Social Welfare Series. Institute of Health Studies, University of Hull

Tribe D, Korgaonkar G 1991 Medical manslaughter. Journal of Medical Deficiency 7(1): 10

Turnbull J 1994 Facing up to the challenge: a view of the capacity of services to meet the needs of people with challenging behaviour. Journal of Psychiatric and Mental Health Nursing 1: 67-75

Tyler V O, Brown G D 1976 The use of swift, brief isolation as a group control device for institutionalised delinquents. Behaviour Research and Therapy 5: 1-9

United Kingdom Central Council for Nursing, Midwifery and Health Visiting 1989 Exercising accountability. UKCC, London

United Kingdom Central Council for Nursing, Midwifery and Health Visiting 1992 UKCC Code of Conduct, 3rd edn. UKCC, London

United Nations Organisation 1971 Declaration of the Rights of the Disabled. UNO, Geneva

Werry J 1988 Conclusions. In: Aman M G, Singh N N Psychopharmacology of the developmental disabilities. Springer-Verlag, New York

Wharton F 1992 Risk assessuent: basic concepts and general principles. In: Ansell J, Wharton F (eds) Risk: analysis and management. Wiley, Chichester

William P 1978 Our mutual handicap: attitudes and perceptions of others by mentally handicapped people. Paper given to the International Cerebral Palsy Society's seminar, Idealism and Reality: Mental Handicap in the 1980s. University College, Oxford, 5-9 April 1978

Wolfensberger W 1975 The origins and nature of institutions. Syracuse University, Human Policy Press, Syracuse, New York

Wolfensberger W 1977 Principle of normalisation: a foundation for effective services. Values into Action. John O'Brien, London

Wolfensberger W 1980 A brief overview of the principle of normalisation. In: Flynn R J, Nitsch K E (eds) Normalisation, social integration and community services. University Park Press, Baltimore

Wong S E, Woolsey J E, Innocent A J, Lieberman R P 1998 Behavioural treatment of violent psychiatric patients. Journal of Clinical Psychiatry, North America 11: 569–580

Wright K, Haycox A, Leedham I 1994 Evaluating community care: services for people with learning disabilities. Open University Press, Buckingham

Seven therapeutic interventions used in behavioural distress

4 Nonviolent (compassionate) Communication   79
   Jane Gear

5 The arts therapies   107
   Marian Liebmann

6 Chemotherapy and other physical treatments   131
   Ibrahim Y. A. Turkistani

7 Gentle Teaching   159
   Siobhan O'Rourke and Jane Wray

8 Structured teaching   185
   Owen Barr, David Sines, Ken Moore and Gillian Boyd

9 Behavioural interventions   215
   Michael McCue

10 Cognitive behavioural interventions   257
   John Turnbull

Each of the seven chapters in Section 2 presents a detailed overview of different therapeutic interventions that might be used with people who are experiencing behavioural distress. The rationale for the choice of interventions described here was to offer readers a sample of therapeutic approaches born of a wide spectrum of theoretical perspectives.

Chapter 4 provides an overview of the use of Nonviolent (compassionate) Communication. The subject of this chapter is a language for 'conscious connection' with self and others as a means of reducing behavioural distress. Chapter 5 provides an overview of the four main arts therapies – art, drama, music and dance movement therapy – and describes how they are used with people experiencing different types of behavioural distress. By way of contrast, Chapter 6 outlines chemotherapeutic and other physical treatment approaches that are used in medicine when working with people in behavioural distress. Chapter 7 describes Gentle Teaching, a therapeutic approach based on the unconditional valuing of others, which places relationships at the centre of learning and development. Chapter 8 gives a detailed account of the use of structured teaching from the TEACCH 'Treatment and Education of Autistic and Communication Handicapped Children' programme, used with people who lie within the spectrum of autistic disorders. Chapter 9 outlines and discusses ways in which behavioural approaches can assist in the identification, understanding and management of behavioural difficulties and distress, either individually or as a conjunctive component of therapy. Finally, Chapter 10 describes the use of cognitive behavioural interventions and the theoretical and philosophical assumptions that underpin this approach. The chapter focuses on how emotional and behavioural problems are understood from a cognitive behavioural viewpoint.

Each of the chapters in Section 2 is supported with research findings and/or references to literature that documents the evidence we have at our disposal concerning the efficacy of each approach. Each chapter also has a section of additional information/resources and an annotated further reading list.

4 Nonviolent (compassionate) Communication

Jane Gear

Key issues
- Nonviolent Communication (NVC) is a language and means of communication that helps us reframe how we express ourselves and hear others; it clarifies intentions, observations, feelings, needs and requests
- The NVC model and process guide us away from habitual and automatic reactions towards 'conscious connection' with self and others; and can be used as a means of defusing confrontation, mediation and conflict resolution
- NVC operates at a core level of communication and relationships to affect self-esteem and behaviour
- APM-A theory is consistent with NVC, facilitates a compassionate attitude towards people, and provides substantial theoretical support for the NVC process and model

Overview
The subject of this chapter is a language for 'conscious connection' with self and others, as a means of reducing behavioural distress. The language is Marshall Rosenberg's Nonviolent Communication (1983, 1999). Nonviolent Communication (NVC) is Rosenberg's original and preferred name for his process and model sometimes called compassionate communication because of its reliance on empathy. NVC shares values with APM-A theory (also known as orientation theory (Gear 1985, 1989), outlined in Ch. 1). While the APM-A viewpoint facilitates a compassionate attitude towards people who behave in ways we do not like, NVC provides a language and a means of communicating in a compassionate way. This chapter outlines some of the background and development of NVC and offers examples of the approach in action. Powerful influences on the development of this language included Rosenberg's early experiences of racial discrimination, bullying and violence in Detroit, research with Carl Rogers, exposure to radical perspectives in psychology, and working with civil rights groups. NVC has been used in conflict situations, and people have been trained in NVC in many different kinds of institution around the globe for more than 30 years, often in war-torn countries. Case illustrations, research and work in schools exemplify changes in behaviour that are attributable to NVC. The chapter ends with a brief discussion of the usefulness and boundaries of the

approach, as well as further reading and information about training, resources and contact addresses.

What is Nonviolent Communication?

Nonviolent communication (NVC) is a means of communication and 'connection' that works both within and between people. It can be used as a powerful way of defusing aggression and violence, a means of clarification or reconnection when communication 'goes wrong', or as an everyday language that helps to build secure relationships and reduce stress. It is a language that helps us to meet our own needs while staying aware of the needs of others and 'to remain human, even under trying conditions' (Rosenberg 1999, p. 3). Essentially, NVC works through a particular way of offering empathy and by helping us to be as clear as possible about our own and others' feelings, needs and wants. The process can be used in any situation, whether other people are familiar with it or not:

> *NVC guides us in reframing how we express ourselves and hear others. Instead of being habitual, automatic reactions, our words become conscious responses based firmly on an awareness of what we are perceiving, feeling, and wanting. We are led to express ourselves with honesty and clarity, while simultaneously paying others a respectful and empathic attention. In any exchange we come to hear our own deeper needs and those of others. NVC trains us to observe carefully, and to be able to specify behaviours and conditions that are affecting us. We learn to identify and clearly articulate what we are concretely wanting in a given situation. The form is simple, yet powerfully transformative.*

[Rosenberg 1999, p. 3]

NVC allows us to move away from communication that might be heard as criticism, blame or judgement (of ourselves as well as others) to being able to express observations, feelings, needs and requests in ways that are likely to be received compassionately. The process and model also allow us to hear pain and offer empathy for the unfulfilled needs that lie behind violent forms of expression and other kinds of behaviour we find difficult to handle. To turn our attention and energy away from interpreting and judging and towards connecting with other people, the model teaches us to pause and give empathy to ourselves first.

Personal growth and the development of NVC

The story of the development of NVC is intimately bound up with the biography of its creator, Marshall Rosenberg. The biography offers insight into Rosenberg's own personal struggle against discrimination. The struggle turned into hatred of physical violence, hatred of self, and even anti-Semitism. The last two were eventually difficult to *un*learn, and Rosenberg's account of his own process of growth and change lends insight into NVC. The biographical detail describes learning self-empathy, growth in self-acceptance and self-respect, empathy for others and recognition of his own power and needs. These are all elements of Nonviolent Communication.

The words 'violent' and 'nonviolent' in NVC refer to verbal, emotional and spiritual 'violence' as well as physical violence. These kinds of non-physical violence are often unintentional, and an outcome of deeply ingrained habits of speech: words and phrases that either contain or imply judgements, criticism and blame of others.

An account of the development of Rosenberg's thinking about NVC is contained in transcripts of tape-recorded interviews by a biographer, Marjorie Witty (1990). The thinking about the model developed through early involvement in radically different communities. These ranged from studying clinical psychology and research with Carl Rogers, and working in academic institutions and private practice, to working with people on the streets of St Louis, Oakland and Washington DC, with 'spirit people' in California, radical Catholics, and with other movement groups. However, when talking about his first preoccupation with trying to define the difference between violent and nonviolent communication, Rosenberg starts with his childhood.

Learning about hatred and suffering

Rosenberg begins by recalling his family's move to Detroit, a move made in order for his father to find work; this involved his own move from the familiarity and safety of a small town school to one in the inner city. He says that it was there that he learnt about suffering, and for the first time found that he could be hated for a characteristic of himself that he had no control over. He remembers being asked by another child if he was a 'kike' (a term for Jew that he had never heard before) and being attacked after school. At that time (1943) there were race riots in America, while in Russia, where most of his family came from, Jews were being persecuted, as they were in other parts of Europe. His grandparents aunts and uncles told him horror stories of what it would be like if the family were still there. He realises now that the family, already struggling to care for two very sick, and one learning disabled, members, did not know how to deal with his pain other than to tell him 'you think you have it bad' stories. Because his father was a migrant worker the family were not part of a Jewish community; in fact, the young Rosenberg came to hate his Jewishness. In his own words, he 'grew up to be absolutely, virulently anti-Semitic and to hate myself'.

Learning the roots of violence and compassion

Rosenberg came to realise that the attempts he had made to deny part of his identity, and his hatred of himself, were powerful learning experiences. On the other hand, he also talks of learning to appear stony-faced and tough. He became very violent himself (he says 'vicious') and found all of these behaviours very difficult to unlearn. The pain of humiliation through experiences such as having a crowd of children around him laughing and enjoying his torment had overwhelmed his initial fear of fighting.

He describes himself as having been 'not only living in a war zone but living in a minority group in a war zone'. One outcome of this was to spend many years 'trying to figure out *why* people caused each other to suffer, and to have some control over it, something I could *do* in the face of it'. Another outcome has been spending most of his adult life travelling around the globe visiting war zones and being able to do things 'in the face of it'.

At the time when he was learning to inflict pain in his own defence, he was also learning about deep love and compassion from members of his own family. He talks particularly of his grandmother, who although having nine children and living in 'hard core poverty' in her younger life, ran her home like a settlement, always taking in hungry people. He learned too from an uncle who was a pharmacist in an all black neighbourhood, but was never robbed because he showed everyone who came into the store the same strong compassion. The stark contrast between what he experienced inside and outside his home fuelled obsessive curiosity about violence rooted in prejudice, and how it was that some people could be so cruel to others.

Unable to get into fraternity at the University of Michigan because he was Jewish, and having to work and wait on wealthier students, Rosenberg continued to feel an outsider, alone and lonely, feeling what he called a 'slow burning rage' while he studied psychology. During that time he continued to confront his own violence when he felt upset with people. He says that he dealt with that, and feeling what he calls being 'obnoxiously depressed', by getting drunk and spending a lot of the time thinking of killing himself. The only thing he says that sustained him was how deeply he wanted to learn ways to help him deal with people's suffering. He graduated quickly, for economic reasons, and went on to study clinical psychology at the University of Wisconsin. At that stage he was strongly influenced by Michael Hakeem, his tutor on a course in social disorganisation, and in 1960 he was a member of a research project headed by Carl Rogers.

Radical perspectives in psychology

The radical perspectives in psychology that began to emerge at the beginning of the 1960s became strong influences on NVC. Rosenberg's tutor Michael Hakeem was also seen as a radical thinker and Rosenberg received this basic message: psychology and psychiatry are very dangerous because they do not differentiate between scientific and value judgements. It was also Hakeem who Rosenberg says enlightened Thomas Szasz, the author of *The Myth of Mental Illness* (Szasz 1960), and who in turn enlightened him. The work of Szasz had a very profound impact on Rosenberg, who especially liked Szasz's quotation from Joseph Conrad decrying medical approaches: 'Don't cure us. Teach us how to live'. Another influence on Rosenberg and NVC, through Hakeem, was Goffman's book *Asylums* (Goffman 1961). Goffman talked about how 'crazy-making' the system could be. This reinforced Hakeem's own view of the possibility of psychiatry being used as a tool of oppression. The encounter with Hakeem was a turning point in several ways, including growth in Rosenberg's political awareness.

Results of the research project headed by Carl Rogers contributed largely to the development of the process of NVC. Rosenberg first met Rogers in a group where the chairs had been put in a circle. He did not know he was sitting next to Rogers and was amazed when he said, 'I'd like to get things started', and even more amazed that he did not say anything else! This was a powerful introduction to Rogers's non-directive approach, and Rosenberg was deeply impressed with the power of that way of allowing things to evolve without being didactic.

Another strong influence on NVC was a journal article by Bandura (1961) called 'Psychotherapy as a learning process'. The effect of this article was to lead Rosenberg to think, 'What if we did just get clear about what people need, and try to teach them how to do stuff, rather than therapize them?'. This was reinforced by Hakeem pointing Rosenberg towards literature that drew attention to how effective psychiatry was at the beginning of the century. At that time the standard approach to therapy was not to think so much of people as sick, but as down on their luck. In those early days therapists seemed to have acted more in the manner of kindly and supportive ministers and were described as more successful in helping people than Rosenberg considered possible by scientific method. However, it was ultimately a book by O. J. Harvey (1962), *Conceptual Systems and Personality Organization*, that provided the conceptual framework for the NVC model.

Family therapy

Private practice in St Louis led Rosenberg towards what was then a radical paradigm, and what we now know as family therapy. At that time he was criticised for seeing children with their families, and he had huge difficulties trying to explain to other psychiatrists what he was doing. Their whole way of looking at distress was based on the conception of 'mental illness'. By then Rosenberg had begun to find it helpful to commit himself to discovering which skills people needed to resolve their problems and to 'getting beyond professionalism and treating people as human beings'. His approach was to think in terms of skills and to get clear the skills that people do not have.

Disenchantment with formal institutions and conventional practice began to coincide with recognition of his own power. This happened when family therapy started to come into vogue and he talked about his own approach to a conference in St Louis. When people found out that he was already working with families, and even teaching them how to communicate with one another, he was invited to do workshops and began to see his work differently. He could see that he was not just a troublemaker, but someone who had ideas that the mainstream valued.

Community psychology

At this time Rosenberg was working in a private practice and saw scores of children who were not doing well in school. He decided to educate himself in learning disabilities and by 1962 he was regarded as an expert, and decided to educate the educators. By 1965 he was looking beyond psychotherapy and beginning to notice the work of George Miller, then president of the American Psychological Association, who talked of developing ways of distributing psychology differently and 'giving it away to the masses'. Rosenberg began to look at how he could become more of a community psychologist. He was already teaching his model (though never using the word 'model' or anything like it) in workshops on 'diagnostic teaching' based on research that in 1968 became a book of the same name. By this time he had started travelling and doing workshops around America. He also became aware of the political power, in the Freirean sense (Freire 1970), of being the kind of community psychologist he wanted to be.

Rosenberg became involved in a project with a street gang called Zulu 1200. He was later to describe the gang leader, Al Chappelle, as one of the most important influences in his life. Rosenberg had joined in the work of a poverty programme in St Louis, called the Block Partnership, which brought together white people from the suburbs and black people from the inner city with the purpose of sharing power and working on projects together. In fact the project nearly collapsed because of the inability of the people within the partnership to communicate, and Rosenberg's new role was to teach communication skills to the white people.

At a citizens' group meeting Chappelle had walked in uninvited and sat just outside of the group staring at Rosenberg. Eventually Chappelle said:

> *We don't need no great white father come down here and tell us how to communicate.*

Rosenberg was tired and found himself 'getting into a nice competitive interaction and all of a sudden could see this was leading to disaster'. He paused, and was then able to empathise to the point where Chappelle became fascinated with what had happened, and later asked, 'What the fuck did you do to me in there?' and then to Rosenberg's astonishment asked him to come and teach the street gang. Chappelle had said:

> *We need to learn that shit ... we will never get to beat the police at the violence.*

This breakthrough led to years of travelling together, with Chappelle helping Rosenberg to access the groups he wanted to work with. Over the next 4 years they trained hundreds of people in minority groups in the skills of NVC and had the satisfaction of seeing the skills being used.

Global mediation and training

Rosenberg wanted to introduce social change 'without infuriating the opposition'. This eventually led to world-wide mediation work and training people in the skills of NVC, and a global network of certified trainers. In 1984 Rosenberg founded the Center for Nonviolent Communication in America, closely followed by centres in Switzerland (see resources at the end of this chapter) and Israel. There are now 30 centres around the world, and NVC has been used for transforming conflicts into peaceful dialogues on all five continents.

Evidence base

For the past 30 years the major focus for Rosenberg has always been – and still is – training people in NVC in order to alleviate suffering. Only since the mid-1980s, and the setting up of the American and Swiss centres in particular, has there been any attempt to disseminate wider knowledge of NVC other than via training, either by Rosenberg himself or by certified trainers. The training has taken place in many different environments, including school communities (parents, pupils and staff), postgraduate and professional settings in colleges, and universities, prisons, hospitals and other health care settings, families and businesses. In recent years papers have been published in journals, while Rosenberg's own creative energy has been pulled mainly towards providing materials for the training. Seeking evidence to support work that seemed to Rosenberg and to people who learned NVC skills, self-evidently helpful, and in many cases transformational, has been a lower priority. Hence, most evidence of the effectiveness of NVC is still experiential and anecdotal, and devising methods of formal evaluation of the work is currently a high priority. Whereas there is scant research evidence to date, the anecdotal evidence world-wide has now accumulated to a stage where it might be impossible to log.

However, there are currently bids being made for funding for research in medicine, health care and education, and there have been investments by both UNICEF and the European Union (EU) for work in schools. Since 1993, NVC has been part of a UNICEF funded 'Program for Supporting and Promoting Child Development' in primary and secondary schools in Serbia, Montenegro and Kosovo. This 'Smilekeepers' programme was originally designed to help children traumatised by war, and has now been incorporated into school curricula and experienced by more than 12 000 children and 600 teachers in Serbia alone. The original programme was offered to teachers, principals, school psychologists and parents, as well as to children. Outcomes included significant improvements in mood and behaviour of the children who took part: depression and anxiety scores decreased, and scores for cooperation and confidence increased; at the same time, a control group showed significant increases in aggression and decreases in cooperation (Ignajatovic-Savic 1995).

Since the completion of the original 'Smilekeepers' programme in 1995, a programme based wholly on NVC, 'Mutual Education: Giraffe Language in Kindergarten and Schools', has been running in Yugoslavia. In this programme teachers, principals and school psychologists who had already taken part in the 'Smilekeepers' programme undertook a further 6 days training in NVC, 3 days learning the 'basics' of NVC and a further 3 days applying this learning to education.

NVC in schools funded by the European Union started in Israel in 1995. The programme there has been extended and is still running with extra funding for schools in two European countries to be involved alongside four Palestinian and four Israeli schools. These programmes have now started in Serbia and Italy. Video-taped evidence of the success of the project shows, for example, children as 'peace-keepers' helping peers resolve conflicts with one another. Formal research into the outcomes of the EU funded work is still in progress. During 1999, the NVC programme was extended by volunteers into underground cellars and shelters in Yugoslavia and Kosovo, and to communities of displaced persons in adjoining countries.

An NVC project that started as a peace movement in 1993 in Wajiri in north-eastern Kenya has resulted in transformation of how a community is being run (telephone interview with D. Ibraham, 30 April 1999). After 35 years of the community being ruled by armed violence, government officials and community elders have learned that they can do things differently, and now sit down and plan together. A local proverb, 'If we talk we can also agree', has been given new meaning. Since 1998 the NVC training has been extended to primary school, secondary school and youth work. This new focus is communally funded by the people who were formerly involved in the peace movement from 1993. This work has changed warring clans to people at peace, linking and working for a purpose, having moved from investment in the munitions trade to investing in people.

A quite different kind of evidence, in the form of independent theoretical support comes from the coincidence and overlap between aspects of APM-A theory (Gear 1985, 1989; see also Ch. 1) and Nonviolent Communication. The common elements of NVC and APM-A are listed in Box 4.1, and some of

Box 4.1
Consistency and overlap between APM-A theory and NVC

NVC and APM-A share the following:
- Concern with human vulnerability
- Concern with safety and congruence
- Concern with compassionate understanding of inner states of self and others
- Concern with quality of attention and consciousness (in different ways)
- A view of feelings arising from needs
- Similar perceptions of the relationship between unmet needs and violence
- Rejection of 'labelling' and using 'static' descriptions of people
- Rejection of absolute values (sometimes prefaced by 'shoulds' 'oughts' and 'musts')

the ways in which APM-A complements and offers theoretical support to NVC are illustrated in the case study 'A husband's violence' (see p. 95–101), and listed on pages 101, 102 and 103.

The NVC process

NVC facilitates both expressing and receiving messages, connecting empathically in a specific way with other people, and connecting empathically with ourselves. The process involves developing skills in perceiving, expressing and exchanging information about how we are, and what we are feeling, needing and wanting at any given moment. For training purposes the metaphors of 'jackal' and 'giraffe' (see reflection box below) often help people to distinguish between habits of communication that our culture 'trains' us in, and a different style of communicating which comes from keener awareness and a deeper place inside us.

The metaphors of jackal and giraffe are used for training purposes only, and are not meant to imply duality, values of 'good' and 'bad', or to encourage labelling people. Capacities for 'jackal' and 'giraffe' continue to coexist internally, even after training. With practice we can recognise the habitual and defensive 'short cuts' to communication described as jackal, and choose to express ourselves verbally as part of a present encounter, as opposed to being subject to habits and rituals of speech.

Jackal and giraffe

The habitual 'jackal' language that we grow up with in Western cultures can contain subtle expressions of control, 'put downs', sarcasm, accusations and interpretations of the behaviour of self and others that we may be unconscious of, or even mistake for simple expressions of our own feelings and needs, until we develop greater awareness of words and their impact. This is the language referred to as 'life-alienating'. Rosenberg describes it more fully as language that blocks compassion: a language that contains moralistic judgements, diagnoses, analyses, criticisms, comparisons, denial of responsibility for our actions and conclusions about who 'deserves' what and (consciously or not) making demands rather than requests.

On the other hand, the symbolism of the giraffe carries with it an image of elegance and nonviolence in itself. Giraffes also have the largest hearts of any land animal; this symbolises the benefits of speaking to others 'from the heart' and sharing feelings and needs, as opposed to speaking 'from the head' in the sense of a tendency to offer analyses and diagnoses. The long neck of the giraffe symbolises 'far-sightedness' as well as offering a metaphor for taking risks: the neck can be 'stuck out' either to reveal and admit vulnerability, or to say 'no' when it seems difficult, or request something that feels difficult to ask for.

Above all, however, NVC is an inner process that involves keeping in mind the purpose of the model in order to be able to practise the skills. The purpose is to connect with other people, and to communicate 'in the moment' in relation to immediate situations, feelings and needs, rather than allowing unexpressed tension to build up and block communication.

Rosenberg draws a contrast between this way of communicating that he calls 'life-enhancing' and communication that he sees as 'life-alienating' (Rosenberg 1983, 1999): as described more fully below, life-alientating communication is 'disconnected' from self and/or others, usually because its conscious or unconscious intention is to defend or attack.

In order to keep in mind the purpose of the model – primarily 'to connect with other people' – the inner process of NVC also involves effort to connect with ourselves and monitor our own thoughts, feelings and behaviour without self-judgement, blame or criticism. For example, at times, frustration, disappointment, anger or other negative feelings get in the way of relating empathically to others, usually because we are in need of empathy ourselves. At these times it is possible to use NVC skills to be in touch with ourselves, to stop, recognise our own feelings and needs, give self-empathy, and then be able to look outwards again.

Self-empathy consists of being able to recognise and take time to acknowledge internally our initial reactions to our own or others' diagnoses, analyses, criticism or blame. Having acknowledged our own needs, we can then translate initial judgements, and eventually find positive language about whatever it is specifically that we, or others, might like to happen. At this stage it becomes possible to move back into empathic connection before eventually being able to express or receive concrete requests, so that each person can have needs met.

To use the model without keeping its purpose of *connection* in focus (as opposed to simply expressing and receiving feelings, needs and making requests) would be to experience a rather mechanistic exercise. We might achieve a temporary and static connection with another person, but dynamic and creative relationships require the momentum and energy of an ongoing intent and awareness. Experience of connection depends on developing moment-to-moment consciousness of what is going on inside ourselves, as well as guessing, and checking out, what the other person is feeling and needing in order to be able to stay in a continuous loop of interaction (Fig. 4.1).

The NVC model

Whether we are reflecting on our own behaviour or that of others, NVC requires that we learn to communicate four different kinds of information. They are:

- Making clear distinctions between observations and evaluations
- Identifying feelings that are distinct from interpretations of behaviour or mixed with needs
- Recognising deep needs that have inner connections to the feelings they drive, as opposed to what we want others to do
- Expressing clear, specific and 'do-able' requests.

Distinguishing facts from perceptions and evaluations

NVC acknowledges how difficult it is to express clearly the four different kinds of information we need – observations, feelings, needs and requests – and to communicate compassionately. Habitually, and inadvertently, we tend to mix observations, feelings, needs and requests with one another, and with evaluations of other people and their actions. However, the first piece of information used in NVC is a clear and objective observation, a factual statement that is free of evaluation, sensed directly through sight, hearing, touch, smell or taste. To say, for example, 'Mary is good at catching the ball'

Fig. 4.1
NVC as a 'dance' of interaction between people (from Marshall Rosenberg, with permission, personal communication)

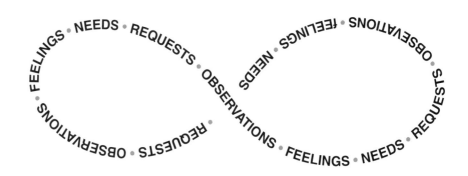

would be an evaluation, whereas 'Mary has caught the ball every time' is a clear observation, as is using a direct quotation such as 'Hugh said, "Mary is good at catching the ball"'. It can be helpful to start observations with the word 'When' and then refer directly to what it was we saw, heard, or otherwise experienced that triggered whatever feelings and needs are currently alive within us. Rosenberg (1976) cites six different ways in which observations and evaluations become confused. These are:

- Using the verb 'to be' (in the sense that a person is of a particular type, e.g. as in 'Clare is lazy') without indicating consciousness that an evaluation is taking place, and the use of verbs that in themselves have evaluative connotations (as in saying that someone procrastinates) without indicating any consciousness that this is a personal view, and that an evaluation is taking place
- A confusion of prediction with certainty (as in, 'If you don't drink milk your bones will not be strong')
- A failure to be specific about a person or situation
- The use of words denoting ability or inability, without indicating that a judgement or evaluation is being made
- The use of adjectives and adverbs that do not signify that an evaluation is being made (as in 'Jill is pretty' rather than acknowledging an evaluation in a form such as 'I find Jill pretty')
- Using other forms of generalisation and/or exaggeration that obscure observations with evaluations, including words such as 'always', 'never', 'frequently' and 'too'.

Compassionate communication starts with an objective statement because when people hear interpretations of what they have said or done they are likely to divert energy to being defensive, and so disconnect from whatever it is that we would really like them to hear. With this first piece of information we direct attention to whatever it is that we like or dislike that has stimulated awareness of more specific feelings and needs.

Distinguishing feelings from thoughts and interpretations

The second piece of information used in NVC is about feelings. Again, being as specific as possible is important. Using specific feeling words such as 'excited', 'hopeful', or 'tender', when needs are fulfilled (as opposed to saying 'I feel good'), and choosing specific terms such as 'bitter', 'resentful', or 'frightened' when needs are not met (rather than saying 'I feel bad') conveys more information and is easier for other people to connect with. If it is a feeling that is being expressed, rather than an interpretation of someone else's behaviour (such as feeling 'let down'), it usually consists of just one word. Unfortunately, use of the word 'I feel' does not guarantee that it is a feeling that we are expressing or that we are referring to our inner states only. In English we can say, 'I feel . . .' and follow it with a thought or judgement rather than a feeling. This is usually the case if we say 'I feel that . . .' or 'I feel as if . . .' or, with even greater risk of there being an interpretation of someone else's behaviour, 'I feel you have/do/should . . .'. There are also many words we use for feelings that in themselves contain interpretations – words such as: cheated, rejected, humiliated, abandoned, patronised and intimidated.

Identifying the needs that drive feelings

The third piece of information refers to needs. Identifying needs is core to the whole NVC process because needs are intimately linked to both feelings and requests. We are alerted to needs by our feelings and, in turn, clear requests are dependent on defining needs as accurately as possible. Identifying our own needs and guessing needs of others based on hearing feelings can be the most difficult aspect of learning NVC. Reasons for this are likely to be that cultural 'training' leads us to avoid recognising, let alone showing, emotional states, and because needs are unconscious most of the time. For example, acknowledging needs that are difficult to meet, or are in conflict with one another, can be painful. It is sometimes easier to convince ourselves that we need something that is available, possible or attractive (or even things that are apparently none of these) and then, if we succeed in getting what we 'wanted', be surprised because we still feel dissatisfied or unhappy.

NVC emphasises the importance of making *inner* connections between feelings and needs, otherwise it is easy to believe that our feelings are attributable to the actions of others.

To help us remain aware that our feelings are generated by connections we make ourselves, NVC recommends that we use the form, 'I feel . . . because I need . . .'. For example, saying, 'You upset me when you refused to come out with me' is likely to impact on another person quite differently from, 'When you said "No" when I asked you to come out with me I felt upset because I needed company, and I would have liked that company to have been yours.' In the latter case the speaker is taking full responsibility for his or her feelings as opposed to blaming the other person.

Rosenberg has described several ways in which, linguistically, we can attribute responsibility for our feelings to others. These include:

- Following the statement 'I feel as I do because ...' with some word other than 'I', as in: 'I feel disappointed because you ...'
- Expressing feelings in the passive voice, as in: 'It really annoys me when people ...'
- Stating only what others do and feelings not associated with needs, as in: 'When you tap your foot, I feel irritated'.

Needs, as opposed to wants or desires, are usually universally recognised and can affect us deeply, both psychologically and physically, when ignored. They come under many different headings. Some examples of headings used by Rosenberg (1999), and some needs that fall under them, are set out in Box 4.2 below.

Box 4.2
Some examples of universal human needs

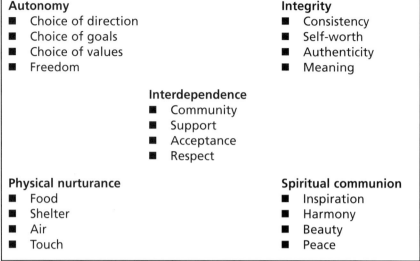

Autonomy
■ Choice of direction
■ Choice of goals
■ Choice of values
■ Freedom

Integrity
■ Consistency
■ Self-worth
■ Authenticity
■ Meaning

Interdependence
■ Community
■ Support
■ Acceptance
■ Respect

Physical nurturance
■ Food
■ Shelter
■ Air
■ Touch

Spiritual communion
■ Inspiration
■ Harmony
■ Beauty
■ Peace

Making requests

Finally, we need to be able to express requests that are clear, concrete and 'do-able'. Learners of NVC are sometimes surprised at how much practice this takes, and how much confusion can result from lack of specificity. A graphic example used by Rosenberg is of a cartoon showing a man who has fallen into a lake and who shouts to his dog, 'Lassie! get help!' The next picture shows the dog on a psychiatrist's couch. We also need to learn to say what we *do* want rather than what we *do not* want: for example, if we say to a child pulling a cat's tail 'Don't do that', we are likely to find to our cost that the child can find many other ways of handling the cat that can cause pain or distress. One of the first lessons in making requests is to use positive action language.

Another skill that is required is the ability to distinguish between requests and demands. This is not simply a matter of prefacing what we want with 'Would you be willing to . . .'. Sometimes the distinction between a request and a demand only becomes clear in the original speaker's response when a request is turned down. A classic kind of response that changes a request into a demand happens when 'No' is followed by the reactions 'You would if you cared' or 'I'm hurt'.

In responses like these the speaker is interpreting the feelings, needs and reaction of someone else as a rejection or deficiency of some kind. A possible outcome of this is that the more it happens the more likely requests are to be heard as demands so that eventually neither party is able to hear the other accurately. Another key difference between a request and a demand is that, in NVC, requests are preceded with empathy with whatever is currently 'alive' in the other person that may block our needs from being heard, let alone met.

The outline of NVC offered above is a brief overview. Learning to use NVC requires training, practice and working with live examples to develop skills and change habits of perception and speech. The three descriptions of NVC in use in the case studies that follow are intended to offer more insight into the process and model.

Case illustrations of NVC in use

The three examples in the case illustrations (below) are of NVC used in quite different circumstances and at different levels of proficiency. The first is a short account about the effectiveness of NVC used by a teacher with relatively little knowledge of the tool. The second is an example that includes some of the inner communication of a father (already practised in NVC) attempting to connect with his son. The third example is of NVC used alongside other tools and APM-A theory (see Ch. 1) in a counselling situation.

A teacher's use of NVC in the classroom

This is an account of the first use of the Nonviolent Communication model 'live' by a teacher who had just experienced his first 2 days of training in NVC. The teacher was working in an inner city primary school on a council estate in the north of England. The estate has a very high crime rate and high levels of drug abuse, and 60% of children at the school had been diagnosed as having 'special needs'. Members of staff at the school expressed feelings of despair about the children's behaviour on a daily basis. This teacher's class was Year 5 and the children were between 9 and 10 years old.

Because of concern about behaviour in the school, any activity seen as holding potential for positive change was given priority, even in an already crowded curriculum. In this case, the teacher also felt able to devote class time to telling the children about NVC because training was currently taking place elsewhere in the school; first, he used NVC himself.

The teacher had an urgent need to find 5 minutes of quiet time to do a small administrative task and, on past experience, anticipated difficulty. He decided to use NVC to explain his needs. He started by telling the children that he had the task to do and said he felt anxious because he needed absolute quiet in order to concentrate fully. He then made a request for the children to do a specific exercise for 5 minutes without talking at all. To his surprise two children came forward to set a timer kept in a cupboard, and then everyone was silent. Not every child stayed on task, but no one spoke and he completed his work without interruption.

The following morning the teacher decided to tell the children how using NVC had contributed to the positive atmosphere of their class the day before. He explained the model and then asked them if they thought it might be helpful to them to tell people about their feelings and needs, rather than simply reacting from habit when something happened that they did not like. The children liked the idea, and as a class thought about problems that they were experiencing where NVC might be useful.

The first issue brought up was about a child being 'bullied' by an elder sibling. Alan said that his brother was 'always telling lies and getting me into trouble'. He went on to say how he hated his brother for it, because there was nothing he could do. The teacher and the rest of the class helped him to translate this into an observation that referred to a particular incident involving his sister; then they helped him to express his feelings and needs at the time it had happened. Eventually, the boy arrived at what he might say to his sister:

> *When my brother said I took money from your purse, I felt angry because I need to be seen as honest. If Darren says again that I have done something wrong will you please check it out with me?*

Alan felt secure enough with this to say that he would try it out that evening.

A teacher's use of NVC in the classroom *cont'd*

The second problem was brought up by a boy, Ben, whose mother the teacher had an appointment with that lunchtime. Ben belonged to a group of children who used drugs and he was a smoker. In class he habitually disturbed other children by 'baiting' them with imaginary accusations.

Ben brought up the issue of his anxiety about his mother coming to school, and after help in choosing his words from other children in the class, Ben eventually said:

> *When my mum has to come to school because I have been so naughty, I feel ashamed, and whenever a letter has to be sent home I feel sad.*

After more exploration and discussion amongst his peers he decided his need was to feel proud of himself.

As a class, the children decided that he might make a request concerning what form of sanction could help him best. They listed possibilities. Ben dismissed three of them as not having worked for him in the past. He was eventually quite firm in his choice of 'daily report'. (This involved having teachers sign a statement about his behaviour at the end of lessons and discussing these reports with his class teacher and the headmistress. This system also allowed him to earn points for the five areas of behaviour represented in the classroom rules.) After making his decision Ben happily accepted other ideas and suggestions by his peers for using the opportunity as fully as possible.

This session of sharing problems, exploring feelings, needs and requests and telling the children more about the language of 'giraffe' went on for the whole 1 hour lesson. (The children became so interested that they wanted to use the CD-Rom encyclopedia to find out just how much bigger a giraffe's heart is than a human heart.)

When Ben's mother, older brother and baby brother came to join Ben and the teacher for the meeting, the teacher gave Ben's mother a brief account of what had taken place. He told her that without the model he would now have been giving her a list of disruptive behaviours, and probably excluding her son from school. He explained how the daily report system worked, and her own responsibility in its positive use. She expressed her willingness to give it a try and the three of them said how happy they felt about the outcome of the meeting.

That afternoon the class gave Ben support, usually in the form of reminders when he 'lost the thread'. Initially Ben was very happy to accept this. Unfortunately, in the last quarter of the day he threw his books on the floor and left the room slamming the door, but then came back. After that, and for at least another 6 weeks, he was happy to use the report system, and wanted to explore where he was losing points. He had yet to reach his own target figure; however, he had lost his fear of taking even the disappointing reports home.

Father and son (an example of 'NVC in action', from Marshall Rosenberg's *Nonviolent Communication* (Rosenberg 1999), with permission)

In this situation, 15-year-old Bill took a car without permission from Jorge, a family friend. He went on a joy ride with two friends and returned the car undamaged to the garage, where its absence had not been detected. Since then, however, Jorge's 14-year-old daughter Eva, who had gone along for the ride, told her father what had happened. Jorge then informed Bill's father, who is now approaching his son. The father has just recently been practising NVC.

Father: So I hear you, Eva and Dave took Jorge's car without asking.

Bill: No we didn't!

Father and son *cont'd*

Father: (*in a loud voice*) Don't lie to me; it will only make it worse! (*Then remembers to first connect with his own feelings and needs in order to stay in connection with his son.*) You just sit there for a minute; I need to think. (*Going inside himself, he sees how angry and scared he is. He's angry because he is telling himself, 'Bill should have known better! What a liar he has become!' He's scared when he thinks of all the potential consequences not only of Bill's action, but his own misjudgement of what his son might do. 'That was stupid of me to assume he knows better.' 'Someone could have gotten killed in this!' He catches himself, 'Oops, I need to translate the labels 'stupid' and 'liar' into feelings and needs. For stupid, I guess the feeling is disappointment in myself: I would have liked to think I knew him better. And as for 'liar'. I'm feeling pretty scared because I want to count on getting accurate information to deal with this situation.' Silence while he mulls over how to begin talking.*) Bill, are you worried that if you give me accurate information, you'd be punished?

Bill: Yeah, you're always so mean when I do anything you don't like.

Father: Are you saying you'd like more understanding and fairer treatment for what you do?

Bill: Oh, sure, like I'm really gonna get fair treatment and understanding from you!

Father: (*silently to himself, 'Boy, do I get angry when he says that! Can't he see how hard I'm trying? I really need a little respect for how hard this is, and I guess also a little caring for how scared I'm feeling.'*) Sounds to me like you're worried that no matter what you say, you won't be treated fairly?

Bill: What do you care about treating me fairly? When something happens, you just want someone to punish. Besides, what's the big deal? Even if we did take the car, no one got hurt and it's back where it was. I mean this is no major crime wave.

Father: Are you scared there will be harsh consequences if you admit to taking the car, and you're wanting trust that you will be treated justly?

Bill: Yeah.

Father: (*allowing time for silence and the connection to go deeper*) What could I do to give you that reassurance?

Bill: Promise to never punish me again.

Father: (*Aware that punishment will not help Bill develop consciousness around potential consequences of his own behaviour, but will only contribute to greater disconnection and resentment, the father expresses willingness to agree to Bill's request.*) I'd be open to that agreement if you'd agree to stay in dialogue with me. That is, we talk until we're satisfied that you are aware of all of the possible consequences of your having taken that car. However, in the future, if it happens that I'm not confident that you see the potential danger of what you are in for, I might still use force – but only in order to protect you.

Bill: Wow, great! It really feels great that I'm so stupid you have to use force to protect me from myself!

Father: (*Losing touch with his own needs, says silently; 'Man, there are times when I could just kill the little . . . I'm so furious when he says things like that! It really doesn't seem like he cares . . . Damn, what am I needing here? I'm needing to know, when I'm working this hard, that at least he cares.'*) (*out loud, angrily*) You know Bill, when you say things like that, I get really pissed off. I'm trying so hard to stay with you on this, and when I hear things like that . . . Look, I need to know if you even want to keep talking with me.

Bill: I don't care.

Father and son *cont'd*

Father: Bill I'm really wanting to listen to you rather than fall back into my old bad habits of blaming and threatening you whenever something comes up that I'm upset about. But when I hear you say things like, 'It feels good to know that I am so stupid' in the tone of voice you just used, I find it hard to control myself. I could use your help on this. That is if you would rather me listen to you than blame you or threaten. Or if not, then, I suppose my other option is to handle this the way I'm used to handling things.

Bill: And what would that be?

Father: Well, by now, I'd probably be saying, 'Hey, you're grounded for two years: no TV, no car, no money, no date, no nothing!'

Bill: Well, guess I'd want you to do it the new way then.

Father: (*with humour*) I'm glad to see that your sense of self-preservation is still intact. Now I need you to tell me whether you're willing to share some honesty and vulnerability.

Bill: What do you mean by 'vulnerability'?

Father: It means that you tell me what you are really feeling about the things we're talking about, and I tell you the same from my end. (*in a firm voice*) Are you willing?

Bill: Okay, I'll try.

Father: (*with a sigh of relief*) Thank you. I'm grateful for your willingness to try. Did I tell you – Jorge grounded Eva for three months – she won't be allowed to do anything. How do you feel about that?

Bill: Oh man, what a bummer; that's so unfair!

Father: I'd like to hear how you really feel about it.

Bill: I told you – it's totally unfair!

Father: (*realising that Bill is not in touch with what he is feeling, decided to guess*) Are you sad that she is having to pay so much for her mistake?

Bill: No, it's not that. I mean, it wasn't her mistake really.

Father: Oh, so are you upset she's paying for something that was your idea to start with?

Bill: Well, yeah, she must have went along with what I told her to do.

Father: Sounds to me like you're kind of hurting inside seeing the kind of effect your decision had on Eva.

Bill: Sorta.

Father: Billy, I really need to know that you are able to see that your actions have consequences.

Bill: Well, I wasn't thinking about what could have gone wrong. Yeah, I guess I really did screw up bad.

Father: I'd rather you see it as something that did not turn out the way you wanted. And I'm still needing reassurance about your being aware of the consequences.

Bill: I feel really stupid, Dad . . . I didn't mean to hurt anyone.

Father: (*translating Bill's self-judgments into feelings and needs*) So you're sad, and regret what you did because you'd like to be trusted not to do harm?

Bill: Yeah, I didn't mean to cause so much trouble. I just didn't think about it.

Father and son *cont'd*

Father: Are you saying you wish you had thought about it more and gotten clearer before you had acted?

Bill: (reflecting) Yeah . . .

Father: Well, it's reassuring for me to hear that, and for there to be some real healing with Jorge, I would like you to go to him and tell him what you just told me. Would you be willing to do that?

Bill: Oh man, that's so scary; he'll be really mad!

Father: Yeah, it's likely he will be. That's one of the consequences. Are you willing to be responsible for your action? I like Jorge and I want to keep him for a friend, and I'm guessing that you would like to keep your connection with Eva. Is that the case?

Bill: She's one of my best friends.

Father: So shall we go see them?

Bill: (*fearfully and reluctantly*) Well . . . okay. Yeah, I guess so.

Father: Are you scared and needing to know you are safe if you go there?

Bill: Yeah.

Father: We'll go together: I'll be there for you and with you. I'm really proud that you are willing.

A husband's violence

This third case is about the use of NVC in a counselling situation in conjunction with other tools and APM-A theory, otherwise known as orientation theory (Gear 1985, 1989), introduced in Chapter 1. Some of the counsellor's inner reflections are in italics.

First session
Peter and Jill had intended to go to relationship counselling together. Jill had now left the marital home with their three young sons. Peter said that he accepted Jill's criticisms about what she had perceived as a long-term inability to listen to her, and admitted both physical and verbal violence, especially after drinking. He said he felt an urgent need to talk, so kept the appointment alone.

As Peter talked about his distress he shifted in his seat, clenching and unclenching his fists; he seemed to stop only to take breath. He talked about his 'terrible behaviour' and of guilt and regret. The counsellor noticed what seemed like tension in his body, and his apparent need to externalise energy in gestures as well as his almost continuous talk. It was at least 10 minutes before there was space for her to empathise other than non-verbally. Then she began, tentatively, translating his expressions of guilt and regret into empathic responses, checking the feelings and needs she guessed were behind his words:

Peter: I can see it all now, how I have taken her for granted, and how I got things in the wrong order by putting work first, but I have been a good 'provider'.

The counsellor tentatively translated what she had heard as his self-blame into an observation (which in this case was an inner reflection), feelings, and needs:

Counsellor: When you think about Jill, do you feel regret, because you would have liked to show her how much you valued her, and, maybe some relief, because you know that you met your need to be a good provider?

A husband's violence
cont'd

Peter: Yes, that's right. But I've given her all this anger and now she's using it to frighten me. She is playing the divorce card.

Counsellor: *(translating and checking)* And now you are recognising Jill's anger are you feeling really afraid, because you want to stay married and fear losing her completely?

Peter: Yes, that's right.

At this point the counsellor checked out with Peter whether he was meaning to blame himself for everything that had happened:

Peter: I hadn't seen it like that, but, anyway, I am to blame.

Counsellor: *(translating into observation, feelings and needs)* When you think back to Jill leaving with the children, did you feel devastated because you really needed to cherish what you had?

Internally, the counsellor was observing that Peter hardly stopped moving and talking, and (via APM-A) read these and other gestures as signs of stress and heightened arousal. She was interpreting what he had described as his violence towards his wife as expressions of his own heightened feelings and unmet needs; and she was wondering what experiences might have triggered what seemed to her like deep frustration and anger, and what buried pain might be at its root. She saw his self-blame as another aspect of his need for some way of understanding what had happened, and, as yet, probably his only way of recognising his wife's feelings. She looked forward to his being able to recognise Jill's likely feelings and needs, as opposed to simply seeing her as justified in leaving.

She also believed that, by eventually helping him to identify the deeper source of so much eruptive feeling, he could acknowledge it, understand it, and as he found congruence, let go of his pain. In APM-A terms, she saw the possibility of moving from the disorientation that she inferred from his gestures and words, to re-orientation. She saw his need to talk as an urgent physiological as well as emotional need. The counsellor sensed multiple needs for orientation as he talked about his new situation: all of these needs were ultimately emotional. However, she saw some as being more physically and socially oriented and some more clearly as psychological needs, the latter included a need to understand, as he talked of needing 'to get his head around what had happened'.

The counsellor hoped that, as what she perceived as his general level of stress and tension changed, so would Peter's attention, perception, and levels and kinds of needs. The likelihood of stress spilling into violence when triggered by any extra, apparently minor, irritations was also likely to be lower.

Peter talked more about his relationship and his outbursts of violence. The counsellor guessed, and checked with Peter, feelings of hurt, shock and devastation, as well as fears. After more rounds of translating what sounded like self-criticism and blame into empathy, she saw his body language changing and he seemed to feel less tension than before. Eventually, Peter expressed relief about having someone listen to him, and his attention seemed freer to turn outwards. The counsellor commented that Peter had repeated that he understood why Jill had left, without mentioning how she might have felt. She asked Peter whether he could guess any of Jill's feelings at that time:

Peter: I don't blame her for leaving, when I behaved as I did.

Counsellor: I am noticing that you are still telling me why you thought Jill left. Are you able to guess any of her feelings at that time?

Peter: I am not surprised that she went.

A husband's violence
cont'd

Counsellor: I would still like to move away from your guesses of why Jill went, and hear something about her feelings.

Peter: (*pausing to think before speaking*) Probably unloved, frightened, lonely, insecure, hurt.

When the counsellor wondered what needs might have been underneath Jill's feelings, Peter's guess was that she needed to feel safe and to have a husband to be proud of.

As the session was coming to its close, the counsellor reflected on Peter's needs from the counselling. The APM-A 'orientation needs' she had inferred included a need to use the counselling as a means of finding direction, to acknowledge the things he had said and done, to try and understand his own behaviour, and to change.

She checked out whether it was Peter's wish to change his behaviour, and that he did not know how. She then asked whether he would be interested in learning nonviolent ways of expressing his feelings and needs, and a way of giving empathy to himself as well as to other people. He said he was very keen to start.

Second session
Although Peter had said that he wanted very much to learn and use NVC, the counsellor also sensed a still urgent need for expression, as words seemed to well up and flow from him in an outpouring of feelings and apparent need for empathy. Over the course of the session the counsellor was able to use NVC herself, to connect and empathise with Peter's expressed feelings of loss, rejection, shock and anger; to help him recognise needs; and to frame possible requests to himself as well as others. At the same time she used APM-A to guide the direction and pace of their exploring. APM-A also helped her to stay connected, by giving her a framework of understanding that helped her to keep her energy and attention free to concentrate on Peter's feelings and needs.

Peter spoke of how Jill had 'made' him 'frustrated and angry'. As part of translating his notion that anyone can actually 'make' anyone feel anything, the counsellor asked Peter when it was that he used to 'experience this frustration and anger':

Peter: When she whinged and moaned about not getting out during the day. I used to say to her, 'If you had learned to drive your life wouldn't be like this'.

Counsellor: (*translating what he said from evaluation into observation, feelings, and needs, and checking her understanding*) When Jill said how unhappy she was, because she wanted to go out more often, were you feeling frustrated and angry because you would have liked her to take her own initiative to do that?

Peter: Yes, something like that.

Peter guessed that Jill had felt lonely and bored at home, and by the end of the session he realised that maybe she also wanted him to hear her feelings and needs and have empathy from him. They explored how he might still be able to try and connect with her feelings when he picked up the children at the weekends. Peter also thought through and rehearsed a possible request, taking care to make it clear and specific: 'Would you be willing to come with me on Saturday morning to a driving school to explore the possibility of your learning to drive?'.

He described Jill as lazy, passive and lethargic, and gave the example of wanting to clear the kitchen, and finding the dishwasher full, when he would say, 'Oh Christ, the dishwasher's still loaded!' The counsellor helped Peter to translate his view of Jill into language that expressed his own

A husband's violence
cont'd

feelings and needs, before framing an observation (rather than an exclamation) that he might have used to start talking about wanting the dishwasher emptied. Peter came up with: 'When I go into the kitchen to clear up and see the dishwasher still full, I feel disappointed and frustrated because I need chores to be shared. Would you be willing to unload the machine each time you finish with it?'.

Peter then said that they both found parenting hard and had many arguments, especially when Jill had been suffering from postnatal depression. He said he feels ashamed now when he remembers saying,'Christ, you belong in mental hospital!'

He went on to talk of some of the differences between Jill and himself. He said: 'Whereas I am confident and outgoing and like feeling in control, with order around me, Jill has low self-esteem. She's quiet and shy, more relaxed than me, a bit scruffy, and disorganised.'

The counsellor again helped him to notice and translate his judgements of himself and Jill into observations, feelings, needs and preferences. She also reflected on how helpful it might be gradually to help Peter appreciate (via APM-A) their apparent very different natural ways of attending, perceiving, thinking and behaving that gave rise to so many other differences between them.

Peter said he now recognised that Jill's need had been for empathy, and to be heard. He could see that, had he guessed her feelings and needs until she had shown signs of relaxing, and then asked whether there was anything specific that she had wanted from him, she might have felt supported. He could also see that, had he been connected with his own feelings and needs (as opposed to analyses and judgements), these could have been expressed after Jill had been heard, and that he might have been heard compassionately too.

Third session
Peter talked about having seen his wife and having been able to express some empathy and demonstrate having at last heard some of her feelings and needs. He was also gradually needing less help in translating his 'self-jackaling' into a form that he could use as self-empathy.

Peter also realised that his needs included finding a means to communicate his remorse, and wish to change, to Jill's parents as well as to Jill. The counsellor asked him whether his intention had ever been to connect with them in a heart-felt way, and if not, what it had been. He saw that his intent in the past had been to show his disapproval, and added that he could not hide that. Peter was surprised when the counsellor said that it was not necessary for him to hide his feelings. All he needed to do was to change his intentions towards Jill's parents. If he really wanted to connect with them, it was likely that he would find himself interested in what they were feeling, needing and wanting; and if he still had negative feelings, these could be expressed, but in a different way from how he might have expressed them before.

After guessing that Jill's parents may sometimes have felt uneasy and insecure, and had needs to feel welcome in his presence, the counsellor and Peter explored what they might be feeling and needing now that they knew about his violence towards Jill. Peter thought they may feel disgusted, devastated and despondent, because they needed to know that their daughter was being cherished and was safe with her husband. He also wondered if there was anything that they might be wanting from him now.

Fourth session
This session became a turning point for Peter. The counsellor explored with Peter what triggers there had been for his violence, and a theme of feelings of humiliation emerged. As they explored his background Peter also mentioned being 'bullied' at school, that his father had been crippled with

A husband's violence
cont'd

polio, and that his mother had been 'bullied' by his father. He expressed surprise about the feelings he was experiencing as they talked, and that the bullying was still a source of huge pain and anger. In APM-A terms, this seemed to be the pain that filled him to a point of 'overflow', until he externalised bursts of undirected energy when he felt other, apparently minor, frustrations.

At school Peter had been liked by teachers, seen as bright, liked art, writing, and drama, and had stood out as different from other children. He was taunted with: 'You're gay!', and 'Gay boy, gay boy, we will give you a good kicking!', 'We will stop picking on you if you admit you're gay.', 'Say it over and over "I love men", "I hate women".' They would also shout, 'Your sister's a slag!', 'Your Dad's a spaci', and imitate his father's limp.

Peter was surprised at how clear and strong these memories were and how deeply he still felt. He had thought that he had got over it all and put it behind him. Now he realised how much it still hurt and how angry he still felt:

Peter: If I saw them now . . . If I saw them now I would do real violence.

Counsellor: (*translating*) Thinking about ever seeing them again, are you feeling so much humiliation and anger that you want to show them that you can express yourself, and that you can match their strength?

The counsellor helped Peter to recognise feelings he identified as loneliness, despair, and other pains, particularly of denial of friendship and needs for acceptance. These feelings were still present as were so many apparent self-judgements: 'Why did I take it for 2 years when I was so lonely and insecure? To think I just took it!', 'If it happened now I would deal with them a good deal better. I would give them as good as I got.' The counsellor translated again and wondered how long it might be before Peter might see the boys' actions as expressions of their own unmet needs.

The counsellor continued to concentrate on helping Peter to move away from self-blame and helping him to learn self-empathy, as a stepping stone towards being able to turn his attention to what feelings and needs may have been active in the boys.

Fifth session
Peter arrived in a more positive mood having recognised that as a result of his painful experiences he now took bullying seriously, whereas many of his colleagues in the police force did not. He also said that he was beginning to recognise that he was 'still stuck with judging myself'. Examples included: 'I let it develop when I could have stopped it. I was weak.', 'Why did I stand there like a weak kid?', 'Why didn't I have the balls to stand up for myself?', 'I wish that I had had the skills to deal with it then.', 'I wish I could have hurt one of them.'

The counsellor expressed her appreciation of the fact that he was now recognising what he was doing, and helped him to find the feelings and needs driving his self-criticism. He gradually identified feelings of helplessness and shame, and expressed needs to see himself as strong and someone who could look after himself, to have self-respect and acceptance from others.

After practising self-empathy again, the counsellor asked him to express his feelings towards the boys in 'jackal' terms before translating them into empathy. She explained too, how, in a live situation, this part would happen as an inner process until he felt ready to be able to turn his attention outwards and towards the boys' needs.

Peter gradually began to see the possible envy, embarrassment and insecurity felt by the boys who had taunted him. He began to link the feelings to needs that could have driven them (maybe to see themselves as

A husband's violence
cont'd

clever, to see all boys as like them, to be in control, and have power) and framed some possible NVC responses.

Peter said that he could see that it might be helpful to him to go through a similar exercise with reference to some of his teachers whom he had seen as weak when they heard his complaints but did not help him.

Sixth session

Peter seemed to be making gradual changes in his habits of thinking, feeling and expression. His language contained noticeably fewer critical and self-critical words and phrases, and he sometimes stopped himself as he lapsed. He also wanted to practise his new NVC skills.

He told the counsellor how he could now appreciate the embarrassment he had triggered in Jill, on more than one occasion, but particularly when (he now recognises) his need for acceptance and approval from peers had been so high that he accepted a drunken challenge to do the 'full Monty' in a restaurant at a Christmas party.

The counsellor noticed that Peter was shifting his perceptions from seeing Jill as 'lacking' because she was different from him, to being able to see that she was a different kind of person from him, with different ways of 'coping and defending' in APM-A terms, and different needs predominating.

As well as looking forward to trying to reconnect with his wife, Peter was now looking towards connecting for the first time with her parents, and guessing their feelings and needs. He was going to risk sending a birthday card to his father-in-law, although he feared it would be thrown away. He talked of pleasure at still seeing his ring on Jill's finger and seeing her in new clothes to meet him when she collected the children. The counsellor helped him see how he could express these kinds of positive feelings directly to his wife too.

Then Peter expressed his fear that Jill would not come back and said how he was going to carry on trying to get her to come for joint counselling. The counsellor asked him whether he thought that Jill felt a need to attend counselling with him. He thought not, and remembered guessing earlier that her need was for connection. He then also realised that they actually shared this need, but experienced it in different ways.

By the end of the session he could see that he and Jill were more likely to get both sets of needs met if he focused on the intention to connect. He could also see that carrying this intention into action by keeping his attention on Jill's inner states, and demonstrating that he could listen to her, rather than focusing on his own goals (of persuading her to come to joint counselling and return home) was also necessary to getting needs met; his goals were not inner needs but strategies and 'requests' that were going to be dependent on Jill feeling connected. These requests could be expressed at a later date, but, for the present, would be disconnected from the deeper needs of either of them.

The interaction of APM-A (orientation) theory and NVC

Although NVC can be a therapeutic and transformational tool in itself, depending on many factors, in formal counselling and therapy it is the author's view that its prime use is as a fundamental and facilitating language. It can be used effectively to facilitate other interventions as well as acting as a key to identifying deep feelings and needs.

In the case illustration 'A husband's violence' (p. 92), it was used in tandem with other tools and APM-A theory (described in Ch. 1). The purpose of APM-A is to offer awareness of what is likely to be happening to the whole person – past as well as present, and in heart, mind and body – and to give insights into means of moving from disorientation to reorientation. In this example, APM-A complemented and reinforced NVC in several different ways:

- Whereas recognition of feelings is an important part of all counselling and therapy practice, both NVC and APM-A highlight the significance of linking feelings to needs.

- APM-A offered particular awareness of the client's need to understand his situation, and his need to express feelings in ways other than words, as well as his need for verbal expression.

- Focus on feelings and needs was helped by:
  — the APM-A view of the ultimate predominance of emotion over cognition
  — awareness of the interactive effects of APM-A (attention, perception, memory and arousal)
  — awareness of the effects of unfulfilled emotional needs on physiological, as well as emotional and psychological 'balance'.

- Awareness of the APM-A framework of general 'orientation needs' helped the counsellor to identify more specific needs at cognitive, social and physical levels.

- The focus of APM-A on levels and kinds of arousal, and their effects on the experience of stress and needs to externalise tension, helped the counsellor recognise physical signs of emotional pain and unmet needs, as well as give time and space to allowing externalisation when needs were high.

- Using APM-A, the counsellor was alerted to possible unconscious as well as conscious factors, so that the significance of background events and stressors were also taken into account; the counsellor was also alerted to explore triggers that raised inner tensions and feelings of treat that heightened vulnerability.

- The 'unitary model of regression' and its alternative (see Ch. 1, Figs. 1.8 and 1.9) sharpened awareness of the client's need for empathy and self-empathy before he was able to shift his focus outwards to the needs of others.

- APM-A helped to identify individual differences, beyond gender differences. The theory also alerted the counsellor to the fact that 'orientation needs' are heightened under stress. The APM-A view of fundamental needs being universal, *and* of different needs predominating in different people, also helped the counsellor to recognise an individual pattern of needs: some clustered as being likely to be 'core' and attributable to 'personality', and others that could have been heightened by trauma.

- The theoretical framework also helped to find ways of helping the client acknowledge fundamental differences in style between his partner and himself.

- As a theory of adaptation and change, APM-A also interactive with NVC to add a dimension of learning and development (Gear 1987, 1996).

■ APM-A offered a deep understanding of stress and a holistic view of its effects on individual experience and behaviour that guided the pace and direction of the counselling and shifts from disorientation to reorientation. Additionally, the process and model of NVC itself were understood at a deep level within the framework of APM-A theory. Other, more general implications of APM-A are discussed in Chapter 1 (pp. 27–28).

The qualities and uses of NVC

Usefulness

Two major aspects of the usefulness of NVC are the simplicity of the concept and its universal applicability as a fundamental language. Another aspect is its 'graininess', and the fact that it operates at a deep level, and can act as a tool of transformation.

NVC can be used in many different ways and, as a 'core language', can facilitate other interventions. It is useful even with limited skills (as in the first case illustration) and has been used as an effective tool for behavioural change and conflict resolution around the globe. As mentioned already as a core language, NVC also facilitates other kinds of intervention because the model marries easily with other tools and concepts.

Use of the model has been experienced as effective in very diverse situations (see above). The kinds of behavioural distress it has relieved range from extreme violence in war zones, to facilitating compassionate communication in many different settings, including hospitals and other medical fields and schools and colleges. It has also been used alongside other tools in counselling and therapy, in other professional practices, with families, and in organisations and business environments to improve cooperation, morale, team-work and efficiency.

Challenges and boundaries

In common with the learning of any language, to achieve fluency and transformation (i.e. breaking long-term habits of perception, thought and expression), NVC learners are likely to need regular opportunities for practice, and experienced support. Although NVC can be used effectively with very limited skills (as described in the first case illustration above), and the eventual pay-off of fluency is high (see above), communication can feel slower than we are used to at first. With support and practice, however, the use of NVC eventually speeds up the exchange of information and resources as a result of increased clarity about our own and other people's needs and requests, as well as greater clarity of expression itself.

The only other potential limitation of NVC perceived by the author arise from possible misunderstandings of its nature and purpose.

Possible misconceptions

NVC is a fundamental language that works at a deep level to enable connection between people. It can be mistakenly seen as a complete therapeutic intervention in itself, rather than what it is – a tool which can have highly therapeutic effects. Seeing NVC used as a therapeutic tool by experts who are not working in formal settings, when background experience and professional knowledge are invisible, can lead to misconceptions about outcomes attributable to NVC alone (see case study 'A violent husband', and pages 101 and 102). The power of NVC can mask needs for wide knowledge, understanding of human nature, self-awareness (especially of one's own defences) and awareness of ethical issues in therapeutic settings.

The emphasis on feelings and needs and on speaking 'from the heart', rather than 'from the head', to achieve connection via empathy, is sometimes misread (particularly in early stages of training) as placing a negative value on analysis, evaluation, thinking and social and psychological theory and knowledge in general. In fact it places a negative value on mixing these with the expression of observations, feelings, needs and requests. This kind of misconception and others might be avoided by NVC being linked to a complementary theory of human nature such as APM-A. Understanding the process and model in the context of a general understanding of mind facilitates differentiation, for example between analysis, evaluation and judgements necessary to perform tasks and roles necessary for survival, and their effects mixed up with interpersonal communication as described above.

Box 4.3 identifics some ways in which APM-A holds potential for broadening the theoretical base of NVC (in addition to points already mentioned in Box 4.1, and on pages 101 and 102).

Box 4.3
Potential for broadening the theoretical base of NVC via APM-A theory

- Clarifying the relationship between Nonviolent Communication and other aspects of thinking and expression
- Placing clear value and adopting a wider stance on the significance of the relationship between skills and understanding in helping people
- Recognition and understanding of the relationship between perception, cognition and feelings and needs
- Recognition of the roles and value of thinking and theory, while still seeing emotional needs as ultimately dominating experience and behaviour
- Recognition of the relationship between met and unmet needs, and other factors in experience and behaviour in general
- Recognition of individuality *as well as* universality of needs
- Introduction of the concept of needs relating to 'psychological survival'
- Relating biochemical and evolutionary explanations of emotion and the expression of unmet needs to psycho-sociological explanations of disaffection and violence
- While sharing with NVC dismissal of labelling and any view of people that is 'static', APM-A sees dynamic and informal analyses and assessments as important to choice of 'tools' in helping people
- The notion of 'biological alternatives'(see Ch. 1, p. 25) as a way of understanding how the same needs being met in psychologically and socially disruptive ways can be met in ways that display sensitivity to the needs of others
- Offering models in support of self-empathy (see Ch. 1, Figs. 1.8 and 1.8)

Training   Training is from authorised and certificated NVC trainers, and comprises introductory training (usually in 1 day workshops), foundation training (usually 2 days), and longer workshops lasting 5 or 7 days. International intensive training is usually 10 days long, and takes place in many different countries, mainly in Europe and America. Support from practice groups is also recommended. At the time of writing there are no formal qualifications required, nor is any particular kind of background experience needed in order to become a certified NVC trainer; current training and criteria include approximately 100 hours of training, including international intensive training, and written and oral tests. Existing certified trainers reflect experience across many helping roles and professional fields, for example medicine, other health care fields, education, theology, counselling and therapy, psychology, personal development, social work, the probation service, and backgrounds in voluntary work, community development, peace activity and mediation, among others. There is a current focus on the significance of training for trainers world-wide, and requirements for authorisation and certification are under review at the time of writing.

Further reading

Rosenberg M 1999 Nonviolent Communication: a language of compassion. Del Mar, California
Learners of NVC express appreciation of the accessibility of this recent description by Marshall Rosenberg of his process and model.

Rosenberg R, Molho P 1998 Nonviolent (empathic) Communication for health care providers. Haemophilia 4: 335—350
A recent journal article of particular interest to health care providers. The purpose of the presentation on which the paper was based was 'to offer tools to deal with feelings and restore effective, compassionate and fulfilling communication' between health care providers and patients.

Myers W 1998 Nonviolent Communication: the basics as I know and use them. Wayland Myers, California
This is a short primer and text of elementary principles of NVC written to help people understand the 'basics'. It is available from the American and European Centres for Nonviolent Communication (for addresses see resources list, below).

Freire P, Shor I 1987 A pedagogy for liberation. Bergin and Garvey, Massachusetts
Issues addressed in this book include power relationships within education, and the tensions between 'direction' and 'liberation': for example, teasing out the difference between the meaning of 'authority' that offers freedom and 'authority' as control.

The following two books are about techniques and skills that facilitate learning NVC skills:

Gendlin E 1978 Focusing. Living Skills Media Center, Portland, Oregon
A book that Carl Rogers called 'original, innovative and exciting' when it was first published. Focusing is based on research at the University of Chicago. It offers a technique that 'guides people to the deepest level of awareness' in the body where 'unresolved feelings actually exist and only on this level actually change'. The technique helps people to be in touch with feelings on a physical level.

Dass R, Gorman P 1988 How can I help? Stories and reflections on service. Alfred Knopf, New York
The authors have backgrounds in psychology and philosophy, and experience as therapists and in politics. The book considers what is common to the 'helping professions', self-help groups and voluntary service, and has a strong focus on listening to others and 'listening' to self.

Greenberg D, Jacobs M 1999 (first published 1966) How to make yourself miserable. Vintage Books, Random House, New York
A humorous approach to alerting us to the variety of kinds of negative thinking and language we use in messages we give ourselves and how we disempower ourselves and each other: valuable insights for learners of NVC.

References

Bandura A 1961 Psychotherapy as a learning process. Psychology Bulletin 56: 2

Freire P 1970 Pedagogy of the oppressed. Seabury Press, New York

Gear J 1985 Perception and the evolution of style: a unified view of human modes of learning and expression. PhD thesis, University of Hull

Gear J 1987 Attention, affect and learning. Newland Paper 13, Department of Adult Education, University of Hull

Gear J 1989 Perception and the evolution of style: a new model of mind. Routledge, London

Gear J 1996 Bringing the theories together: an integrating and integrated theory. Paper presented to the International Colloquium 'Bringing Theory to Life', Campaign for Learning, Royal Society of Arts, Westwood Hall, Leeds

Goffman E 1961 Asylums. Doubleday/Anchor, New York

Harvey O J 1962 Conceptual systems and personality organization. Harper & Row

Ibraham D 1999 Interview by telephone from Birmingham, April 30

Ignajatovic-Savic N 1995 Expecting the unexpected: a view on child development from war affected social context. Psihologija: Journal of the Serbian Psychological Association 28 (special issue): 27–47

Rosenberg M 1976 From now on. Community Psychological Consultants, St Louis, Missouri

Rosenberg M 1983 A model for nonviolent communication. New Society Publishers, Philadelphia

Rosenberg M 1999 Nonviolent communication: a language of compassion. Del Mar, California

Szasz T 1960 The myth of mental illness: foundations of a theory of personal conduct. Hoeber-Harper, New York

Witty M 1990 Life history studies of committed lives. PhD Thesis, UMI, Ann Arbor, Michigan, vol 3

Resources

Website: www.cnvc.org

Lists of books and tapes are available from the Swiss and American Centers and through the CNVC contacts below.

CNVC USA, PO Box 2662, Sherman, TX 75091, USA
Tel: +1 (903) 893-3886
Fax: +1 (903) 893-2935
Email: cnvc@compuserve.com

CNVC Switzerland, Orchidea Lodge, Postfach 232, 4418 Reigoldswil, Switzerland
Tel: 061 941 20 60
Fax: 061 941 20 79
Email: wasserfallen@access.ch

NVC in the UK

For further information about NVC, or NVC training in the UK, contact the author, Dr Jane Gear, at the time of writing Chair of the International Educational Materials Committee, member of the CNVC UK Co-ordinating Team and a certified NVC trainer.

Contact the Institute for Learning, University of Hull
Tel: 01482 346311 *or*
Tel: 01482 844330
Fax: 01482 840060
Email: j.gear@ifl.hull.ac.uk *or*
janegear@justconnect.org.uk

5

The arts therapies

Marian Liebmann

Key issues
- The four major arts therapies are: art, drama, music and dance movement therapy
- Arts therapies are used therapeutically in a diverse range of settings including mental health, learning disabilities, child and adult education and social services
- Arts therapies are considered to have particular therapeutic potential for those people who have difficulties with verbal communication
- Arts therapies involve active methods working in a holistic way both with individuals and in groups
- Research into the processes involved in arts therapies have indicated positive therapeutic impact, although little work has been conducted in terms of outcome measures

---

Overview

This chapter covers the four main arts therapies: art, drama, music and dance movement. These four therapies all have established frames of reference and recognised training courses. There are the beginnings of other forms of arts therapies, such as phototherapy and creative writing, but these are very much in their infancy and, consequently, not covered here. This chapter is also unable to cover specialist areas such as eurythmy and the work of Rudolf Steiner. The whole field is one which is changing and expanding rapidly, and there are many influential thinkers who are now saying that it is time for arts therapies to 'move from the margins to the mainstream' (Times 1998) in the healing professions. The chapter includes case illustrations from each of the four therapies described, a brief discussion of the limitations of arts therapies, and notes on training and resources.

Introduction

There has been an enormous increase in the use of the arts therapies over the last 20 years, and also a growth in the range of activity. Arts therapies are now used in a wide range of settings, including mental health, learning disabilities, education, social services, voluntary organisations, and for children in distress and physical illness. The case studies in this chapter are drawn from a variety of contexts, but represent a small part only of the wide variety of work being done.

Arts therapies are very useful as non-verbal interventions, especially (although not only) for those who find verbal communication difficult, for whatever reason. They are active methods which involve the whole person, and can be used with individuals or groups.

Arts therapists can work from a variety of theoretical viewpoints, such as psychoanalytic (e.g. Freudian, Jungian, Kleinian), or cognitive and humanistic approaches (e.g. Gestalt, brief therapy, solution-focused, personal construct psychology). Many arts therapists work in an eclectic way, selecting from different approaches, or use more than one approach, depending on the client group and the work to be done.

The evidence base for arts therapies has been gathered in a number of different ways. These include traditional outcome studies and 'new paradigm' methods which look at the process of arts therapies, integrating the subjectivity of the process into the research methods. Although the arts therapies are young disciplines, there is now a growing body of research to draw on.

History

The histories of the four arts therapies have several common themes, as well as differences linked partly to the nature of the particular therapy and partly to external events of social history. A strong influence has been the emergence of child-centred education during the first half of the 20th century. This emphasised children's self-expression and development, and began to use the arts in this way rather than for the achievement of external standards. Some arts practitioners (who have often found it difficult to make a living practising their art) also turned to teaching adults and on occasion, by chance, found themselves teaching in psychiatric hospitals. They found that their teaching developed into therapy. Although this was already taking place in the 1930s, the Second World War gave new impetus to this trend, and the arts played an important part in the search for ways of helping the many men who were physically injured or psychologically traumatised by their wartime experiences.

Some of the arts therapies developed first in the USA, and then later in the UK, which has in turn led the way in Europe. In other cases there have been parallel developments, with early establishment of some arts therapies in the Netherlands. However, they have not been simply 'transplanted', but have acquired their own histories and flavours. For example, in the USA there is a greater emphasis on the use of the arts therapies in diagnosis, and research is based on the scientific model, whereas in the UK there is more emphasis on the use of the arts therapies as a personal process, and much of the research is based on a humanistic model.

Although the arts therapies in the UK have their separate professions, they may work together with clients, and a recent conference ('Borderlands', held in Newport, Gwent, in 1997) brought all the professions together in a very fruitful way.

Another important development took place in 1997, when state registration was achieved for art therapy, music therapy and dramatherapy as part of the Council for Professions Supplementary to Medicine. This means that these professions are now officially recognised in the UK: qualified arts therapists can practise under their own standards, rather than, say, as a nursing assistant or occupational therapy helper as has sometimes been the case in the past. It also means that unqualified practitioners can no longer call themselves arts therapists. State registration has brought with it new responsibilities which the arts therapy professions have welcomed.

From their early beginnings in child-centred education and mental health, arts therapists now work in many different settings, including education, social services, probation, prisons, hospitals, day centres and hospices, to name but a few. Client groups too are very varied: they may be children, adults with learning disabilities, people with mental health needs, clients with terminal illnesses, people with eating disorders, and people addicted to alcohol or drugs or with problems of other kinds.

It is impossible here to do justice to the full history of each arts therapy, so this chapter concentrates on the UK history, without comment on developments in other parts of Europe and with only brief mentions of the history of arts therapies in the USA.

Art therapy

The roots of art therapy lie in 'child art', and started from work done by a progressive art educator in Austria, Franz Cizek, in about 1900 (Waller 1991). Cizek believed in children having 'free expression' in art, and arranged an exhibition of child art in 1908. As his ideas spread, he brought the exhibition to London in 1934–35. In England, Marion Richardson promoted the idea, and spontaneous work in children's art classes became widespread during the 1940s.

In 1922, Hans Prinzhorn published *Bildernei der Geisteskranken*, translated into English as *Artistry of the Mentally Ill* (Prinzhorn 1922), based on art produced by people living in asylums. Three psychiatrists who had emigrated to England from Nazi persecution in the 1930s were inspired to try to obtain a further collection of paintings for research. This led to the appointment of Edward Adamson as artist at the Netherne Hospital. His brief was to facilitate patients in drawing and painting without any intervention, using an open studio approach in which patients paint on their own, but in the company of others with the therapist on hand. He effectively became the first art therapist working with people suffering from mental health problems.

Meanwhile Adrian Hill was the artist who first used the term 'art therapy' in his book *Art Versus Illness* (Hill 1945). He had used his art to pass the time while convalescing from tuberculosis in 1938, and was then asked by doctors to help others, especially, later, soldiers returning from the Second World War.

Many other pioneers were involved in the early days of art therapy, often working as artists, teachers or occupational therapists. They came together to form the British Association of Art Therapists (BAAT) in 1963. In the early days there were strong links with teaching, but as more art therapists found themselves working in hospitals, BAAT looked more towards the National Health Service (NHS), achieving recognition in 1982. State registration was achieved in 1997. Therapists working in the field of visual arts form the largest group of therapists from all of the arts in the UK.

Music therapy

There is a long tradition of the use of music as a healing force (Bunt 1994, Boyce-Tillman 1996). In more modern times, one of the first known uses of music as a therapy was by the Guild of St Cecilia, founded in 1891 to play sedative music to patients in London hospitals. In the early 20th century, music was generally used in hospitals to boost morale and to entertain. In a similar way to the rise of art therapy, the needs of Second World War veterans led to musicians being employed regularly by hospitals. In the USA, the first association for music therapy was formed in 1950, and the British Society for Music Therapy started in 1958, followed by the Association of Professional Music Therapists in 1976 (music therapy in the UK differs from the other arts therapies in separating the general and professional organisations).

Juliette Alvin was one of the pioneer music therapists in the UK. Already a well-known concert cellist and teacher, she started the first music therapy course in 1968 at the Guildhall School of Music and Drama, London. She worked with children with autism and/or other learning disabilities, and the early history of music therapy has many links with special education. A second course was started by Paul Nordoff and Clive Robbins in 1974, specifically for music therapists to work with people with learning disabilities. Although music therapists now work with many other client groups, people with learning disabilities still form their largest single client group. This is in part because music therapy provides another (aural) avenue of communication for those with poorly developed verbal communication skills (Durham & Zallik 1998). Music therapy was recognised by the NHS in 1982 at the same time as art therapy, and achieved state registration in 1997.

Dramatherapy

As with music, there is a long history of theatre and drama being linked to healing processes (Jones 1996). There are records of European asylums which had their own theatres, and several 19th century asylums, such as Broadmoor, were built with theatres included. Recreational and occupational uses of drama were introduced into hospitals during the mid-20th century, again often in connection with war casualties.

Several pioneers in theatre used techniques now familiar to dramatherapy. In Russia, between 1915 and 1924, Nikolai Evreinov developed 'theatrotherapy', based on theatre as a therapy for actors and audience. Vladimir Iljine developed 'therapeutic theatre' between 1908 and 1917, based on improvisation training and scenarios for impromptu performances. Moreno developed the 'theatre of spontaneity' in Vienna in the 1920s, then had to emigrate to New York, where he created his first psychodrama theatre. This led to the inclusion of psychodrama theatres in hospitals in the early 1940s.

There were also parallel developments to the 'child art' movement in drama education. Several educators, such as Caldwell Cook and John Dewey, advocated children 'learning by doing' and using drama to express themselves and develop creativity. Peter Slade was the most famous pioneer of 'child drama' in the UK from 1930 onwards. The coming together of child drama and hospital theatre led to the beginnings of dramatherapy, with Sue Jennings as one of the prime movers in developing the Remedial Drama Group in 1962 and Marian Lindkvist founding Sesame in 1964 (British Association for Dramatherapists 1994). The British Association for Dramatherapists started in 1976, and dramatherapy achieved state registration in 1997 at the same time as art and music therapy.

Dance movement therapy

Dance was first used in psychiatry in the 1940s, and later began to be used in special education, in family work, with older people and with people with learning disabilities (Payne 1992). There was only isolated use of dance movement therapy in hospitals in the UK, until a small group of therapists began to meet in the late 1970s and early 1980s. Guest teachers from the USA were invited to join them. In America dance movement therapy was already more established, having grown there out of modern dance and 'dance for communication' developed by Marian Chace, who took her work into psychiatric hospitals (Stanton-Jones 1992). Another influence on many dance movement therapists was Rudolf Laban, who developed a system of movement notation called Laban Movement Analysis. One of the pioneers in the UK has been Helen Payne, who developed the first training course in the UK. The Association for Dance Movement Therapy was formed in 1982, and dance movement therapy is becoming more widely known, although as yet there are fewer practitioners than in other arts therapies.

The theoretical basis

This section commences with brief definitions of the different arts therapies, as described by their associations or by well-known authors.

Art therapy

Art therapy involves the use of different art media through which a patient can express and work through the issues and concerns that have brought him or her into therapy. The therapist and client are in partnership in trying to understand the art process and product of the session.

[Case & Dalley 1992]

Music therapy

The following definition is based on a synthesis of organisational definitions:

Music therapy is the use of organised sounds and music within an evolving relationship between client and therapist to support and encourage physical, social and emotional well-being.

[Bunt 1994]

Dramatherapy

Dramatherapy has as its main focus the intentional use of healing aspects of drama and theatre as the therapeutic process. It is a method of working and playing that uses action methods to facilitate creativity, imagination, learning insight and growth.

[British Association for Dramatherapists 1994]

Dance movement therapy

Dance movement therapy is the psychotherapeutic use of movement and dance through which a person can engage creatively in a process to further their emotional, cognitive, physical and social integration.

[Association for Dance Movement Therapy UK 1998]

Using all the arts therapies

All the arts therapies provide verbal and/or non-verbal means of communication that can help people to express themselves or become aware of feelings and thoughts not accessible through words – although they can of course also include words. This experience can then be used to help make changes in their behaviour and lives. All the arts therapies can be used with individuals or groups.

Often only one form of arts therapy, if any, is available in a particular setting. However, where two or more are available, it is worth thinking about the special attributes each one has to offer. Art therapy is especially good at providing a very concrete way for people to express themselves, and the durability of the products can help people to see patterns over a period of time. It is also useful for client groups for whom quiet individual time is helpful. Music therapy is especially helpful as a means of developing communication for those with poorly developed verbal communication skills. It can involve listening to, playing and creating sounds. Dramatherapy is particularly useful for enacting situations and participating actively in them. Dance movement therapy is helpful in working with 'mind and body together', and helping people become aware of how ways of moving and being can affect, and be affected by, feelings.

In those fortunate places where several arts therapies are available, it is not only possible to choose the most appropriate form, it is also possible to combine the different arts therapies. For example, in a day unit for clients with mental health problems, art therapy was used on one day to raise awareness of feelings, and the following day dramatherapy helped them to work with feelings in an active way.

The philosophical basis

History has played an important part in the development of different perspectives on arts therapy; some of these differences are common to all arts therapies.

One perennial debate is between arts therapies as activities in their own right and arts therapies as adjuncts to psychotherapy. Those who support the first point of view see the activity of engaging in the art form as the therapeutic agent of change – whether it be painting a picture, playing music, or engaging in movement or drama – and any incidental verbal activity or discussion as less important. Those who support the second point of view see the arts activity as one important part of therapy, but incomplete in itself, needing verbal discussion to make any therapeutic change. The latter group often adhere to a particular school of verbal psychotherapy, such as Freudian, Jungian or object relations, involving central use of the concept of 'transference' in the psychoanalytical field; or Gestalt, person-centred, psychosynthesis and brief therapy (to name but a few) in the field of humanistic psychology. Many arts therapists strike a balance and adopt an eclectic approach to the psychological theories they use, recognising that arts therapies can be used within a wide variety of theoretical frameworks.

There is also a more recent view expressed by some arts therapists (Bunt 1994, Jones 1996, Liebmann 1990) that arts therapies do not need to be built on other psychological theories, they have their own unique identity and can stand on their own merits.

Arts therapies need to be distinguished from arts activities. In general, arts activities have as their main aim an external product, such as a mural or a concert or play, though participants may gain great benefit from being involved. Arts therapies are concerned with the personal processes leading to learning and change – any work produced is less important than the process. There is obviously a continuum between these two stances, and it is sometimes difficult to see where an activity shades into therapy. Usually, it is the context that makes this explicit.

Central to all arts therapies is the concept of empowerment, especially for those clients disenfranchised by lack of verbal communication. With the support of a trained specialist, arts therapies can provide another world, another frame of reference, and the opportunity to be a whole person through the ability to express emotions and thoughts in a more immediate way.

Colour plates

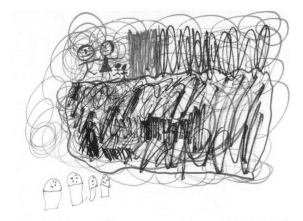

Fig. 5.1
House on fire
(Ed Kuczaj, Phoenix Trust, with permission).

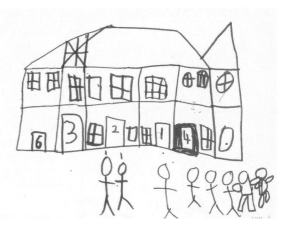

Fig. 5.2
House left intact
(Ed Kuczaj, Phoenix Trust, with permission).

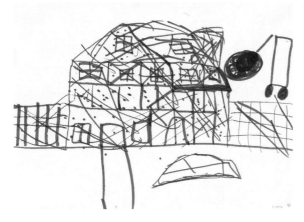

Fig. 5.3
House with demolition ball
(Ed Kuczaj, Phoenix Trust, with permission).

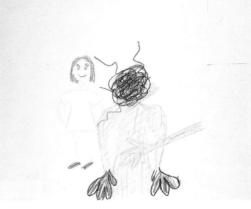
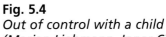

Fig. 5.4
Out of control with a child
(Marian Liebmann, Inner City Mental Health Service, United Bristol Healthcare Trust, with permission).

1

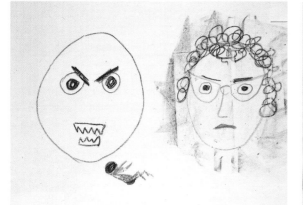

Fig. 5.5
Self and mother
(Marian Liebmann, Inner City Mental Health
Service, United Bristol Healthcare Trust, with
permission).

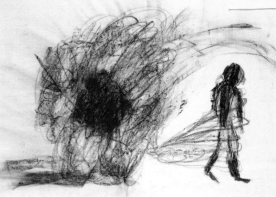

Fig. 5.6
The baggage (1)
(Marian Liebmann, Inner City Mental Health
Service, United Bristol Healthcare Trust, with
permission).

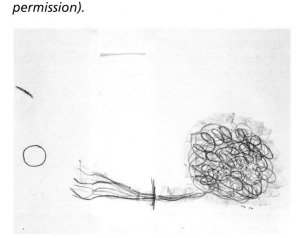

Fig. 5.7
The baggage (2)
(Marian Liebmann, Inner City Mental Health
Service, United Bristol Healthcare Trust, with
permission).

Fig. 5.8
The baggage (3)
(Marian Liebmann, Inner City Mental Health
Service, United Bristol Healthcare Trust, with
permission).

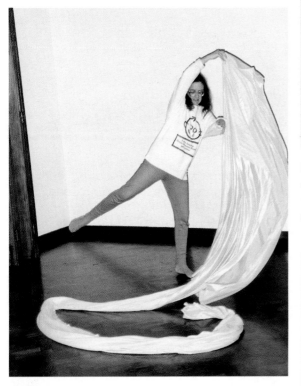

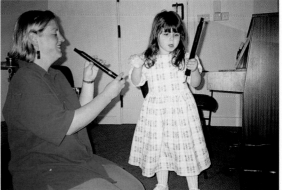

Fig. 5.10
Individual music therapy with an autistic child (Bristol MusicSpace and Michele Scott, with permission).

Fig. 5.9
Dance movement therapy: working with imagery of water – and my feelings flow (Dance Voice, with permission).

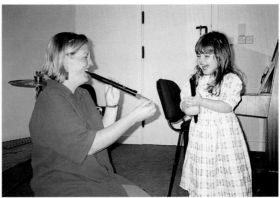

Fig. 5.11
Making communicative contact (Bristol MusicSpace and Michele Scott, with permission).

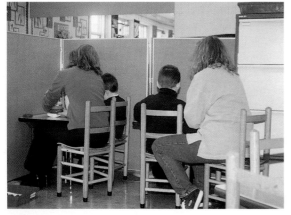

Fig. 8.1
Structure of the immediate physical environment.

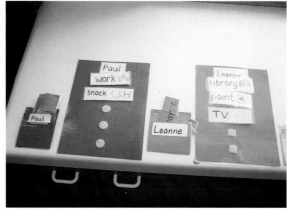

Fig. 8.2
Two individualised timetables using word and symbol prompts provide directions for the children. The child removes the prompt from the timetable and takes it to the appropriate workstation.

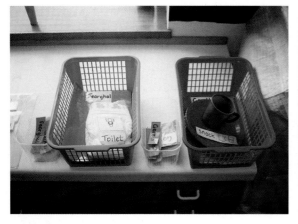

Fig. 8.3
These workboxes contain object and symbol prompts that provide direction for children.

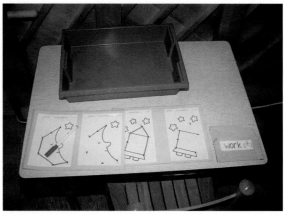

Fig. 8.4
These workboxes contain templates and jigs that may be used to assist the child complete tasks and are developments of those shown in Figure 8.3.

The evidence base

With any intervention, it is natural to ask 'Does it work?', to ascertain its efficacy before opening oneself to it (as a client) or spending scarce resources on its implementation (as a manager). There is increasing emphasis in health services on 'clinical effectiveness' (Tolley & Rowland 1995, Muir Gray 1997, Welsh Office 1995) and this is to be welcomed. Arts therapists too are keen to evaluate their work and provide the best service possible to their clients.

However, 'Does it work?' is not a simple question to answer for the arts therapies. This broad question is about as meaningless as the question 'Is conversation effective?' (Bannister 1980, p. 13). We need to ask what criteria for effectiveness we are using – and there is also the question of who selects these criteria. The arts therapies are not external pills or ointments to be applied to passive subjects by anonymous agents; they are human endeavours requiring active engagement in a subjective experience, in a relationship with a therapist.

Case illustrations as evidence

Arts therapists are used to describing their work in order to demonstrate the benefits for clients, as is shown by the case illustrations given below (pp. 115–125). Case studies are often evidence of a process that has worked, either for an individual or for a group, in particular circumstances, with a particular therapist, using a particular arts therapy, and in a particular way. Thus case illustrations can demonstrate effectiveness in a personal and subjective way – which is important for such a personal and subjective process.

Now that arts therapies are becoming better known, another general indicator of 'effectiveness' is their increasing popularity with clients. This has been demonstrated by surveys of clients' needs in some health trusts (Osborn 1998) and by waiting lists in others. Clients see arts therapies as opportunities to be treated as whole persons in a creative way, especially if they find verbal communication difficult or insufficient.

Outcome research

This is the kind of research most often used by scientists, managers, resource planners and others outside the arts therapies, who want to know which are the most effective (and cost-effective) treatments for particular disorders. However, rigorous outcome studies often require considerable resources in terms of time and money to achieve results on a large enough scale to be scientifically valid. The other difficulty is that traditional scientific method treats subjects as objects, and assumes that the researcher can investigate the situation without altering it – which is not the case. In the arts therapies these methods have also been criticised by many for being too inflexible to provide useful information, and for ignoring the important subjective process and meaning. These factors may explain why there are few outcome studies in the arts therapies.

Nevertheless, some arts therapists have undertaken outcome studies to demonstrate the effectiveness of arts therapies. Music therapy has the largest body of such knowledge. A series of studies undertaken by Leslie Bunt in 1980–81 on the effectiveness of music therapy with children used analysis of videotapes to demonstrate that music therapy helped children with no speech to develop concentration, vocalisation, communication and turn-taking. Although some of these gains could be achieved through play therapy, music therapy was particularly effective at developing vocalisation and the ability to take turns (Bunt 1994, Ch. 5). Another illustration demonstrated that music therapy was effective in encouraging participation, capturing attention and cutting down confusion during sessions (Wigram et al 1995).

Payne showed gains in children's ability to make and sustain relationships through dance movement therapy (Payne 1993b) by using a control group, rating scales and Laban Movement Analysis. Jones (1993) demonstrated the effectiveness of a dramatherapy group in decreasing stereotyped, withdrawn and solitary behaviour, while increasing responsive and self-initiated behaviour.

Gilroy (1995) explored changes in experiential art therapy groups attended by art therapy students in training. She used a mixture of quantitative and qualitative methods, including a questionnaire administered to two groups on three occasions: early in the year, at the mid-point and just after completion of the group work. The highest overall change scores were in students' self-perceptions.

The recent availability of video recording facilities to record sessions (and the use of independent observers to analyse the videotapes) has made it possible to measure more accurately behavioural changes occurring over a period of time. This is particularly helpful for music therapy, dance movement therapy and dramatherapy, where the process is timed-based and therefore very elusive. Art therapy differs from the other arts therapies in having a visible and concrete record of at least part of the process, in the pictures or sculptures made. This makes it possible to carry out research on a single case study, by reviewing all the pictures within a particular framework (e.g. Schaverien 1993). It is also possible to try to correlate particular features of paintings with other variables, although this kind of research is more common in the USA than in the UK (Gilroy & Lee 1995b, Wadeson 1980).

In Wales, arts therapists have been part of the therapy advisory team (along with chiropody, nutrition, occupational therapy, physiotherapy and speech therapy) of the Clinical Effectiveness Initiative (Wales). They have developed ways of moving towards evidenced-based practice (Welsh Office 1995), so that evaluation and research become part of their work. Their method is to form a clinical question, find evidence, appraise the evidence, apply it in practice and evaluate practice (Manners 1998).

Process research   The largest bulk of research in the arts therapies consists of systematic enquiries into aspects of arts therapy processes. These illustrations provide much useful information, usually using research methods drawn from the arts, art history, sociology or philosophy (Gilroy & Lee 1995a).

Many such pieces of research have also used 'collaborative inquiry' methods developed by Rowan, Reason and Parlett (Parlett 1981, Reason & Rowan 1981, Reason 1988). Collaborative inquiry fully acknowledges the subjective nature of arts therapies; and researchers and participants design the research process together. These methods may use questionnaires and statistics, but also make full use of journals, discussions, active participation and critical analysis by those being researched. Research in this mode does not remain fixed by the starting point, but evolves as it proceeds.

This kind of research covers a wide spectrum of topics, as the following examples show: Pavlicevic (1995) explained the distinction between musical and emotional processes in music therapy; Rees (1995) investigated clients' use of physical space in art therapy and its potential symbolic significance; Dokter (1993) used social anthropology methods to study different cultural perceptions of dramatherapy and its implications for dramatherapy training; and Meekums (1993) used 'new paradigm' methodology (involving collaborative inquiry and use of subjective evidence from participants and therapists) to investigate dance therapy as a way of working with mother–child interactions. Clearly this kind of research has contributed greatly to knowledge of the process in arts therapies, and has led to a greater understanding of what is happening and how practice can be improved.

Gathering interest from arts therapists led in 1988 to the establishment of the National Arts Therapies Research Committee, which has coordinated two conferences on arts therapies research, in 1989 and 1990. This committee has recently been reconvened and meets regularly in Birmingham. The conferences led to the publication of two collections of work: *Handbook of Inquiry in the Arts Therapies: One River, Many Currents* (Payne 1993a) and *Art and Music: Therapy and Research* (Gilroy & Lee 1995a). Two summaries of past and current research in the arts therapies have also been compiled (Payne 1993c, Kliendienst 1998). Music therapy has had its own *European Music Therapy Research Register* for several years (Rogers 1998).

Case illustrations of arts therapies in use

The case illustrations in this chapter (below) are selected from a variety of settings. Although they do not cover the whole range of uses of arts therapies, they give a flavour of the possibilities. Some of the case studies show work over a long period of time, others concentrate on just a few sessions. Both individual work and group work are described. The client groups covered include children, adolescents, adults with learning disabilities, adults with mental health problems and women survivors of childhood sexual abuse. All clients have given their permission; their names have been changed to preserve confidentiality. The case illustrations are written from the point of view of the therapist.

The art therapy pictures (Figs 5.1–5.8, see plate section, between pages 112 and 113) are all from the case illustrations described, whereas the photographs of music therapy and dance movement therapy (Figs 5.9, 5.10 and 5.11, see plate section) do not depict the clients or sessions described in this book, in order to ensure confidentiality.

When working with clients who present us with 'challenging behaviour', the primary issue for both the client and the therapist is one of control or power. The first case ('Art therapy: an adolescent with learning disabilities and challenging behaviour') illustrates the way art therapy offers clients a way to express feelings in complex and changing situations, and also how to use power and control in a positive way.

Art therapy: an adolescent with learning disabilities and challenging behaviour (Ed Kuczaj, Phoenix Trust, with permission)

Alan was a 14-year-old young man with moderate/mild learning disabilities who, along with his siblings, had been placed in care when he was aged 4, as a result of neglect and possible abuse. After various residential placements, Alan was now living in a local authority home, the least able in a mixed group of adolescents with emotional and behavioural difficulties. Concern about his behaviour revolved mainly around his targeting of younger children in an aggressive and sexual way, and his excessive cruelty to animals. The art therapist saw Alan over a period of 18 months for individual sessions.

The sessions were held in the school he attended, and because of his difficulty in forming positive relationships with adults, the therapist focused initially on forming a trusting relationship with him. At each session he offered Alan a choice of materials, ranging from paint to play materials, including play figures.

The first few sessions were taken up with boundary setting and testing. Alan found it almost impossible to stay within the boundaries of the room

Art therapy: an adolescent with learning disabilities and challenging behaviour *cont'd*

and the materials available. The room became an extension of his excited mind, and he wanted to use everything at once. His need to push boundaries led to the therapist's need to negotiate and set boundaries. Alan developed a pattern of using play figures in a story, sometimes including the therapist, and then moving on to art materials to paint or draw a picture. The sessions always ended by (joint decision) with a story read by the therapist. This final story became a cooling off period and a bridge back to the ordinary world. Formerly, there had been a number of occasions when his excitedness had spilled over into the classroom, to the dismay of his teacher!

In his play, family figures (not his family, he said), with a dominant male father figure, acted out family life. Father told the children off, becoming more and more aggressive until he finally killed them. Alan ritually destroyed the figures so many times that they literally fell apart.

Figure 5.1 (plate section) shows an image produced after several weeks. Houses with people inside had become a constant theme in his pictures, but usually, after drawing them Alan scribbled over them, so that they looked like uninhabitable ruins of houses with smashed windows and doors. Alan explained as he drew, that there were four children in the bedroom in the house, when a fire broke out downstairs. 'Will they get out?' asked the therapist. 'No', he replied, 'the fire will go along the bottom of the house and then upstairs until finally they will die.' He then drew four graves below the house. Although a fantasy on paper, the drawing contained some truth, in that when he was 4 years old and still living with his family there had indeed been a small fire in one of the children's bedrooms.

Slowly Alan became able to feel and express emotions in very small ways. He first acknowledged being unhappy or sad indirectly through the play figures. Using objects or images to represent himself gave him the control to relate to emotions closer to himself.

Gradually the sessions became less destructive to the point where (see Fig. 5.2, plate section) he was able to construct a house and leave it whole and intact.

In another similar picture (see Fig. 5.3, plate section), Alan first drew a house and then drew a crane with a huge demolition ball to the side. This then demolished the house so that no one could live inside. If he could not live in the house, then he did not want anyone else to either. This was an expression of his disappointment when his hoped-for move to another house had fallen through.

After nearly 18 months and a good deal of planning, Alan did move to a more permanent residential community, where he continued to progress. Through image making and play Alan was able to explore his world, test boundaries and create his own. He was then able to meet the therapist in the middle ground of trust and possibility, to start to gain a sense of his 'self'.

Art therapy: a client's use of drawings as metaphors
(Marian Liebmann, Inner City Mental Health Service, United Bristol Healthcare Trust, with permission)

This case illustration is an excerpt of 5 sessions work with a client (Barbara, aged 41) who was suffering from depression and also many other symptoms of behavioural distress: she shut down and went 'blank' if things became too stressful, could only concentrate for short periods of time, was unable to be near children because she felt she might damage them, and was unable to cope with any activity beyond her weekly therapy sessions. After a year's work, she felt more confident in many ways, could concentrate for the whole art therapy session, and led a fairly active life.

Session 1
Barbara drew a picture (see Fig. 5.4, plate section) of a situation when she felt out of control with a friend's child. The friend rescued her when he saw the look on her face, which spelt 'danger' (he knew her very well). The picture shows Barbara struggling to keep her hands to herself, and

Art therapy: a client's use of drawings as metaphors *cont'd*

her friend's hand on her back reassuring her. This event distressed Barbara a lot, as she felt she could not go into any situations where children were likely to be, for fear of hurting them. She was near to tears. In discussion, she felt the picture reminded her of herself and her mother.

Session 2

After looking at the previous week's picture again, Barbara drew a picture of her mother, face only (see right hand side of Fig. 5.5, plate section), with herself very small on her back, helpless (bottom left). She felt her mother always thought the worst of her, and remembered when she was small being accused (she felt unjustly) of deliberately hurting others. She ended up 'being a good girl' and fulfilling expectations of others, but found her mother still hated her, and she felt very angry about this. When Barbara finished the picture she was shaking. The therapist asked her what she could say to her mother to redress the balance and lower the fear. She could not think of anything to say, but drew another face the same size, to represent herself (upper left), with staring eyes and jagged teeth to protect herself.

Session 3

Barbara had felt very depressed and nauseous for a whole week, and said she felt as if she were dragging a huge weight behind her. She did a picture of this (see Fig. 5.6, plate section). The 'baggage' was messy, scribbly and very heavy in the centre, and was joined to Barbara by thick ropes. Once again, this seemed to represent baggage from her mother, but at least here it was separate from Barbara and a little distance away.

Session 4

Barbara had visualised her picture quite a lot during the week between sessions, but when she looked again at the actual picture, she realised her visualisation was not quite the same, so she drew it out (see Fig. 5.7, plate section). This time the tangle was smaller and lighter, and further away from Barbara. She even drew a tiny pale unthreatening figure of her mother at the top right of the picture, almost invisible apart from the black stick in her hand.

Session 5

There was a month's gap in therapy because Barbara was ill, so we reviewed the pictures from the previous weeks. Then Barbara did another picture of herself and the 'baggage', to see where she felt she had got to. She used the same colours, but the ball of 'mess' was quite small now, and the space between it and her had lengthened considerably (see Fig. 5.8, plate section). Also, bits of Barbara's internal 'mess' could be taken off and dealt with in small manageable chunks along the way. Barbara portrayed herself (right hand side) as a channel which could process this 'stuff' and then be rid of it.

Barbara also recounted a small moment – a split second – when she realised she no longer cared what her mother thought of her. This was a very freeing thought, experienced for the first time in her life, and brought with it a feeling of a whole fresh perception of the universe. She was with a good friend at the time, and found herself laughing out loud. She described it as her 'Walt Disney moment' which kept her going through her 3 weeks of illness.

This sequence shows how pictures can use metaphors to describe situations – in this case a piece of heavy baggage attached by ropes – and then work can be done with the metaphor itself to mirror an inner process of change.

Dramatherapy: group work with a woman with learning disabilities
(Rachel Matthews, with permission)

Linda was part of a small dramatherapy group for people with learning disabilities. She was referred for therapy because she was seen as being very volatile, often angry, sometimes distressed, and abusive at her day centre. It was hoped that dramatherapy could help Linda to be calmer, improve her communication skills, and help her develop more satisfying relationships with others.

In the group, Linda found it very hard to allow time and space for other people. Arriving late, she interrupted whatever was going on. She needed to tell the story of something which had distressed her, either an incident she had been involved in, or a news item.

Linda found it difficult to join in with the active parts of the group, although when she did, she used the theatre process well. When the group was doing warm-up exercises or dramatic activities, she sat out until she was clear what the activity was. In improvisations or role play, she waited and then came in midway. Invariably, her character – however it had been set up – was angry and intransigent.

On one occasion two members of the group were being small babies, rolling on the floor, making some contact with each other, alternating between laughing and crying. When one of the babies started to cry, Linda came rushing in, shouting at the baby to stop crying, and miming hitting her as well.

As the group progressed, it became apparent that Linda was mirroring her home life, where she was consistently put down, verbally abused, and blamed and punished inappropriately. It seemed that her family was almost perpetually shouting at her, and at each other. She was not encouraged to do things which were well within her capabilities.

Linda appeared confident and assertive in most of her social interactions, because she was demanding, articulate and tended to dominate others. In the group, through the use of character, improvisation, developed story work and role play, Linda began to show her extremely vulnerable and wounded interior. Her self-esteem was extremely low, she had no confidence in her own abilities, and had enormous fears about abandonment, people's opinions of her (which she saw as universally bad) and punishment. She shared parts of her history which showed how some of those feelings and responses had evolved.

Over a period of $2\frac{1}{2}$ years, Linda was able to make changes within the group, as her patterns and behaviour were reflected back to her, and through her deepening relationships with other group members. However, the therapist did not think this change had translated into any change outside the group. The group had acted in a diagnostic way for Linda, showing where her needs were.

Substantial change in Linda's emotional well-being and behaviour could only be achieved if her home circumstances changed. However, Linda was not willing to even consider leaving home – she was afraid of the ramifications if she even raised the subject there.

At the day centre, staff were encouraged to treat her with more compassion, to realise that she was vulnerable, and not the resilient, feisty woman that she appeared to be, and to keep the subject of leaving home alive. This cut through the vicious circle of transference and counter-transference, where Linda replicated her home situation with the clients and staff in the day centre.

Further therapy was not recommended as it would be totally outweighed by her home situation; it could even be damaging, touching on painful material which could not be effectively worked on without a more supportive environment.

Linda's case history reflects a common problem in therapeutic work in the public sector, especially with clients with learning disabilities. Clients behave in a way which causes problems for their support services, and

Dramatherapy: group work with a woman with learning disabilities *cont'd*

Dramatherapy: group for women survivors of childhood sexual abuse (Cass Moggridge, with permission)

therapy is seen as a way of changing the clients' behaviour. In therapy, it becomes clear that the behaviour is an adaptive response to circumstances, and it may be that the environment, or the way in which the client is treated, needs to change. Then there may be an opportunity for therapeutic work to address the emotional issues which lie behind the problematic behaviour.

Dramatherapy in groups can be very powerful. The aim of the group in this case study was to enable clients to 'move on' from their time-limited 10 sessions of individual counselling by sharing their experiences within a group of women with similar difficulties. The dramatherapy group ran for 10 sessions with 10 clients, and this account follows the experience of one member, Belinda.

The activity was based on the story 'The Woman from the Stars' (in Gersie 1991), chosen for the beauty of its imagery and the relevance of its themes. It was read out at each session, usually towards the end (except for the first session), so that members could distance themselves from their painful feelings by focusing on the story before leaving the group.

The story
A farmer worries that milk from his cows is being stolen at night. He watches. Young women climb down a cord from the stars. All but one return. She has a beautiful basket. She tells the farmer not to look inside without her permission. He agrees. She lives with him. One day he breaks his promise. He laughs, saying, 'There is nothing inside!' The woman leaves.

Session 1
Belinda admired the woman's decision to leave. If she had been in the same situation, she would have worried about leaving the cows and whether the farmer could manage without her. She related how, as a child, she had cooked for her family at home, and said her mother could not have managed without her. She added that she now wanted to learn to care for herself rather than look after others.

Session 2
Group members had been asked to bring something that gave them comfort, but Belinda did not bring anything. She was interested in what other people had brought.

Session 3
This session started with the opportunity to draw feelings on pieces of paper. Belinda drew large swirls of black (her despair) with red swirls on top (her bubbling rage). She felt angry with the farmer for not being trustworthy, but when other women spoke of their rage towards their abusers, Belinda said her rage was with herself.

Session 4
Each person was asked to make a statement starting 'I trust myself to . . .'. Belinda said she could trust herself to muck things up. Finally, with help from the group, she said she could trust herself to keep going. The positive response from the group touched her.

Session 5
Belinda said she felt like a basket into which everyone chucked their rubbish. Someone suggested she was also the kind of basket that held things safely. Belinda realised that both these aspects were true.

Dramatherapy: group for women survivors of childhood sexual abuse *cont'd*

Session 6
Belinda did not attend this session.

Session 7
Several members of the group wanted to vent their rage. As part of this, Belinda decided to build her 'pile of shit'. She piled books, cushions and chairs, giving a name to each object as she told the story of her abuse. She sat down, exhausted. Suddenly, someone else kicked the pile over, saying it represented her wall of secrecy that she had to knock down. A stunned silence followed. There was concern for Belinda seeing her work demolished, but she (predictably) only showed concern for the other person. The ensuing discussion focused on the difference between privacy and secrecy.

Session 8
Following on from the previous week's session, Belinda reported that she had never before seen her abuse as a whole. Later the group returned to the story and wondered whether the woman took her basket with her. Belinda thought she·did.

Session 9
The group challenged Belinda for telling other members they were not responsible for their abuse, while continuing to blame herself.

Session 10
This was the final session, in which members were asked to reflect on what they had gained from the group. Belinda said she had been weighed down by 'baggage' when she joined the group, but had become so used to it that she had ceased to notice it. Now she wanted to attend to it properly, and said she wanted to get further counselling for herself.

This case illustrates how the dramatherapy group helped Belinda to include herself in the sensitive caring she had previously only offered to others. The group also helped her to shift her perception of herself from unlovable to lovable.

Dance movement therapy: a man with depression and alcohol dependency
(from the work of Marie Ware, Dance Voice, with permission)

Dance Voice runs a weekly session at the local psychiatric hospital, reminding all the wards just beforehand, so that new in-patients can take part if they want. On this occasion, Philip, in his early 30s, suffering from depression and recovering from alcohol addiction, came over very tentatively to the room where the session was held. He felt very low, and came in and sat down near the door in a slumped posture. The therapist welcomed him and said it was fine for him to take part or just to be there.

Five other people had also arrived from different wards. One of them chose some music and the group warmed up with some coloured streamers, making light-hearted movements. To his own surprise, Philip joined in and did not sit down again for the rest of the session. Someone else was choosing two lengths of silver-grey fabric for the next activity, when Philip remembered he had not taken his medication. He dashed back to the ward to do this and returned within 5 minutes.

By this time the group was using a multicoloured parachute, lifting it up and down with a lot of energy, over one member lying on the floor. Soon Philip asked for a turn. Next, people took it in turns to lie on the parachute while the rest of the group made waves from the rest of the material. Philip enjoyed the feel of this, as he lay on his back with gentle waves, rough waves and big waves washing over him – he said it felt cool and refreshing, and very good. Each person gave a signal when they wanted the group to stop, and Philip said later that having this control

Dance movement therapy: a man with depression and alcohol dependency *cont'd*

over the experience was also something new for him, which had helped him to enjoy it.

In another exercise, members of the group were asked to stretch up, as if reaching for an imaginary £10 note floating above their heads, then let their arms relax, and feel the resultant posture. 'This posture – you can feel really confident, can't you?' Philip commented.

The movement part of the session always ended with a foot or hand massage. Philip asked for a foot massage, which he directed, and for an additional forehead massage because he felt so tense. Again, it meant a lot to him that he was in control of the massage.

The whole session finished with a cup of tea and discussion. Philip spoke about having always had to look after other people, so that he felt guilty about nurturing himself. He had formerly used drugs to avoid dealing with issues and more recently had turned to alcohol. He found social contact difficult and often isolated himself.

Philip was only an in-patient for 1 week, so this was the only session he attended. However, he was able to experience how he could change his feelings and lack of self-care, just by using his own body in a different posture and by feeling in control of this. He began to see other strategies for dealing with his problems and for living his life.

Dance movement therapy: young woman with learning disabilities
(Marie Ware at Dance Voice, with permission)

Lucy was a young woman of 27 with learning disabilities, who went into residential care because her parents could no longer cope with the challenges she presented. She ran around all the time, never stopping, even to eat or drink. At home she grabbed food on the run, then threw it away as soon as she had tasted it. Dance Voice already worked with several others in Lucy's residential home and agreed to include her in the sessions, held three times a week.

For much of this work, a ratio of one-to-one help is needed, so in this group the therapist worked with several assistants. At first they just observed Lucy and allowed her to be there in her own way. They noticed that her pattern was to engage with others by pushing them, then withdrawing and circling round the room, looking over her shoulder and making eye contact. To show that they approved of her, the therapist and the helpers all gave her the 'thumbs up' sign whenever she made eye contact.

Then the therapist started to initiate new patterns of behaviour very gradually. As Lucy became aware of other people's stillness, her pace began to slow down. Exercises using people to model different spatial patterns gave Lucy a greater sense of her own body, the space surrounding her and the greater variety of movements she could make. To give her the idea of sitting on a chair, the therapist did not expect Lucy to come to the chair, but took the chair to Lucy. Gradually she learned to sit on a chair, sit on the floor, stand quietly and pause, and to stand on a series of boxes as they gradually became higher. One week she actually sat on a vaulting box, lay down on it (showing great trust) and allowed herself to do a backwards somersault with the therapist's help. She was very surprised and smiled at her achievement.

After 4 months, Lucy was able to be still and watch others, and could be approached by others without running off. She was able to stay for whole sessions without being disruptive, and sat down to eat her meals. She was less jerky and 'puppet-like' in her movements, and seemed able to cope better with many situations.

Figure 5.9 (see plate section) shows a different example of dance movement therapy – working with the imagery of water, and allowing feelings to flow.

Music therapy: a child with autism
(Cathy Durham, with permission)

Joe was a child of 8 who had autism and epilepsy, which affected his concentration quite severely. He was a very anxious child who constantly asked what was happening next. He became fearful several times a minute, even in familiar situations; if he was not reassured that 'x' will happen next' within a few seconds, he would start screaming and throwing objects.

Joe started school in an autistic unit attached to a mainstream primary school when he was 8. He was referred to individual music therapy by his teacher, who felt that music therapy might offer him a focus for his attention and an outlet for creative expression. Although Joe was able to talk in simple sentences, his speech was often muddled, and he referred to himself as 'him' or 'Joe' instead of 'me'. He rarely interacted with other children, but would talk to the member of staff who worked with him. As Joe was demanding, and often violent, no member of staff was able to work with him for more than half a morning.

Early sessions

During his assessment for music therapy, which took place over a 4-week period, the therapist worked non-directively with him, allowing him time and space to explore the room and to play instruments. At first Joe was unable to stay in the room for more than 5 or 6 minutes at a time. He also found ways of testing boundaries so strongly that the therapist found it was she who was stopping sessions.

In the initial session, Joe sat and played a drum with a regular pulse with one beater for about 6 seconds. The therapist joined him by playing guitar chords at the same speed and singing his name. Immediately he stopped and began turning light switches near him on and off, looking at the therapist to gauge her reaction. Next, he banged on the radiator and after the therapist quietly asked him to stop, he picked up a drum and tried to throw it through a plate glass window. At this point the therapist stopped the session.

The second and third sessions were just as traumatic: Joe flung wooden bars of a xylophone about; he constantly asked to go to the toilet; finally he urinated on the drum and the therapist had to disinfect it. She decided to change her approach.

Several children with autistim on the unit had responded well to a non-directive approach. They found the space to explore instruments in their own way, without intervention from an adult, quite liberating, and became increasingly keen to attend sessions. When the children felt safe, they would ask the therapist to join their activities. Another way of making a connection with the children was vocally. The therapist would sing about what they were doing, or imitate and respond to their own vocalisations. In this way, non-verbal and more expressive communication began to develop.

However, this approach clearly did not suit Joe. He needed a way of helping focus his attention every few seconds, and a way of being contained, so the therapist enlisted the help of a classroom assistant, who sat next to him in subsequent sessions, saying little, but stroking his arm as soon as he became anxious, and pointing back to instruments when he lost his focus of attention. She needed to do this several times a minute at first. (It transpired that this support for Joe was also necessary in almost all activities in the classroom.) The therapist removed all instruments from the room except the guitar, sat in front of Joe and held it for him to play. He smiled, reached out and played one strum, then immediately frowned and asked in a high, anxious voice 'When can I go to the toilet?' The therapist said that once he had finished playing the guitar, he would be going. The assistant pointed to the guitar and he strummed once again. The therapist then began singing a highly structured song, with his name at the end of every phrase. She asked him to sing his name together with her each time.

Music therapy: a child with autism *cont'd*

He managed once every four lines, and there were frequent interjections in his high voice, asking to go to the toilet. After 5 minutes, the therapist sang a goodbye song, again with his name mentioned frequently in it, always at the end of the phrase.

The following week, he sang his name at the end of each phrase. All the therapist needed to do was to leave a gap, and the beginning of each phrase acted as a cue for him. This session again lasted 5 minutes, and had a 'hello' and 'goodbye' song in it.

The next week, he managed to strum fairly constantly throughout the song, and also sang verses for the therapist and assistant when gaps were left. Sometimes he muddled the names, but he consistently used the musical cue to sing in the predictable place. He still needed reminders to re-focus on the guitar but these were needed slightly less frequently than before.

Later sessions

As the weeks passed, Joe was able to stay in the sessions for longer periods of time (between 20 and 25 minutes) before he asked for the 'goodbye' song; and it became rare that his anxiety escalated to the point where he had to leave.

After 15 sessions, Joe was singing full lines of the songs and only needed re-focusing about three times a session. (This compared to Session 4, when he had needed re-focusing about 30 times.) He also began to explore playing instruments in different ways, such as running the beaters back and forth across the xylophone bars, rather than hitting them with a very fixed and rigid beating pattern, as he had done previously. He began to smile when producing different sounds, and started looking at the therapist to share his experience. The therapist's music continued to be extremely structured and predictable, 'holding' him, but his playing began to develop some promise of creativity. As he lost interest in one instrument, he would say 'finished' and hand it back to the therapist, who then offered him a different choice from two others. In order to help him learn the names of the instruments, and to focus on tasks, one of the songs involved repetitions of the line 'Joe is playing the *drum*', or whatever instrument he had chosen.

After a further 10 sessions, he was remembering names of instruments, and asking for them before they were offered. In this way he developed control over the course of the session in a positive way, rather than influencing the session only by forcing it to end.

Group work

Joe also attended a small music therapy group which met weekly. This consisted of himself and two other children who were non-verbal and autistic. The purpose of the group setting was to encourage all three children to develop awareness of each other's music, and to develop their listening and waiting skills. There was also the possibility of using non-verbal creative expression from vocalising and playing instruments.

In order to 'contain' Joe within the group, his adult support continued. His assistant was particularly helpful in the greeting song, when it was not his turn to perform. Joe was able to choose by name each person's turn, but only concentrated when it was his turn. The turns were kept very short, and always travelled around the group in the same direction, so that each child began to be able to predict his or her own turn. Joe participated very vigorously when everyone played together in the group, seemingly conscious of a strong beat, and able to join it. He began to set the pulse for different group improvisations. As he was beginning to explore and notice different ways of making sounds on the same instrument, he began to develop this in the group and began to smile frequently when this was happening.

Joe's progress was not always smooth, and sometimes he became too anxious to continue a particular session. In fact, the ease he developed in the group setting only became apparent when one of the other children in

Music therapy: a child with autism *cont'd*

the group began hitting others at the end of his turn. The therapist realised that Joe was no longer the child that demanded most support and constant attention. As he settled, another child seemed to take over his former role.

Joe came more and more eagerly to the sessions, and started improvising on the slide whistle, drum or xylophone for up to 4 minutes at a time. He was also singing the full lines of songs, and was able to stay for a 30-minute group session. His behaviour had settled in class over the year, and this was partly due to the consistent and structured approach of the school. Joe's mother and the school staff also acknowledged the role music therapy had played in helping Joe reduce his anxiety and begin to develop his self-confidence in a positive way.

Music therapy: man with learning disabilities
(Cathy Durham, with permission)

Frank was a man in his 50s who had spent most of his adolescent and adult life in institutions, and was now living in a shared home with live-in carers. Frank had a profound learning disability, no verbal language, and seemed reluctant or unable to communicate with anyone around him. His behaviour involved frequent and severe self-injury, including a tendency to hit his face and head very hard with his fists. Unless distracted, this hitting could continue for several hours at a time. Frank's disfigured face showed the effects of these injuries. He had two 'cauliflower ears', extremely pronounced cheekbones and permanent scabs on his cheeks. It was even thought possible that years of self-harm had also resulted in brain damage. Frank's episodes of self-harm resulted in bleeding, and were wearing and distressing, for both him and his carers. This sometimes warranted physical interventions.

Frank was referred to music therapy by his dedicated case coordinator, to see if Frank could find a more positive way of channelling his energy, and also to develop his communication with others. The team of carers was very keen to find any intervention which might reduce his self-harming.

Early sessions
When the therapist first met him, Frank hummed and rocked from foot to foot. He avoided eye contact, and moved quickly away when the therapist moved slowly towards him. She was hoping to encourage him to walk with her across the grass to the room where the music therapy session was to take place. It actually took three meetings before he would go with her to the music therapy room. However, in these first sessions, he began to approach her and ask for things. For example, he took her hand and led her to the kitchen, clearly wanting a drink. She hummed gently with him, at a similar pitch, when walking somewhere, allowing him to lead. His humming intensified in volume when she did this. He always vocalised on one note. The therapist began to start on this note, and then raise the pitch suddenly in quite a dramatic way. At this point Frank looked up at her, and for the first time, smiled. She then joined him again on his note. A few seconds later she tried singing the change in pitch, and again he looked at her curiously. In the third session he tried to raise the pitch himself. He looked at the therapist, smiled, and then moved away.

By this time, the therapist felt that Frank trusted her enough for her to lead him to the music therapy room. He took some time to come in the same direction with her, and stopped when they reached the room. Then he turned back and walked away from her, showing no more interest in further contact.

The following week, he came into the room and sat in a chair, twiddling a bright red plastic skittle he had been carrying. He did not look at any instruments, but rocked backwards and forwards in the chair in time to heavily rhythmic music played by the therapist on the piano or guitar. He was reluctant to leave at the end of the session, even after the therapist had packed away all the instruments as a clear indicator that it was time to finish.

Further sessions

Frank continued to spend most of his contact each week testing out whether the therapist was going to listen to him, before allowing himself to be led to the room. There he responded vigorously to any rhythmic aspect of music played by the therapist, with strong rhythmical and unvarying movements on the guitar and the metallophone (a xylophone with metal bars). He vocalised on different pitches according to the key of the music. Sometimes he spontaneously stood up to dance, rocking from foot to foot in time to a slow musical beat. During these experiences, he showed more awareness of the therapist and evidence of being engaged in the music.

The most significant aspect of the sessions seemed to be the fact that he was slowly gaining some sense of being able to influence the music. At first, the therapist would improvise music to start him rocking. If he stopped, then she would stop the music. In the sixth session he began to start rocking again, then laughed when the therapist joined him musically, and immediately stopped rocking, looking at her. Then he very slowly began to start the rocking again. He had grasped that he was responsible for starting and stopping an experience he really enjoyed. This felt an important moment in the therapy. The therapist wondered how much control he felt he had over the rest of his life.

Frank's responses to new events were always very delayed. However, if given time to respond, Frank could do so. For example, if the therapist speeded up the tempo of her playing suddenly, he stopped rocking, as if he had lost the connection. But if she increased the tempo gradually, he was able to follow it and stay with the beat. He even began to increase the speed of rocking himself, thereby initiating change himself.

Frank never showed any sign of self-injury in the sessions, although occasionally he began to circle his cheeks with his fingers, a sign that the 'boxing' was about to begin. It was always possible to engage him musically in some way so that he stopped doing this. The therapist began to suspect a link between the circling of his cheeks with times in the sessions when he seemed less engaged. This information was useful to his carers, who then tried distracting Frank when it looked as if he was about to self-injure. They also saw the need to wait for Frank's very slow reactions, and to provide meaningful stimulation for him.

This did not eliminate all of Frank's self-injury, but provided some positive ways forward, and also increased his confidence to initiate more communicative contact with others. After a year of music therapy, the therapist worked towards handing over some of the musical experiences she and Frank had shared to others, and helping his carer to understand the basic principles related to Frank's needs.

Figures 5.10 and 5.11 (see plate section) show a different example of individual music therapy, this time with a child with autistic spectrum disorder.

Limitations
Client group

There are no real limitations for arts therapies in this area, as arts therapies have something to offer all client groups, from those with no verbal communication skills to those with excellent verbal skills. However, their greatest contribution may be to those with least verbal communication.

Nevertheless, all clients need to be in the 'right space at the right time' to make the best use of arts therapies (or any therapy) for personal change. So, for instance, clients who are in such a chaotic state that they cannot turn up regularly may not be able to benefit very much. Clients may also have particular things on their minds, such as a family crisis or an impending move, which make it difficult to concentrate on anything else. Clients with severe alcohol or drug problems, or who are on high doses of medication, may not be able to get in touch with any of their feelings. It may be better to wait until such clients are more settled and both able and willing to engage in the arts therapy properly. There are situations, of course, where irregular attendance is part of the client's situation – such as being homeless or a refugee – in which case supportive art therapy can be offered, without expectation of great personal changes.

It goes without saying that clients must be willing to try arts therapies; they cannot be forced. However, no previous experience or skill is needed. Some clients are mistakenly referred to arts therapies when they are looking for arts activities (see above, p. 112). Arts therapists need to explain the difference to them (and to referrers!) and refer clients on to facilities more suited to their needs.

Training and supervision

In the USA and the UK, most arts therapists now start from a basis of a degree in their own art form, and each arts therapy has its own profession and route to qualification; there are several training courses for each profession in the UK, all at postgraduate level (see also resources at the end of the chapter). This contrasts with several countries in Europe, where arts therapists often start by being qualified psychologists or psychiatrists. In several European countries, arts therapists train and practise in all the expressive arts; although there are such courses in the UK, they are not qualifying courses for practising as arts therapists.

All arts therapists undertake postgraduate training in their profession. This includes theory and practice of their particular arts therapy, as well as methods of working with individuals and groups. Therapists should also have regular supervision. In 1997 art, music and dramatherapy achieved state registration, which means that unregistered practitioners cannot call themselves arts therapists.

Physical requirements

Arts therapies require suitable space, equipment and materials. For art therapy, a plentiful supply of good art materials is needed, as well as a room with good daylight. For group art therapy, a separate area with tables for painting and a more comfortable area for discussion are useful (although not essential). Dramatherapy needs a large room, preferably with a carpet, without too much furniture (and with furniture that can be easily moved) and where it is possible to make some noise without disturbing others. Music therapy also needs a room where noise can be made, a variety of good quality musical instruments – often including a piano – and space to play them. Dance therapy needs a large space, either carpeted or with a good quality wooden floor where people can work barefoot and, usually, a cassette recorder to play music.

All these spaces need to be free from interruptions. Arts therapists often have to explain this to other staff, who may see nothing wrong in bringing in messages or requests, or who may use the room as a through-route to another room. Sadly, arts therapists often find themselves working in less than ideal conditions, then have to tailor their work to take this into account. Often this means not attempting any work in depth if it is likely to be disrupted.

Emotional safety

Arts therapies can be very powerful, and can 'open a floodgate' so that clients feel overwhelmed and unable to cope with normal life. It is vital to create safe boundaries and to pay attention to beginnings and endings. In particular, it is important to allow clients adequate time to finish off in a session so that they leave in a fit state to go about their normal lives. Similarly, a series of sessions needs to be rounded off and integrated into clients' lives.

It is important for clients to be able to make their own interpretations, and change and develop in their own ways. For this reason, arts therapists are trained to be flexible, to listen well and to be non-judgemental. Regular reviews with clients can help to check that clients are happy with the therapy, and allow adjustments to be made.

Conclusion

This chapter has given a flavour of the four established arts therapies – art therapy, music therapy, dramatherapy and dance movement therapy – and how they may be applied in different settings. Only a fraction of the possibilities have been glimpsed here, but perhaps enough to help readers find their way to the next stage of exploration.

Arts therapies have demonstrated their benefits for many client groups. With the growing number of applications to different fields of work, the small but increasing body of research providing evidence of effectiveness and their popularity with clients, arts therapies provide an exciting and stimulating whole-person way forward for many who cannot benefit from other therapies.

Note for parents and helpers

Parents and helpers will want to use whatever activities will benefit the children or adults in their care. The arts are natural forms of communication, so many people can help others enjoy using paint, musical instruments, movement and drama. This is not the same as using arts therapies to work with clients' problems and difficulties – which is the work of trained arts therapists. However, there may be occasions, as in one of the music therapy examples described above, where parents and helpers can work with clients under the guidance of a trained arts therapist.

Further reading

Art therapy
Case C, Dalley T 1992 The handbook of art therapy. Tavistock/Routledge, London
An introduction to the theory and practice of art therapy in different work settings from a psychoanalytical point of view, with a variety of examples from individual and group work.

Liebmann M (ed) 1990 Art therapy in practice. Jessica Kingsley, London
An edited compilation of accounts of art therapy with different client groups, from authors based in one geographical area, explaining how art therapy works in each setting.

Rees M (ed) 1998 Drawing on difference: art therapy with people who have learning difficulties. Routledge, London
Collection of chapters covering art therapy work with children and adults with learning difficulties. Also covers links with music therapy and dramatherapy, clinical effectiveness and clinical supervision.

Dance movement therapy
Payne H (ed) 1992 Dance movement therapy: theory and practice. Routledge, London
An introduction to dance movement therapy, with chapters from practitioners working in different contexts.

Stanton-Jones K 1992 An introduction to dance movement therapy in psychiatry. Routledge, London
Covers different models of dance movement therapy used in a psychiatric setting, with examples.

Dramatherapy

Emunah R 1994 Acting for real: drama therapy process, technique and performance. Brunner Mazel, New York
A description of a particular approach to working with dramatherapy, with different methods of application, from an American practitioner.

Jennings S, Cattanach A, Mitchell S, Chesner A, Meldrum B 1994 The handbook of dramatherapy. Routledge, London
A series of introductory chapters on different aspects of dramatherapy, looking at areas such as the relationship between dramatherapy and psychodrama, and different models of dramatherapy.

Jones P 1996 Drama as therapy: theatre as living. Routledge, London
An overview of the core processes in dramatherapy, illustrated with a wide variety of case material and analysis of techniques.

Music therapy

Bunt L 1994 Music therapy: an art beyond words. Routledge, London
A general introduction to music therapy, covering the history, different ways of working, and research, illustrated with case studies.

Nordoff P, Robbins C 1992 Therapy in music for handicapped children. Gollancz, London
Description of the pioneering approaches of Paul Nordoff and Clive Robbins, including case discussions and photographs of music therapy in process.

Priestley M 1994 Essays on analytic music therapy. Barcelona Publishers, Phoenixville, PA
Collection of papers exploring specific analytic techniques in relation to music therapy, with case examples from a variety of client groups.

Research

Gilroy A, Lee C (eds) 1995 Art and music: therapy and research. Routledge, London
Compendium of writings on research in art therapy and music therapy, with sections on the practice of research, examples of clinical research using different research methodologies and on the importance of context and culture.

Payne H (ed) 1993 Handbook of inquiry in the arts therapies: one river, many currents. Jessica Kingsley, London
The first British book on arts therapies research, covering general questions concerning research methods, followed by separate sections on research in art therapy, dance movement therapy, dramatherapy and music therapy. Also contains the first directory of arts therapies research.

Wigram T, West R, Saperston B 1995 The art and science of music therapy: a handbook. Harwood Academic Publishers, Switzerland
Covers recent research, evaluation and literature in this field.

Evidence-based practice

Muir Gray J A 1997 Evidence-based healthcare: how to make health policy and management decisions. Churchill Livingstone, Edinburgh
General text on 'doing the right things right', including skills for individuals and organisational perspectives.

Tolley K, Rowland N 1995 Evaluating the cost-effectiveness of counselling in healthcare. Routledge, London
An example of how data can be collected and applied to gather evidence in a form that is as accessible, accurate and relevant as possible.

References

Association for Dance Movement Therapy UK 1998 General information leaflet. Association for Dance Movement Therapy UK, London

Bannister D 1980 The nonsense of effectiveness. New Forum Journal of the Psychology and Psychotherapy Association (August)

Boyce-Tillman J 1996 Getting our acts together. In: Liebmann M (ed) Arts approaches to conflict. Jessica Kingsley, London

British Association for Dramatherapists 1994 Information Pack. British Association for Dramatherapists, Swanage, Dorset

Bunt L 1994 Music therapy: an art beyond words. Routledge, London

Case C, Dalley T 1992 The handbook of art therapy. Tavistock/Routledge, London

Dokter D 1993 Dramatherapy across Europe: cultural contradictions: an inquiry into the parameters of British training and practice. In: Payne H (ed) Handbook of inquiry in the arts therapies: one river, many currents. Jessica Kingsley, London

Durham C, Zallik S 1998 Interviews with author, January, Bristol

Gersie A 1991 Storymaking in bereavement: dragons fight in the meadow. Jessica Kingsley, London

Gilroy A 1995 Change in art therapy groups. In: Gilroy A, Lee C (eds) Art and music: therapy and research. Routledge, London

Gilroy A, Lee C (eds) 1995a Art and music: therapy and research. Routledge, London

Gilroy A, Lee C 1995b Introduction: juxtapositions in art therapy and music therapy research. In: Gilroy A, Lee C (eds) Art and music: therapy and research. Routledge, London

Hill A 1945 Art versus illness. Allen and Unwin, London

Jones P 1993 The active witness: the acquisition of meaning in dramatherapy. In: Payne H (ed) Handbook of inquiry in the arts therapies: one river, many currents. Jessica Kingsley, London

Jones P 1996 Drama as therapy: theatre as living. Routledge, London

Kliendienst M 1998 Systematic review of research relevant to outcome measurement in the arts therapies. Unpublished paper

Liebmann M 1990 Art therapy and other caring professions (introduction). In: Liebmann M (ed) Art therapy in practice. Jessica Kingsley, London

Manners R 1998 Arts therapists and the Wales initiative. Handout at Clinical Effectiveness course, 5–6 February

Meekums B 1993 Research as an act of creation. In: Payne H (ed) Handbook of inquiry in the arts therapies: one river, many currents. Jessica Kingsley, London

Muir Gray J A 1997 Evidence-based healthcare: how to make health policy and management decisions. Churchill Livingstone, Edinburgh

Osborn J 1998 Letter to R Thornton, art therapist, Bristol Patients' Council, United Bristol Healthcare Trust, Mental Health Directorate, Bristol

Parlett M 1981 Illuminative evaluation. In: Reason P, Rowan J (eds) Human inquiry. John Wiley, Chichester

Pavlicevic M 1995 Music and emotion: aspects of music therapy research. In: Gilroy A, Lee C (eds) Art and music: therapy and research. Routledge, London

Payne H (ed) 1992 Dance movement therapy: theory and practice. Routledge, London

Payne H (ed) 1993a Handbook of inquiry in the arts therapies: one river, many currents. Jessica Kingsley, London

Payne H 1993b From practitioner to researcher: research as a learning process. In: Payne H (ed) Handbook of inquiry in the arts therapies: one river, many currents. Jessica Kingsley, London

Payne H 1993c Directory of arts therapies research. In: Payne H (ed) Handbook of inquiry in the arts therapies: one river, many currents. Jessica Kingsley, London

Prinzhorn H 1922 Bildernei der Geisteskranken. Springer Verlag, Berlin Translated by E. von Brockendorff 1972 Artistry of the mentally ill. Springer Verlag, Berlin

Reason P (ed) 1988 Human inquiry in action. Sage, London

Reason P, Rowan J (eds) 1981 Human inquiry. John Wiley, Chichester

Rees M 1995 Making sense of marking space: researching art therapy with people who have severe learning difficulties. In: Gilroy A, Lee C (eds) Art and music: therapy and research. Routledge, London

Rogers P 1998 European music therapy research register, 3rd edn. Child and Adolescent Research and Therapy Trust, Suffolk. Obtainable from P.O. Box 8, Saxmundham, Suffolk, IP17 1RW

Schaverien J 1993 The retrospective review of pictures: data for research in art therapy. In: Payne H (ed) Handbook of inquiry in the arts therapies: one river, many currents. Jessica Kingsley, London

Stanton-Jones K 1992 An introduction to dance movement therapy in psychiatry. Routledge, London

Times 1998 Arts therapy will have role in NHS. The Times, 24 March 1998

Tolley K, Rowland N 1995 Evaluating the cost-effectiveness of counselling in healthcare. Routledge, London

Wadeson H 1980 Art psychotherapy. John Wiley, New York, Ch 21

Waller D 1991 Becoming a profession: the history of art therapy in Britain, 1940–82. Tavistock/Routledge, London

Welsh Office 1995 Towards evidence based practice. Central Office of Information, London

Wigram T, West R, Saperston B 1995 The art and science of music therapy: a handbook. Harwood Academic, Switzerland

Resources

Association for Dance Movement Therapy UK
c/o Arts Therapies Department
Springfield Hospital
Glenburnie Road
London SW17 7DJ
Email: query@dmtuk.demon.co.uk

British Association of Art Therapists
5 Tavistock Place
London WC1H 9SN
Tel: 0207 383 3774
Fax: 0207 431 2450
Email:boat@gateway.net

British Association of Dramatherapists
41 Broomhouse Lane
London SW6 3DP
Tel/Fax: 0207 731 0160

Association of Professional Music Therapists
Chestnut Cottage
38 Pierce Lane
Fulbourn
Cambridge CB1 5DL
Tel: 01223 880377
Fax: 01223 881679
The professional body of qualified music therapists in the UK.

British Society for Music Therapy
25 Rosslyn Avenue
East Barnet
Herts EN4 8DH
Tel/Fax: 0208 368 8879
Promotes the use and development of music therapy, membership open to all who have an interest in music therapy.

National Arts Therapies Research Committee
Birmingham Centre for Arts Therapies
The Friends' Institute
220 Moseley Road
Highgate
Birmingham B12 0DG
Tel/Fax: 0121 440 4455
Email: ccc@cableinet.co.uk

Training courses

There are postgraduate qualifying courses at the locations given below. For the addresses, readers are advised to contact the relevant professional association (see above). In addition there are many introductory courses for those who want to find out about arts therapies. These are often organised by local universities or adult education colleges.

Art Therapy: Bath, Edinburgh, Hatfield, London (Goldsmiths), Sheffield
Dance Movement Therapy: Hatfield, London (Laban Centre), London (Roehampton Institute)
Dramatherapy: Hatfield, London (Sesame/Central School of Speech and Drama), London (Roehampton Institute), Manchester, Torquay, York
Music Therapy: Bristol, Cambridge, Cardiff, London (Guildhall), London (Nordoff-Robbins Centre), London (Roehampton Institute)

6 Chemotherapy and other physical treatments

Ibrahim Y. A. Turkistani

Key issues
- Chemotherapeutic interventions are one of the oldest, and arguably fastest, ways of controlling and treating behavioural distress
- Historically, chemotherapy has been used for centuries, however modern psychopharmacology has only developed since the Second World War
- Overuse of chemotherapy has occurred. This is often due to the fact that psychological treatments are time-consuming, there are waiting lists to see therapists, and in some developing countries chemotherapy is the only treatment available
- Chemotherapy has been successfully used to treat a range of disorders such as schizophrenia, depression, mania and obsessive-compulsive disorder

Overview

The use of chemotherapy is one of the oldest, perhaps easiest, and arguably fastest ways of controlling and treating behavioural distress. As a consequence it is widely used and occasionally misused, sometimes resulting in unnecessary side-effects.

This chapter has a slightly different shape and pattern from other chapters in this book. Broadly, it is divided into four sections. The first section begins with a brief account of the history of chemotherapy usage for people in behavioural distress, and in the second section the chemotherapeutic treatment of a range of conditions that underlie behavioural distress are described. The third section of the chapter is devoted to a classification of medications, their uses and effects, and this is known as pharmacotherapy. In this section both psychotropic and non-psychotropic drugs are discussed, including indications, uses and side-effects. In the final section electroconvulsive therapy (ECT) and psychosurgery as physical treatments are briefly considered. The reader is then asked to consider two case illustrations; the first illustrates inappropriate use of medication, and the second presents some of the unpleasant side-effects that might be encountered when taking medication.

History

Drugs that are used in cases of distressed behaviours are as old as humanity. Alcohol, opium poppy seeds and marijuana or hashish have long been used to elevate mood, and to treat anxiety, phobias and other unwanted behaviours.

Until the middle of the 19th century little scientific attention had been paid to the effects of using drugs for treatment. As a result, the use of drugs remained primitive until Western scientists became interested in exploring their potential for the treatment of disease. By the end of the 19th century, chloral hydrate and morphine became available and shortly after that barbiturates were synthesised. These substances were used heavily during that period for almost all psychiatric and emotional problems. Then there was reasonably slow progress in this field until after the Second World War, when the modern era of psychopharmacology commenced. Most of the psychotropic medications used at present (for example, antipsychotics, antidepressants and benzodiazepines) were discovered in the 1950s.

The discovery of new drugs is often associated with a claim that they are safer and have less harmful effects than the original compound, and this often leads to extensive usage. Often, newly introduced drugs will later show side-effects that will trigger a search for other members of the same chemical class that are more effective, have a broader spectrum of usage and a better side-effect profile than the original compounds.

Generally, the side-effects of drugs range from mild (not serious effects that last for a short period or disappear with discontinuation of medication, for example a dry mouth) to more serious (for example liver disease) and, rarely, fatal effects. The side-effects of such substances and their inappropriate use in managing behavioural difficulties were among the reasons given by scientists for exploring different methods of treatment, for example improving and modifying psychological treatments.

Overuse of chemotherapy at the present time arises from a number of different factors: for example, psychological treatments are time-consuming and the waiting time to see a therapist may be several months, consequently family doctors and psychiatrists sometimes prescribe medication while patients are waiting for appointments with therapists. Another factor is that some clients prefer pharmacotherapy, as they have greater faith in medication than in other therapies. Also, in developing countries pharmacotherapy is often the main, if not the only, treatment in the field of psychiatry, as the number of therapists is very few, and psychotherapy is time-consuming and potentially expensive for providers of health services.

The next section identifies a range of conditions that may underlie the manifestation of behavioural distress, as seen from a medical perspective.

Chemo-therapeutic treatment of some conditions with underlying behavioural distress

This section presents a range of conditions that typically present with behavioural distress and suggests how chemotherapeutic intervention may alleviate, and in some instances assist in the treatment of these disorders. Before any of these disorders can be ascertained it is necessary for the individual concerned to be seen, assessed and diagnosed by a psychiatrist. In determining the classification of the disorder the psychiatrist usually uses one of two widely known diagnostic systems. The first, the Diagnostic and Statistical Manual (DSM) was developed by the American Psychiatric Association. The second, The International Classification of Mental and Behavioural Disorders (ICD), has been produced by the World Health Organization. It is the ICD(version 10) classification system that is used in this chapter (World Health Organization 1992). ICD-10 uses standard and internationally agreed criteria to enable a valid diagnosis to be reached, and assists in determining the prevalence rate of some these disorders. The publication comprises carefully constructed descriptions of a range of behavioural disorders to assist in determining the correct diagnosis for the behaviours that are manifested. Some of the more specific and well-known disorders are outlined below, and this is followed by some more general states of distress that may benefit from chemotherapeutic treatment.

Schizophrenia   This is one of the major mental illnesses, with a lifetime prevalence (calculated in population surveys, in most industrial countries) of approximately 1% (Kendell & Zealley 1993). ICD(version 10) recognises seven varieties of schizophrenia, but in this chapter its clinical presentation will be briefly described as acute and chronic episodes. Acute episodes usually present with florid symptoms such as thought disorders, hallucinations and delusions. Insight into the illness is also usually impaired. The behaviour largely reflects the severity of the symptoms; it may be odd, disruptive, suspicious or aggressive and violent, and this may possibly make the sufferer dangerous to themselves or to others. This phase should be treated with antipsychotic medication which not only controls agitation but also treats psychotic symptoms. In an emergency, and only in certain circumstances, physical restraint or seclusion may be required, both for the client's own and others' safety. The chronic phase of schizophrenia is characterised by social withdrawal, lack of motivation, poverty of speech, attention deficits and flattening of affect (the latter refers to generalised shallow emotional responses to life events). In this phase, although behaviour and other therapies are important, antipsychotic chemotherapy, as maintenance therapy, should be used to minimise the occurrence of relapse.

The dose of antipsychotic medication prescribed in the acute phase is usually much higher than the maintenance dose in stable or chronic cases. In some acute cases for example, a dose of up to 120 mg daily of haloperidol can be given, while the smallest maintenance dose recommended is 2–5 mg of haloperidol daily. Clients need to be reviewed on a regular basis to assess their mental state, look for any side-effects and adjust the daily dose of medication, where necessary.

Depression   This is a common disorder with a prevalence rate of 2.6–5.5% in men and 6.0–11.8% in women (Fara & Davidson 1996). In psychiatry, it is most important to differentiate between depressive illnesses and simple unhappiness. A diagnosis of depressive illness is only made when the presenting clinical features continue for at least 2 weeks. These include: low mood, loss of interest in everything (including sex and appetite), weight loss, fatigability, poor concentration, reduced self-esteem, broken sleep with early morning waking and ideas of guilt with suicidal ideation. About 60% of people with depression have suicidal thoughts and 15% of them commit suicide (Barraclough et al 1974, Robins et al 1959).

According to the ICD-10 there are three types of depressive illness: mild, moderate and severe (World Health Organization 1992). The difference between the three types of depressive illness lies in the severity and duration of the symptoms. The mild form of depressive illness is very common, usually brief, and does not require active treatment. Moderate depression responds well both to pharmacotherapies and to cognitive behaviour therapy (see Ch. 10), but a combination of both is superior to either treatment approach being used on its own. In contrast, severe depressive illness may be associated with psychotic symptoms (for example delusion of sin, hallucinations and severe psychomotor retardation) that may progress to stupor. The main treatment in this phase is to prescribe medication such as antipsychotics and antidepressants. In severe depression, electroconvulsive therapy (ECT) is sometimes the most effective treatment, and in some empirical studies it has been found to be superior to medication (Weschler et al 1965, Greenblatt et al 1962). In people with severe depression supportive therapy may be used with physical treatment, but clinically, cognitive behaviour therapy is generally less effective during this phase. Depressive illnesses progress to be chronic in 20% of cases; this usually affects older people and they are known to respond better to psychotherapy than to antidepressants.

Mania

Presently, this disorder affects about 1% of the general population. Clinically, the features that characterise mania are the opposite to those occurring in depression. Clients are usually euphoric, irritable, overactive, disinhibited, with pressure of speech, flight of ideas and grandiose delusions. There is also marked distractability with almost uncontrollable excitement. These features do not last long and may shift rapidly to a depressive phase. The best way of managing this acute phase is to admit the client to an acute psychiatric unit for the safety of the client and others. In the unit it is necessary to divert the client's energy into less dangerous channels rather than physically restraining them, as this may provoke violence. Antipsychotic drugs are usually the immediate effective treatment. Mood stabilisers are also effective in preventing relapses. Hypomania is a lesser degree of mania and not accompanied by delusions or hallucinations.

Obsessive-compulsive disorder

This was considered a relatively uncommon neurotic disorder, but the current data indicate that the lifetime prevalence rate is 2.5% (Regier et al 1988). It is characterised by recurrent obsessive thoughts or patterns of behaviour, for example repeated checking to ensure that doors are closed, or gas and lights turned off, or repeated washing of hands for fear of contamination. Sometimes there is a fear of harm coming to a member of the family if certain things are not undertaken at certain times for example counting in special ways or saying certain things. However, clients retain insight into their condition and recognise that their fears and behaviours are irrational, but cannot ignore them, otherwise they become increasingly anxious. For diagnosis this disorder must persist for at least two successive weeks, and be a source of distress. In treatment, anxiolytics such as diazepam should be avoided but they can be used in severe cases for a short period, to give immediate relief.

Clomipramine and other selective serotonin reuptake inhibitors (SSRIs) (for example fluoxetine, fluvoxamine, paroxetine) are useful in the treatment of this condition. Various controlled studies have demonstrated that medications are equally as effective as response prevention (a behavioural therapeutic approach) (Kaplan & Sadock 1995). Some studies have found that people with obsessive-compulsive disorder usually relapse on cessation of medication. However, relapse rate is less with response prevention therapy. Using a combination of drugs and response prevention is superior to either treatment alone.

Panic disorder

This is a common disorder with a prevalence rate of 3% in the general population. Its characteristic features are recurrent panic attacks, which can be severe, unpredictable, and not restricted to any particular situations. The symptoms typically include: sudden onset of palpitations, shortness of breath, trembling, sweating, dizziness, flashes and chest pain. These symptoms often present with a secondary fear of dying, losing control or going mad. A panic attack is often followed by a fear of having another attack. Prescribing anxiolytics in high doses (for example benzodiazepines) has been found to be effective, and they work relatively quickly in relieving symptomology. Antidepressants are equally effective but take about 2–3 weeks to work. However, antidepressants are preferable to benzodiazepines, as they are less likely to bring about tolerance and dependence. In a study undertaken by Klein et al (1980), imipramine, an antidepressant, was compared with a placebo for efficacy, in addition to behaviour therapy. They found that imipramine was significantly superior to the placebo, and the addition of behaviour or supportive therapy to the drug significantly reduced the avoidance behaviour that was associated with panic disorder.

Anorexia nervosa

This disorder occurs mainly in girls of school age, with a prevalence rate between 0.1% and 0.5%. The male to female ratio is 1:10. The disorder is characterised by intense fear of gaining weight or becoming fat, despite being underweight (clients' weight is generally 15% below that expected). Clients usually avoid fattening foods and engage in self-induced vomiting and self-induced purging. They may also engage in excessive exercise and use diuretics and/or appetite suppressants. They have a distorted body image, believing themselves to be fat and overweight even when severely underweight. In women, amenorrhoea is common and this occurs in its early stage. The disorder is potentially fatal, with a mortality rate of between 5% and 12%. In up to 50% of cases, clients have episodes of bulimia (see below).

Inpatient treatment is essential, in case the client's weight is dangerously low (less than 65% of standard weight). The immediate aim is to restore the nutritional state to normal. The treatment is mainly cognitive behavioural therapy, weight reinforcement and family therapy. Pharmacologically, chlorpromazine has been used successfully in some cases, but there has been no controlled double-blind study. Amitriptyline, cyproheptadine and placebo in a double-blind study showed that both amitriptyline and cyproheptadine had marginal effects to placebo (Halmi et al 1986).

Bulimia nervosa

This disorder affects mainly young women who are at senior school or college, with a prevalence of 4–15% of the general population; the male to female ratio is 1:10. It is characterised by 'binge' eating to bring some relief from tension, but this is soon followed by guilt and disgust and then the client usually induces vomiting. Clients also abuse laxatives and diuretics to prevent weight gain. People with this disorder are usually of normal weight; 25% of people with this disorder provide a history of sexual abuse.

Many drugs have been tried in the treatment of this disorder, but only antidepressants seem promising; antidepressants are found to be as effective as cognitive behaviour therapy at reducing the frequency of binge eating and induction of vomiting. Combining both therapies (medication and cognitive behaviour therapy) is more effective than either therapy alone in reducing accompanying depression and dietary preoccupation.

Hyperkinetic disorder

The American classification Diagnostic and Statistical Manual (DSM-IV) refers to this disorder as attention deficit-hyperactivity disorder (ADHD). The difference between this classification and the ICD-10 is that in the latter conduct disorders are excluded, whilst in the former conduct disorders are included. As a result of this, a 10-fold difference in prevalence between the two classifications can be found. (In ICD-10 less than 0.1% prevalence is calculated, whilst in DSM-IV it is estimated to be about 1%.)

The disorder may become evident at the age of 1 year but its peak is between the ages of 3 and 8 years. It is characterised by extreme restlessness, severe pervasive hyperactivity and poor attention, with a consequent difficulty in learning. Other features are impulsiveness, aggression, temper tantrums, recklessness, proneness to accidents and social disinhibition. This disorder usually exhausts parents.

Treatment is mainly through the use of behavioural approaches. Medication such as methylphenidate can be very helpful in reducing overactivity, but it should be reserved only for severe cases that are not responding to other therapy. Nevertheless, if medication is essential it should be used in conjunction with behavioural therapy. Undesirable effects of medication include: loss of appetite, reduced growth rate, insomnia, irritability and depression. Treatment with medication usually takes a long period, however, some authors have suggested that medication should be discontinued for periods of time to check whether the drug is still needed and to minimise the side-effects.

Personality disorders

The ICD-10 definition of personality disorder states that it is represented by a severe disturbance in the characterological constitutions and behavioural tendencies of an individual and usually involves several areas of the personality. Personality disorders are nearly always associated with considerable personal and social disruption. The problems tend to appear in late childhood or adolescence and continue into adulthood.

Personality disorders differ from personality changes in their timing and mode of their emergence. As a developmental condition they are not secondary to other mental disorders or brain disease, although they may precede and/or coexist with other disorders. In contrast, personality change is acquired usually during adult life, following severe or prolonged stress, extreme environmental deprivation, serious psychiatric disorder or brain disease or injury.

It is important to ensure that personality disorder is diagnosed as a separate entity from other forms of behavioural distress that might be confused or conflated with it. For example, most neurotic clients do not have a concomitant personality disorder, and many alcohol abusers are premorbidly normal, even though they may present with some apparent form of personality disorder. Standardised assessment of personality should be used in all cases with a provisional diagnosis of personality disorder. The use of chemotherapeutic treatment approaches in personality disorder is generally limited. Antipsychotic medications in relatively small doses are used with some success in reducing the severity of impulse behaviour. Lithium salt and carbamazepine have been used in aggressive behaviour. Benzodiazepines should not be used with this group of people as they can easily become dependent on them.

Post-traumatic stress disorder

This is a relatively common disorder with a prevalence of 0.5% in men and 1.3% in women (Helzer et al 1987). It is caused by extraordinary and major life stressors. The onset of the reactions are usually delayed and may take months, or even years before they are manifested. Post-traumatic stress disorder is characterised by repeated episodes of re-experiencing a traumatic incident. These episodes manifest themselves as intrusive memories or dreams and a numbing feeling that is accompanied by anxiety symptoms and depression. The disorder can be severe and disabling. Different types of treatments have been tried and cognitive and behavioural therapy has been found to be most effective. Nevertheless, anxiolytics can be of value but are only recommended in very severe disabling conditions, and for a short period. Antidepressants have also been tried with good results, especially in chronic cases.

Alcohol dependence

Alcohol dependence is a common problem that affects 2% of the UK population. Several factors are involved in its aetiology: they include genetic causes, certain types of personality (impulsive and rebellious, more extrovert individuals are more at risk of developing alcohol dependence) and environmental influences.

According to the ICD-10 classification system, to arrive at a correct diagnosis, three or more of the following criteria should have been present together at some time in the previous year:

- A strong desire or compulsion to take alcohol
- Difficulties in controlling alcohol-taking behaviour in terms of its onset, termination, or level of alcohol use
- A withdrawal state
- Progressive neglect of alternative pleasures or interests in favour of alcohol use
- Increased tolerance to alcohol
- Persisting with alcohol use despite clear evidence of overtly harmful consequences.

Excessive drinking can lead to physical, psychological and social damage. In this chapter we are concerned with the possible effects on behaviour. Psychological effects which produce behavioural distress, fall into different classes and include:

- Intoxication features (for example outbursts of aggression, acute psychotic episodes and memory blackouts)
- Withdrawal symptoms (for example tremulousness, agitation, nausea, sweating and, later, convulsions and delirium tremens).

Delirium tremens (DTs) is a serious medical condition that usually occurs 3–5 days after cessation of heavy alcohol use. It is characterised by confusion, delusions and hallucinations. Clients become very frightened and agitated and can be physically violent. Other psychological effects include Wernicke-Korsakoff syndrome. This is a thiamine deficiency caused by excessive alcohol intake. The syndrome refers to two conditions that are successive stages of a single disease. The onset usually commences with Wernicke's syndrome, which is characterised by confusion, ataxia and nystagmus. If the client is not treated urgently with high doses of thiamine, he or she may die or progress to Korsokoff's syndrome, which is characterised by confabulation and poor short-term memory.

Treatment for this disorder is highly dependent on the client's motivation and cooperation. Pharmacological therapy is indicated mainly for detoxification. Benzodiazepine is usually the drug of choice; it minimises the withdrawal symptoms and prevents withdrawal seizures and delirium tremens. Antipsychotic drugs should be avoided as they lower the seizure threshold, and may therefore precipitate seizures.

Disulfiram is a drug that is indicated and used as a deterrent to impulsive drinking. It causes unpleasant reactions when taken with even small amounts of alcohol; these include headache, choking sensation, flushing of the face and sometimes an irregular heart beat. Rarely these reactions can be fatal, thus clients must be warned about the danger of combining these two agents together.

More general states of distress
Psychogenic pain

This condition is usually severe and prolonged in nature. There are generally inadequate physical findings to identify a specific cause, and it is characterised by inconsistent neuro-anatomic distribution. It can be disabling, particularly if chronic. It can limit client's movements, causing weakness of the muscles; this can have an impact on the client's social life and as a result clients sometimes abuse alcohol or analgesics. Psychogenic pain has different causes such as depression, anxiety and different emotional disturbances, and its initiation or exacerbation is closely related to emotionally stressful events. As there are many possible causes of psychogenic pain, comprehensive assessment prior to treatment is essential. Although analgesics have little place here and should be discouraged, there are various antidepressant drugs that have been found to be useful in treating chronic pain with or without depression. In addition, anticonvulsants like carbamazepine and phenytoin may also be prescribed with some success. While anxiolytics such as benzodiazepines act rather faster, they should be avoided because they have some potential for dependence.

Insomnia

This condition is a very common disorder and probably the most common complaint presenting to general practitioners, although it is known that most of the people who complain of insomnia, especially older people, have normal sleep. The causes of insomnia are numerous and in 85% of cases this is mostly secondary to other problems such as pain or discomfort, or psychological factors such as anxiety, depression or various other psychiatric disorders. Insomnia also occurs in association with excessive use of caffeine or alcohol, or changing the place where one sleeps. However, in primary insomnia (which accounts for 15%), no cause can be found.

Insomnia typically is manifested in three forms:

- Initial insomnia – difficulty in getting off to sleep
- Middle insomnia – difficulty in maintaining sleep (broken sleep)
- Late insomnia – an early morning waking with difficulty going back to sleep again.

Generally, early insomnia is associated with anxiety, unlike middle and late insomnia which are typical of depressive illnesses. Nevertheless, all the three types of insomnia may be associated with depressive illness.

Treatment focuses on causation, thus it is essential to have a full assessment that includes medical, psychiatric, and social histories. In general, a short course of hypnotics may be prescribed in secondary insomnia. In anxiety and primary insomnia it is important to encourage non-pharmacological methods of treatment and discourage overindulgence in alcohol. The prescribing of benzodiazepines should be avoided, as dependence is particularly likely in these clients.

Learning disabilities (mental retardation)

In the UK the term learning disabilities is preferred to the term mental retardation, the term used in the ICD-10 classification system, although for the purpose of this chapter the terms are used interchangeably. Learning disability itself is clearly not a condition of distress; however, some people with learning disability will present with behavioural distress. Mental retardation (learning disability) is defined in the ICD-10 as a condition of arrested or incomplete development of the mind which is especially characterised by impairment of skills manifested during the developmental period that contribute to the overall level of intelligence, which includes cognitive, language, motor and social abilities.

The causation of behavioural difficulties in some people with learning disability is complex, and may be due to psychiatric and/or non-psychiatric disorders, depending on the severity of learning disabilities. For example, the more severe the learning disability, the more difficult it may be for the client to express emotions. Thus, challenging behaviour and psychiatric disorders appear to be more common in this population than in general populations (Wing 1971, Kushlik & Cox 1973, Gostason 1985). The presentation of psychiatric disorders in people with learning disabilities is often different from that in the general population, especially in people with profound or severe learning disabilities. For example, depression may present dominantly with agitation, violence and aggressive or self-injurious behaviour.

Treatment depends largely on the causes of the behaviour distress. A thorough medical and psychiatric history and any changes in environmental or social lifestyles need to be noted. A careful physical examination, including laboratory investigations and electroencephalogram (EEG) are essential for the development of an effective treatment plan. These are all needed to assist the psychiatrist in ruling out any physical conditions that may account for the behaviour manifested. The treatment of mental illness in this population is similar to that of the general population. Using antipsychotics for behaviour distress 'not caused by mental illness' is still popular, and can be effective in certain conditions, provided this does not expose the client to risks of side-effects that outweigh the benefits of a reduction in unwanted behaviours.

Pharmacotherapy

Above, a range of conditions have been presented that may underlie behavioural distress. This next section describes the use of medication as prescribed by psychiatrists. The section will include indications for prescribing medicines, different types of drugs that are located within a particular class, the pharmacokinetics of the drugs, and lastly undesirable effects of the drugs. In psychiatry, the use of pharmacotherapy for behavioural distress can be divided into two major groupings, psychotropic and non-psychotropic drugs (see Box 6.1). Although it is appreciated that some readers will not have the specialist knowledge to understand every term that is used in this section, details are offered for readers who are familiar with them. Readers not familiar with terms used are recommended to refer to Resources (at the end of this chapter), under the Royal College of Psychiatrists, and seek patient information fact sheets that will explain some of the medical terms and drug categories referred to in this chapter.

Box 6.1
Major drugs used within psychiatry that fall within the psychotropic and non-psychotropic groupings

Psychotropic drugs
- Antipsychotics
- Antidepressants
- Anxiolytics and hypnotics
- Mood stabilisers
- Stimulants

Non-psychotropic drugs
- Beta-blockers
- Antimuscarinics
- Disulfiram

Psychotropic drugs

Antipsychotics

There are many terms used to describe this group of drugs that includes major tranquillisers, anti-schizophrenic or neuroleptic drugs. None of these terms is wholly satisfactory. Major tranquilliser, for example, does not refer to its important clinical action, and anti-schizophrenic suggests use solely for schizophrenics, while neuroleptic refers to the production of a state of neurolepsis or calm indifference which is a side-effect of the drugs rather than a therapeutic effect. The term antipsychotic is used here, as it seems that these drugs are useful for the whole range of psychotic illnesses. Unlike many other drugs, these agents have little or no potential for abuse.

Indications

Antipsychotic drugs generally tranquillise without causing loss of consciousness and without causing paradoxical excitement as the benzodiazepines do. They are useful for all types of psychosis, especially where there are positive symptoms such as hallucinations, delusions and thought disorder. In the short term, they are also used to calm disturbed clients whatever the psychopathological causes may be – mania, agitated depression, brain damage, toxic delirium or acute severe anxiety. They are also used in the short term for acute behavioural disturbances due to non-psychiatric disorders.

Classification of antipsychotic drugs

Antipsychotic drugs are usually classified according to their chemical structures (see Box 6.2). In addition to those listed in Box 6.2, there is also a range of atypical antipsychotic drugs, including amisulpride, clozapine, olanzapine, risperidone, sertindole, quetiapine and zotepine.

Box 6.2
Classification of antipsychotic drugs

Phenothiazines	aliphatic	i.e.	chlorpromazine
	piperidine	i.e.	thioridazine
	piperazine	i.e.	trifluoperazine
Thioxanthenes		i.e.	flupenthixol
Butyrophenones		i.e.	haloperidol and droperidol
Butylpiperidines		i.e.	pimozide

The different types of antipsychotic drugs are equivalent in overall efficacy, and the obvious differences among these drugs are in their relative side-effect profiles, potency, safety and cost. For example, chlorpromazine is the most sedative, and photosensitisation is more common than with other antipsychotics. Thioridazine has fewer extrapyramidal effects, but commonly causes postural hypotension. Trifluoperazine, pimozide and haloperidol are more potent and less sedative, and more likely to cause extrapyramidal effects. The newer atypical antipsychotics have the advantage of fewer extrapyramidal effects and the prolactin elevation may be less frequent than with other antipsychotics. However, clozapine can cause agranulocytosis in 1–2% of people taking this drug. The atypical drugs are more expensive than other antipsychotic drugs, and in most respects their efficacy is equivalent, with the exception of clozapine which is known to be superior in the treatment of those patients who have not responded to other forms of treatment.

Different antipsychotic drugs have different potencies. For example, 100 mg of chlorpromazine is equivalent to doses of the drugs identified in Box 6.3. These equivalents are intended only as an approximate guide (British Medical Association and Royal Pharmaceutical Society of Great Britain vol 38, 1999).

Box 6.3
Approximate equivalent dosages of various antipsychotic drugs to 100 mg chlorpromazine

Clozapine	50 mg
Haloperidol	2–3 mg
Loxapine	10–20 mg
Pimozide	2 mg
Risperidone	0.5–1 mg
Sulpiride	200 mg
Thioridazine	100 mg
Trifluoperazine	5 mg

Mechanism of action

The mechanism of action of antipsychotics is presumed to involve the postsynaptic blockade of the central nervous system's dopamine receptors. There are different types of dopamine receptors in the brain. D_1 receptors are found in the basal ganglia and blockade produces extrapyramidal side-effects. D_2 receptors are found in the limbic system and blockade produces the therapeutic effect of 'antipsychotic action'. Blockade by dopamine receptors D_3 and D_4 also produces therapeutic effects. Atypical antipsychotic drugs, previously listed, also block serotonin and adrenergic receptors.

Pharmacokinetics

Pharmacokinetics refers to the study in time of the course of drug action, and is mainly concerned with drug administration, absorption, metabolism and excretion.

Antipsychotic drugs are generally well absorbed through oral or parenteral administration. In some antipsychotics (e.g. oral chlorpromazine), the majority of the metabolism is completed as it passes through the portal system before entering the systemic circulation – this is called 'first pass metabolism'. This can significantly reduce the drug's bioavailability, as 75% of it is metabolised in this way, but parenteral administration avoids first pass metabolism, and thus increases its bioavailability several-fold compared to the oral route. Other antipsychotics (e.g. haloperidol) are metabolised in the same way, but with much less degree of first pass metabolism. These drugs are largely metabolised in the liver, and are highly lipophilic and protein-bound in plasma and enter the brain easily. Most of these drugs are excreted through the kidneys, by passive diffusion.

Undesirable side-effects

Extrapyramidal side-effects

These are the most troublesome side-effects, and represent a major cause of limitation to their use. These side-effects are very common with traditional 'typical' high potency antipsychotic drugs (e.g. haloperidol, droperidol, trifluoperazine and pimozide). However, with atypical antipsychotics these effects are mild and represent a major advance in the drug treatment of schizophrenia and other psychotic-related illnesses.

Extrapyramidal symptoms include acute dystonias that occur mainly in children and young men, usually within 2 days of treatment commencing. Dystonias are a range of disorders in the form of spasm of the muscles of the head and neck. They constitute some of the most frightening side-effects of antipsychotic drugs. They include: torticollis, a contraction of neck muscles that causes twisting of the neck and an unnatural positioning of the head; oculogyric crisis, a spasm that leads to upturning of the eyes; tongue protrusion; facial grimacing; and dysarthria. This odd clinical presentation can easily be mistaken for histrionic behaviour or seizures. Akathisia is a form of restless legs syndrome with an unpleasant feeling of being unable to keep still. It usually appears after 5–60 days in up to 20% of clients following treatment with antipsychotics. In mild cases, patients may experience subjective restlessness without increased motor activity. Parkinsonian syndrome, clinically indistinguishable from idiopathic Parkinsonism, develops gradually over days to weeks and most commonly affects older people. The syndrome includes akinesia (a generalised slowing of volitional movements, expressionless face, and reduction in arm movement when walking). These symptoms may resemble features of depressive illness and chronic schizophrenia. Other Parkinsonian symptoms include, cogwheel rigidity, coarse tremors, shuffling gait, stooped posture and a positive glabella tap sign (failure to inhibit eye-blinking when the mid-forehead is tapped repeatedly, a reaction which is rapidly suppressed in most normal people). Rabbit syndrome, a rapid pre-oral tremor of the jaw, is rare, appearing late in treatment and possibly confused with tardive dyskinesia, but this often responds quickly to antimuscarinic drugs (Jus et al 1974). Tardive dyskinesia is characterised by mouth and tongue movements which are repetitive, painless, involuntary and quick choreiform movements. These abnormal movements may include lip smacking, chewing, sucking, puckering and grimacing. Other movements may include choreoathetoid-like movements of fingers and toes; these abnormal movements disappear during sleep and are increased by emotional distress. Between 10% and 15% of patients treated with antipsychotics for more than a year experience this syndrome. Elderly people, women and patients with diffuse brain pathology are more at risk of developing this movement disorder.

Tardive dyskinesia is not a progressive nor an irreversible disorder in the majority of clients taking antipsychotic drugs (as was previously thought). Recent evidence has shown that most of the clients with tardive dyskinesia improve despite continually taking antipsychotic drugs (Kaplan & Sadock 1995). Recent studies also showed that when antipsychotics are discontinued, the majority of those clients taking such drugs do recover from this movement disorder (Kaplan & Sadock 1995). Nevertheless, preventing the syndrome, or minimising its occurrence, is the main goal, and advisable. This is achieved by using the minimum effective dose of antipsychotic drugs for long-term therapy, reviewing the medication regularly and closely observing for early signs of this syndrome. Clozapine, an atypical antipsychotic drug, has showed its usefulness in severe tardive dyskinesia. More interestingly, several studies have shown that high dose of vitamin E is beneficial in some cases, particularly for clients who have had tardive dyskinesia for less than 5 years (Akhtar et al 1993, Lohr & Caligiuri 1996).

Antimuscarinic effects These include dryness of mouth, constipation, blurred vision and retention of urine in men. These symptoms are common with low potency antipsychotic drugs (e.g. thioridazine and chlorpromazine).

Antiadrenergic effects These include nasal congestion, inhibition of ejaculation, reflex tachycardia and postural hypotension. These are dose-related, and commonly occur with high doses of thioridazine, chlorpromazine and risperidone, especially in older people.

Weight gain This can be a major problem, especially with female clients. Chlorpromazine, fluphenazine, flupenthixol or olanzapine are the main antipsychotics causing this problem, although dietary restriction sometimes helps.

Cardio-vascular effects Generally, antipsychotic drugs are safe, although they may produce some changes to an electrocardiogram (ECG). Patients on higher doses should have a regular ECG check. The antipsychotic pimozide is one of the drugs that can cause serious arrhythmias, and all patients should have ECG prior to its use.

Neuroleptic malignant syndrome This is rare but serious, affecting 0.2% of those receiving potent and high doses of antipsychotic drugs. Its main features are hyperthermia, muscular rigidity, confusion and autonomic changes. It affects twice as many men as women, and mostly younger people. It is potentially fatal and on diagnosis requires urgent medical management. The mortality rate is about 25% and this may be higher when depot forms of the drug are used. Early diagnosis and treatment can be lifesaving. Testing for high creatinine phosphokinase is a useful single diagnostic aid for this syndrome. Treatment consists of immediate discontinuation of antipsychotic drugs, and clients should be managed at medical departments with dantrolene and symptomatic treatments.

Other side-effects These include sedation, depression, sexual dysfunctions, skin rash, amenorrhoea, galactorrhoea, gynaecomastia, haematological effects and seizures.

Long-acting depot antipsychotics

These are mainly used for maintenance therapy. Depot compounds are oil-based substances that are administered by deep intramuscular injection. The drug is slowly released from the injection site, and can be administered once every 1–4 weeks. Initially clients should receive a test dose as undesirable effects are prolonged. Their mechanism of action is similar to the traditional antipsychotics. The main advantages and disadvantages for the use of depot injections are shown in Box 6.4.

Drug interactions of antipsychotics

One of the problems of taking any drug is that it may interact with other substances or drugs being taken by the patient. Therefore, it is important to be aware of such interactions, especially for carers or relatives who spend a lot of time with people who are being treated for some type of disorder that has manifested in behavioural distress. A list of some of the more common interactions between antipsychotics and other substances are given in Box 6.5.

Box 6.4
Advantages and disadvantages of depot injections

Advantages
- Offers some solution to patients with poor compliance
- Increases contact between the patient and the community team member
- Absorption problems are overcome
- Reduces abuse or overdose

Disadvantages
- Extrapyramidal symptoms are more common
- Side-effects take longer to subside after stopping or reducing the dose

Box 6.5
Drug interactions of antipsychotics

- Potentiate sedative effects of alcohol and all sedative drugs
- Enhance hypotensive effect of antihypertensive drugs
- Administration of high dose of thioridazine and high dose of antimuscarinic drugs may cause toxic confusional state, especially in elderly patients
- Likely to reduce absorption of antipsychotics if taken together with antacid
- Clozapine should not be administered with drugs that potentially cause agranulocytosis (e.g. sulphonamides, trimethoprim, carbamazepine), as the risk of agranulocytosis increased

Antidepressant drugs

There are various classes of antidepressants available that have proved superior to placebo (Ball & Kiloh 1959). Generally it has been found that about 70% of depressed clients improved on antidepressants as compared with only 30% on placebo. There are about 30 different antidepressants in the British National Formulary (British Medical Association and the Royal Pharmaceutical Society of Great Britain vol 38, 1999) to treat depressive illnesses. It appears that all the different types carry equal efficacy and the differences between them are largely in their side-effects and costs.

Indications

Antidepressant drugs are initially indicated to treat depressive illness and prevent relapses, but growing evidence shows that they are as effective as benzodiazepines in the treatment of phobic, panic, obsessive-compulsive disorders (OCD) as well as generalised anxiety disorders. Amitriptyline has also been found to be effective in the treatment of nocturnal enuresis in children, and in some cases, for chronic pain, while fluoxetine and fluvoxamine have been successfully used in the treatment of bulimia nervosa.

Traditionally it was thought that some types of antidepressant (e.g. amitriptyline) were more useful in agitated depression, and imipramine in retarded depression, but there is no evidence to support this.

Clients must be informed that antidepressants take approximately 2-3 weeks before therapeutic effect is reached. It is important to inform clients of this as they may stop taking medication early because of no change in their condition. Informing patients of this expected delay has been found to improve compliance (Drug and Therapeutics Bulletin 1981).

Types of antidepressant

Each class of antidepressants has a different chemical structure and different potencies in blocking re-uptake of one of the central neurotransmitters (e.g. noradrenaline and serotonin), and makes these neurotransmitters more available. Schildkraut (1965) has suggested that in depression there is a relative deficiency of noradrenaline and serotonin. Thus antidepressants do not appear to influence the normal mood, but rather correct the abnormal levels of neurotransmitters – in other words, they do not help non-clinical depression that is related to a transient reaction to social factors.

The main classes of antidepressant are:

■ Noradrenaline re-uptake inhibitors: these include amoxapine, protriptyline, maprotiline, and reboxetine
■ Serotonin re-uptake inhibitors: these include trazodone, fluoxetine, citalopram, sertraline, paroxetine, fluvoxamine, and nefazodone
■ Mixed noradrenaline and serotonin re-uptake inhibitors; these include amitriptyline, doxepin, imipramine, nortriptyline, trimipramine, venlafaxine, and mirtazapine.

Out of these, fluoextine, paroxetine, fluovoxamine, sertraline, citalopram, mirtazapine, nefazodone, and reboxetine are the newer antidepressants.

Other classes of antidepressants are monoamine oxidase inhibitors (MAOIs). It is thought that they work by increasing the availability of neurotransmitters in the brain, for example, noradrenaline and serotonin. Their use is not popular because of their serious interaction with certain foods and drugs (see below, Box 6.6). They are used sometimes for resistive depressive illness not responding to other antidepressants.

When using reversible monoamine oxidase inhibitors (RMAOIs), for example moclobemide, it is possible to reverse the inhibition of monoamine oxidase. One of the differences between RMAOIs and MAOIs is that the former react less seriously when given with certain food or drugs than do the latter (see below, Box 6.6).

Pharmacokinetics

Antidepressants in general are well absorbed when given orally but poorly absorbed when given intramuscularly. They are largely metabolised in the liver. Most antidepressants have a long half-life and need to be given once daily.

Undesirable effects

The side-effects of the older antidepressants typically include dry mouth, blurring of vision, constipation, palpitation, postural hypotension, increased sweating and occasionally ventricular arrhythmias. Tiredness, drowsiness and weight gain may also occur. These side-effects are a frequent source of, and reason for, non-compliance. This group of antidepressants is relatively cheap. These drugs should be avoided in highly suicidal clients as they can produce serious effects on overdose, and avoided for those clients with heart problems. The newer antidepressants are more expensive, have fewer side-effects and have better compliance. The most common side-effects are nausea, abdominal pain and dyspepsia; these side-effects should remit after 1 week following commencement of treatment. This group of antidepressants differ from the old antidepressants in that they are not sedative, do not cause weight gain and are safer in the event of an overdose. Both groups lower the seizure thresholds and precipitate convulsions, and so caution needs to be taken when prescribing to clients with epilepsy. The MAOIs' main side-effects are dizziness and postural hypotension, especially in older people. This group of antidepressants is safer to prescribe to clients with epilepsy. The interactions between antidepressants and other drugs and substances are shown in Box 6.6.

Box 6.6
Drug interactions with antidepressants

- Alcohol enhances sedative effects of antidepressants
- Antipsychotics and antimuscarinic drugs both increase the antimuscarinic effects of old antidepressants
- Due to drying of the mouth, the effects of nitrates are reduced
- Cimetidine increases the plasma concentration of antidepressants
- MAOIs interact seriously with sympathomimetics (i.e., dexamphetamine, ephedrine and phenylephrin), and with food that contains tyramine, such as foodstuffs that are extracted from meat, yeast, cheese, chicken liver, pickled herrings, or from Chianti, red wine and beers. The interaction causes CNS excitation and hypertension. Antidepressants also interact seriously and require at least 2 weeks gap between stopping MAOIs and starting the antidepressant. MAOIs enhance the effect of insulin and oral hypoglycaemic agents

Anxiolytics and hypnotics

Anxiolytics and hypnotic drugs include:

- Benzodiazepines
- Barbiturates
- Buspirone
- Zopiclone and zolpidem
- Others such as chloral hydrate, bromide, paraldehydes, meprobamate.

All the anxiolytics have hypnotic effects when given in large doses at night; equally, hypnotics work as anxiolytics in small doses when given during the day. Since they were first marketed, these drugs have been prescribed widely, often inappropriately, when other treatments, such as psychological treatment, would have been equally effective.

Benzodiazepines

There are a large number of benzodiazepines available. They are divided into hypnotics (e.g. nitrazepam, loprazolam, temazepam, lormetazepam and flurazepam); and anxiolytics (e.g. chlordiazepoxide, diazepam, alprazolam, oxazepam and lorazepam).

Indications

Benzodiazepines are the most effective treatment for anxiety. In the short term they are superior to psychological treatments, but the relapse rate of anxiety and developing tolerance and dependence to the drugs are to be expected. Thus these drugs should only be used for the emergency treatment of anxiety and insomnia.

Other uses of benzodiazepine include treatment of:

- *Epilepsy*. Although benzodiazepines such as clobazam and clonazepam are highly effective in treating all forms of epilepsy, the majority of clients develop tolerance to its effect. Benzodiazepines should only be used when all other treatments fail to control convulsions.

■ *Status epilepticus*. Diazepam is effective both through intravenous (IV) or rectal (PR) routes. However, its absorption is poor and unpredictable through intramuscular routes, whilst lorazepam is highly effective through an intramuscular (IM) route.

■ *In psychosis*. Although benzodiazepines are not indicated for psychotic illnesses, they can be very helpful when combined with antipsychotic drugs in treating acutely disturbed, aggressive and dangerous clients who are not responding to antipsychotics alone.

■ *Detoxification of alcohol dependence*. A loading dose of benzodiazepine (e.g. chlordiazepoxide) is given to prevent or minimise withdrawal symptoms. The dose should be reduced gradually and stopped over a week.

The various types of benzodiazepines have similar pharmacological properties. The main distinction between them is:

Elimination half-life (the time required for the plasma drug concentration to decrease by half, i.e. the longer the half-life the less frequently the drug is given). Long half-life benzodiazepines such as chlordiazepoxide, diazepam and clobazam, have an average elimination half-life of 3 days, whereas short half-life, as in oxazepam, lorazepam, alprazolam, results in elimination in a few hours. The advantage of a long half-life drug is that the drug can be given once daily, and thus produces less severe withdrawal symptoms. The disadvantages are 'hangover', daytime sedation and difficulty with concentration. The advantages of short half-life drugs are that they produce much less 'hangover' and daytime sedation. Their disadvantage is the production of the more severe withdrawal symptoms that clients experience when they cease medication.

Potency. Different benzodiazepines have different potencies (the amount of milligrams (mg) required to achieve a clinical effect). The approximate equivalent doses, according to BNF (British Medical Association and the Royal Pharmaceutical Society of Great Britain Vol 38, 1999), of 5 mg of diazepam is shown in Box 6.7.

Box 6.7
Approximate equivalent dosage of diazepam 5 mg to different benzodiazepines

Chlordiazepoxide	15 mg
Lorazepam	0.5 mg
Loprazolam	0.5 mg–1 mg
Lormetazepam	0.5 mg–1 mg
Nitrazepam	5 mg
Oxazepam	15 mg
Temazepam	10 mg

Absorption of benzodiazepines is poor after intramuscular (IM) injection, except with lorazepam; thus, it is inappropriate to give diazepam intramuscularly in status epilepticus, but it is highly effective if it is given rectally.

Mechanism of action

Benzodiazepines act by potentiating the inhibitory neurotransmitter gamma-aminobutyric acid (GABA) on its receptors (benzodiazepine receptors), so releasing noradrenaline and serotonin so as to produce some sedative, anxiolytic and anticonvulsant effects.

Pharmacokinetics

Absorption (following oral administration) and the duration of response differ between one benzodiazepine and another. For example, diazepam is rapidly absorbed with rapid onset of action (reaching a peak concentration in about 1 hour), while oxazepam is absorbed slowly, taking about 3 hours to reach its peak concentration. These drugs are highly lipid soluble and highly protein bound, they are metabolised in the liver and excreted by the kidneys.

Undesirable effects

Generally, benzodiazepines are safe drugs, and well tolerated when taken in therapeutic dose. Their side-effects include:

- *Sedation.* This is a common side-effect, and in older people may produce poor memory, poor concentration, poor motor coordination and confusion.

- *Next day hangover, drowsiness and light-headedness.* These are also common, particularly with long acting benzodiazepines.

- *Paradoxical effects.* These include an increase in hostility, whilst anxiety may be reported by some clients taking benzodiazepines.

- *Tolerance to the sedative effects.* This is likely to develop, usually after few weeks is use, leading the client to request an increase in the dose to obtain the same effect of the original dose; this usually leads to dependence.

Withdrawal symptoms

Sudden discontinuation of benzodiazepines usually causes withdrawal symptoms, even after only a few weeks usage. These include: anxiety, irritability, insomnia, tremors, palpitations, vertigo, sweating, nausea and panic attacks. Sudden discontinuation of a large dose may cause seizures and paranoid behaviour. The withdrawal symptoms usually begin within 24 hours with short acting benzodiazepines and up to 6 days later with long acting benzodiazepines.

To avoid or minimise the withdrawal symptoms, benzodiazepines should be slowly tapered off, after changing a short acting drug to an equivalent daily dose of diazepam (a long acting benzodiazepine; see Box 6.7, above).

Overdose

Benzodiazepines are safe when taken alone, especially in young healthy adults, but can be fatal if taken with other CNS depressant substances (for example alcohol). Clients who have taken an overdose (e.g. diazepam 100 mg) become drowsy and fall asleep for more than 24 hours. They may develop dysarthria (Hojer 1994). Flumazenil, a benzodiazepine antagonist, may be used, especially in the differential diagnosis of unclear cases of multiple drug overdose.

Drug interactions

Apart from potentiating sedative effects of psychotropic drugs, alcohol and antihistamines, benzodiazepines generally show few serious drug interactions.

Barbiturates   These drugs act in a similar way to benzodiazepines but are rarely used as anxiolytics or hypnotics because of their toxic side-effects, serious drug interactions, potency (causing dependence) and dangers in overdose (causing respiratory depression that cannot be reversed and can be fatal). Currently their use is restricted to anaesthesia, using very short acting barbiturates such as methohexitone in short surgical procedures. Long acting barbiturate phenobarbitone is used in status epilepticus when benzodiazepine fails; some paediatricians still use phenobarbitone for the treatment of epilepsy in neonates.

Buspirone   This is an effective anti-anxiety drug, but it does not alleviate the anxiety symptoms of benzodiazepine withdrawal. It acts at specific serotonin receptors, and usually takes 2–3 weeks to work; thus it is not useful when used on a 'prescribe when needed' basis. This drug is not sedative and it does not appear to cause tolerance or dependence. Side-effects are common but not serious; they include dizziness, nausea, headache, nervousness, lightheadedness and excitement.

Zopiclone and zolpidem   Both are non benzodiazpine hypnotics, but act on the same receptors as benzodiazepines. They are as effective as benzodiazepine and are becoming popular hypnotics. They are well tolerated with mild side-effects, and have short half-life (4–6 hours), thus causing less hangover on the following day. It has been claimed that these two products are less addictive than benzodiazepines.

Other anxiolytics, include:

- Chloral hydrate
- Bromide
- Paraldehyde
- Meprobamate
- Chlormethiazole.

These are not commonly used, as they are less effective than benzodiazepine, more hazardous in overdose, and cause tolerance and dependence. They are not described in this chapter.

Mood stabilisers

These include:

- Lithium
- Carbamazepine
- Sodium valproate.

Lithium   Lithium is a salt, and was first used to treat gout at the end of the 19th century, but its use was soon stopped due to its toxic effects. John Cade in 1949 used it again but in a smaller dose and found it useful in mania. Lithium comes in two forms:

1. Lithium carbonate: e.g. Camcolit (Norgine), Priadel (Delandale), Lithonate (Berk) and Liskonum (Smith Kline Beecham)

2. Lithium citrate: e.g. Litarex (Dumex), Li-liquid (Rosemont), or Priadel (Delandale).

These preparations are equally effective in treating mania, but the bioavailability of different preparations is different. Lithium should therefore be prescribed by brand name.

Indications

Lithium is used in the treatment and prophylaxis of mania, prevention of relapse in manic-depressive illness, in the prophylaxis of recurrent depression, and for aggressive and self-injurious behaviour. In acute cases of mania, a combination of an antipsychotic and lithium is often recommended as the clinical response of lithium may take up to 2 weeks. Lithium should be discontinued after 6 weeks if clients show no improvement.

Before commencing lithium, it is important to check urea and electrolyte levels, undertake thyroid function tests, a full blood count, ECG and pregnancy test as indicated.

After commencing lithium, its serum should be checked weekly (blood should be taken for the test 10–12 hours after the last dose of lithium) until the level is stable. Then the frequency of serum monitoring should be reduced gradually to once every 6 months. The therapeutic range of serum lithium for prophylaxis is different than that for treating acute cases. For the former it should be 0.8–1.0 mmol/l, while for the latter serum lithium should be 0.9–1.4 mmol/l. Immediate checking of the serum lithium is required when there are signs of toxicity, relapse, vomiting and diarrhoea, or when changing the preparation of the drugs. Other tests, such as thyroid function, should be made every 6 months, and if low, thyroxine may be added rather than stopping the lithium. Urea, electrolytes, FBC, creatinine, ECG and calcium levels should be performed once a year.

Undesirable effects

Fine tremors, thirst, polyuria, dry mouth, weight gain, nausea, diarrhoea and poor memory may occur with the serum lithium at the normal range. Hypothyrodism occurs in about 20% of patients, and 5% develop thyroid gland enlargement.

Long-term lithium use is associated with hyperparathyroidism and hypercalcaemia. Persistent impairment of the concentrating ability of kidney occurs in 10% of cases, but this usually recovers when the drug is stopped.

Toxic effects

These are closely related to serum levels, and usually occur at serum levels over 2 mmol/l. The features are vomiting, diarrhoea, dehydration, ataxia, muscle twitching, coarse tremor, slurred speech, nystagmus and confusion; this can progress to coma, convulsions and death. The treatment depends on the severity of toxicity. Lithium should be stopped immediately and the client rehydrated by increasing fluid and sodium chloride intake. If the serum level exceeds 3 mmol/l, renal dialysis is indicated.

Drug interactions and other effects

■ Thiazide diuretics can precipitate lithium toxicity as they reduce the excretion of lithium.

■ Lithium should be stopped at least 24 hours prior to surgery as muscle relaxant effects are enhanced.

■ Vomiting, diarrhoea or excessive sweating all precipitate lithium toxicity.

Carbamazepine

This is an anticonvulsant drug, but recently it has shown that it is as effective as lithium in the prophylaxis and treatment of mania, and other affective disorders. It also appears to be particularly effective in rapid cycling manic-depressive illness (four or more affective episodes per year). It is used alone, or in combination with lithium, in clients unresponsive to lithium alone or in resistant affective disorders.

Undesirable effects

Ataxia, diplopia, dizziness and nausea are common, particularly with rapid dose titration. Thus the dose should be increased gradually, that is, 100 mg daily increased by 100 mg every third day until the client responds or starts having side-effects. A skin rash is a common side-effect and the drug should only be discontinued if the condition worsens or is accompanied by other symptoms.

Drug interactions

- Carbamazepine level can be increased by erythromycin and lithium causing toxicity

- Carbamazepine level decreases when phenytoin and/or theophylline are simultaneously prescribed.

Sodium valproate

This is another anticonvulsant drug that can be used successfully in the treatment of affective disorders. It can be used alone, or with lithium, in cases responding poorly to lithium alone. Its common side-effects are tremor, nausea, sedation and weight gain. Transient hair loss or thrombocytopenia may also occur.

Stimulants

This class of drugs was much used in the past for the treatment of fatigue, depressive illness and obesity but they are no longer recommended to treat these conditions because of their side-effects. Their use became very limited, mainly indicated in adult clients with narcolepsy and in children with hyperkinetic syndrome. The side-effects include insomnia, anxiety, palpitations, restlessness, tremors, poor appetite and weight loss; they can cause cardiac arrhythmias. Large doses can cause schizophrenic-like symptoms, aggressive behaviour, disorientation, convulsion and coma.

Non-psychotropic drugs

Beta-blockers

There are many beta-blockers available to physicians to prescribe and all appear equally effective. However, they have different medical and psychiatric indications. Psychiatrically they have been used for anxiety states dominated by autonomic symptoms (e.g. palpitation, tremors, flushing and sweating). These drugs do not affect psychological symptoms such as fear, worry, and muscle tension. Beta-blockers can be combined with other anti-anxiety drugs in treating chronic anxiety. Other indications include tremors induced by lithium or akathisia caused by antipsychotics.

Cautions and undesirable effects

Beta-blockers should be avoided in clients with a history of asthma as they may precipitate bronchospasms. They should be used with caution in diabetic clients as they prevent recognition of hypoglycaemia. The main side-effects are bradycardia that may precipitate cardiac failure, and fatigue, coldness of the extremities and sleep disturbances with nightmares.

Antimuscarinic drugs

These are also called antiparkinsonian and anticholinergic; they are used both in Parkinson's disease and for extrapyramidal side-effects caused by antipsychotic drugs (but not tardive dyskinesia or akathisia). There are different preparations available that all appear equally effective, and these include benzhexol, procyclidine, benztropine, orphenadrine and biperiden. These drugs should not be given routinely with antipsychotics, as they may increase the risk of tardive dyskinesia. Their side-effects include: dry mouth, constipation, blurred vision and urinary retention in men, and with high doses may cause disorientation, hallucinations and excitement, particularly in elderly people.

Disulfiram (Antabuse)

This drug is used in aversion therapy in alcohol dependence. It causes unpleasant reactions if taken with even small amounts of alcohol. This reaction is caused by an accumulation of acetaldehyde, and may cause flushing, headache, nausea, palpitation, sweating, hyperventilation and dyspnoea. Clients must be informed about this drug in full, and the treatment should be started at least 12 hours after the last consumption of alcohol. This drug should not be given to clients with recent heart disease or who exhibit suicidal impulsive behaviours.

Citrated calcium carbimide is used in the same way as disulfiram, but it has milder reactions when taken with alcohol

Electro-convulsive therapy

Treating some psychiatric conditions by inducing seizures has a long history. The first chemical used in inducing seizures to treat depression was camphor. Then metrazol was used to induce seizures in schizophrenics. This was based on the erroneous belief that schizophrenia does not affect people with epilepsy. Later, in the 1930s, Cerletti and Bini replaced the toxic pharmacoconvulsive therapy by electrical therapy. Initially, it was given without anaesthesia and muscle relaxants, but since then many changes have been applied that have included the gradual modification of the use of anaesthesia, muscle relaxant, oxygenation, and then using unilateral electrode placement and low energy stimuli. Negative images of this treatment remain, despite the development of many modern techniques for the administration of electroconvulsive therapy (ECT).

Indications

The use of ECT is currently limited to depression, mania and catatonic schizophrenia:

- *Depression*. ECT is highly recommended in depression, particularly when there are concomitant psychotic symptoms, stupor, high suicidal risk and when the client is not responding to other treatments. A series of studies comparing real and simulated ECT (anaesthesia and muscle relaxant only) showed a significant advantage for real over simulated treatment. Also, antidepressants were compared with ECT and it was found that ECT was superior to antidepressants (Greenblatt et al 1964, Medical Research Council 1965).

- *Mania*. In mania, ECT is indicated only in cases that are severe, prolonged, and not responding to other therapies.

- *Catatonic schizophrenia*. This type of schizophrenia is characterised by motor symptoms such as stupor and excitement. In stupor, the client is immobile, mute and unresponsive but fully conscious. Often clients change quickly to a state of excitement and uncontrolled activity. This condition is rare, but potentially fatal from exhaustion, dehydration or self-inflicted injury. ECT can be lifesaving when the condition is not responding to antipsychotic drugs.

All the procedures of the treatment must be discussed with the client, including a brief account of ECT, the number of treatments required, and the possible side-effects. There are special requirements concerning people who are detained for treatment and/or assessment under the Mental Health Act (1983) (see also Ch. 3 for a consideration of the ethical and legal aspects of the use of such treatment).

Undesirable effects

ECT is generally safe, and can be safer than antidepressants, particularly in the older population. Its side-effects are usually mild, transient and not serious. They include nausea, headache and bodyache. Amnesia, which can be troublesome, is usually transient and resolves in 1–2 weeks. This effect is less marked after unilateral ECT. The mortality rate is very low, and is mostly due to anaesthesia rather than ECT; it represents about 3 in 100 000 (Barker & Barker 1959), which is equivalent to the mortality found in dental outpatient's anaesthesia.

Psychosurgery

This term refers to the use of neurosurgery to treat psychiatric disorders. This does not include those who have a pathological lesion in the brain causing the disorder, for example epilepsy or tumours.

Psychosurgery began in the 1930s, when Jacobson and Fullon found that destruction of the frontal lobes of chimpanzees produced changes in their adaptive behaviours. This surgery was gradually developed and then applied to human beings to treat severe intractable cases of obsessive-compulsive disorder, anxiety and depression with some success, but had serious postoperative complications. The mortality rate is about 4%, postoperative epilepsy occurs in 30%, while personality changes occur in 40% of cases. In the 1950s, before the discovery of active psychotropic drugs, thousands of such operations were performed in the UK and the USA.

As the active psychotropic medications are only effective in 60–70% of psychiatric cases, and also have serious short- and long-term side-effects, and some of these are serious, surgeons who were interested in psychosurgery developed a modern technique called stereotactic technique by inserting probes under X-ray guidance to destroy the chosen site of lesion in the brain. The postoperative complications of the newer techniques are minimal compared to the older forms. The mortality rate is very low, the epilepsy rate is about 1% and personality changes are unlikely to occur, but the efficacy of the technique is not clear as there are no randomised controlled studies to test its value. Psychosurgery is therefore only indicated for a minority of chronic, severe intractable cases of obsessive-compulsive disorder, depression and anxiety that have failed to respond to prolonged and vigorous treatment.

Compliance with treatment

Non-compliance is a common problem and this is often underestimated. Many clients do not take their medication as they should. It has been estimated that half of outpatients and a quarter of inpatients were not complying with their medication regimes (Kaplan & Sadock 1995)

The causes of non-compliance are numerous and include:

- Side-effects, particularly when the patient is not counselled
- Multiple medications with different doses and different frequencies of uses
- Those living alone
- Maladaptive personality traits
- Presence of psychiatric disorders such as schizophrenia and depression
- The expense of treatment.

The Drug and Therapeutics Bulletin (1981) recommended informing the clients of the following:

- Name of the drug
- The importance of its use

■ How to tell if it is working and what to do if it appears not to be working
■ The frequency of its use, before or after food
■ What to do if a dose is missed
■ The duration of its use
■ The side-effects and what to do about them
■ Possible effects on driving, work, etc., and what precautions to take
■ The interactions with other drugs and alcohol.

It is helpful if this information and the Royal College of Psychiatrists' patient information fact sheets (see resources at the end of the chapter) are collated in a series of leaflets and given to every client diagnosed with mental illness where there is underlying behavioural distress.

Conclusion

The use of chemotherapy is, as said at the outset of this chapter, one of the easiest ways of controlling behavioural difficulties. With the exception of their use in emergencies, drugs should only be used after a thorough assessment by a psychiatrist and after clients have been counselled about the possible short- and long-term side-effects and the approximate duration of the use of the medication.

The use of antipsychotic medications is essential in schizophrenia and other related psychotic illnesses. In neurotic disorders such as generalised anxiety, phobias, post-traumatic stress disorder (PTSD) and obsessive-compulsive disorder (OCD) the use of medications can be helpful, but they should be used with other psychological therapies, as the relapse rate is high on discontinuation of the drugs.

Finally, all clients on long-term use of psychotropic medication require regular follow ups to monitor their mental state and review the dose and the side-effects of the medication they are receiving.

Two case illustrations showing the use of medications follow; the first illustrates inappropriate use of medication, and the second presents some of the unpleasant side-effects that might be encountered when taking medication.

Man with learning disability

A 62-year-old man with moderate learning disability was admitted to a long stay hospital 6 years ago, as his mother, his main carer, was unable to look after him. His behaviour gradually deteriorated into abusive shouts and screaming, physical aggression towards the staff and other clients, and throwing things. He became slightly withdrawn and isolated. There was no problem with his sleep pattern or appetite. No abnormality was found on physical examination or on basic blood tests. The cause of the learning disability was anoxia at birth. He had no history of mental illness, epilepsy or behavioural difficulties, nor had his family. The initial diagnosis of this man was challenging behaviour due to the change in his place of residence, and probably missing his mother. Various supportive and behaviour therapies were applied but failed to improve his behaviour. This client was tried on several antipsychotics and benzodiazepines to control his behaviour for a number of years with minimum effect. An antidepressant drug was then prescribed, and he responded dramatically and in 2 weeks was back to his 'normal' self. The antipsychotic and the benzodiazepine were then discontinued gradually with no deterioration in his condition.

Man with learning disability *cont'd*

Comments
Behavioural difficulties in people with learning disabilities are common, affecting about 15% of the adult population. The causes are numerous and include discomfort or physical pain, which may then lead to behavioural distress. Some clients may be unable to communicate their feelings and this may consequently affect their behaviour. Psychiatric disorders are four times more common in this population than in the general population. Disorders are often underdiagnosed, particularly depressive illnesses, as their presentation is not always typical. Medication such as benzodiazepine may promote a paradoxical increase in hostility and aggression. Various unpleasant side-effects of antipsychotic or other drugs can precipitate behavioural difficulties, especially when clients are unable to complain about such effects. Thus the management of behavioural difficulties always requires particularly thorough investigation, as mentioned earlier in this chapter.

Woman with chronic anxiety

A 35-year-old woman suffered from severe chronic anxiety. Her symptoms fluctuated, being sometimes slightly better or slightly worse, depending on various emotional and/or external stimuli. She was experiencing anxiety symptoms, with dominant autonomic symptoms such as palpitations, sweating and shakes that were more marked on the lower extremities. She was on a small dose of trifluoperazine (2 mg three times a day) for a number of months with little effect. The dose of the trifluoperazine was then increased further to 5 mg three times daily with a view to control her anxiety and agitation, but the shakes became even worse. Reassessment of the condition paid special attention to the physical symptoms, their severity, and any change in the nature of her problems. The assessment revealed that this lady suffered from marked akathisia on top of her mild anxiety state.

Comments
Akathisia is one of the extrapyramidal side-effects of antipsychotic drugs. It occurs in up to 20% of clients, usually after a week or two (possibly longer) of treatment. It is characterised by motor restlessness, usually affecting the lower limbs. Clients describe it as an unpleasant feeling, and they cannot relax or keep still. In severe cases, clients find it difficult to fall asleep, as they are unable to lie still long enough. The mild form of akathisia involves a feeling of inner restlessness only.

To differentiate between akathisia and anxiety or other psychiatric disorders it must be noted that in akathisia clients usually have difficulty describing feelings of discomfort and they are unable to understand why they feel distressed. Akathisia is also closely associated with antipsychotic treatment. It becomes worse with an increase in the dose of the antipsychotic drug, and better with a reduction or discontinuation of the drug. Akathisia does not respond to antimuscarinic drugs such as procyclidine.

The best way of treating this condition is by stopping or reducing the dose of the drugs. If the client requires antipsychotic treatment, then atypical treatments should be tried. Benzodiazepines and beta-blockers have also been reported to be of benefit in some cases (Ratey & Salzman 1984, Adler et al 1989).

Further reading

British Medical Association and the Royal Pharmaceutical Society of Great Britain 1999 The British national formulary. BNF Number 38. British Medical Association and the Royal Pharmaceutical Society of Great Britain, London

This is one of the best books for rapid reference concerning all drugs that are licensed for prescription in the UK. It provides doctors and other health care professionals with brief but valuable information about the use of medicines. Six-monthly joint updates are prepared by the British Medical Association and the Royal Pharmaceutical Society of Great Britain.

Freeman C P 1995 The ECT handbook: second report of the Royal College of Psychiatrists special committee on ECT. Council Report CR39. Royal College of Psychiatry, London

This useful handbook has been approved by the council of the Royal College of Psychiatrists. It focuses on the main clinical indications, as well as providing clear guidelines for psychiatrists who will be prescribing or administering ECT. It is an up-to-date publication that produces appendices covering developments in this field which are periodically reviewed.

Kaplan H I, Sadock B J 1998 Synopsis of psychiatry, 8th edn. Williams and Wilkins, Baltimore

This useful textbook is detailed, easy to read, global in depth and scope, and covers most subjects in psychiatry, including behavioural sciences, clinical psychiatry and therapeutics. It is designed for psychiatrists and those who work in the field of psychiatry.

Lader M, Herrington R 1996 Biological treatments in psychiatry, 2nd edn. Oxford University Press, Oxford

A good psychopharmacology book, full of useful information. It provides clear guidelines about the use of drugs in psychiatry. This book can be an essential guide for those involved in the care of clients taking psychotropic medications.

Read S G 1997 Psychiatry in learning disability. Saunders London

This relatively new book for the field of learning disabilities covers most aspects of psychiatry. It presents a range of psychiatric disorders and how they are managed in learning disabilities.

Reiss S, Aman G (eds) 1998 Psychotropic medications and developmental disabilities: the international consensus handbook. Ohio State University, Ohio

This excellent publication provides a most authoritative account of mental disorder in learning disabilities. The book comprises three parts that cover aspects of diagnosis, epidemiology, drug interactions, and specific medications used in the field of learning disabilities.

References

Adler L A, Angrist B, Reiter S, Rotroson J 1989 Neuroleptic-induced akathesia: a review. Psychopharmacology 97: 1–11

Akhtar S, Jajor T R, Kumar S 1993 Vitamin E in the treatment of tardive dyskinesia. Journal of Postgraduate Medicine 39(3): 124–126

Ball J R B, Kiloh L G 1959 A controlled trial of imipramine in the treatment of depressive states. British Medical Journal ii: 1052–1055

Barker J C, Barker A A 1959 Deaths associated with electroplexy. Journal of Mental Science 105: 339–348

Barraclough B, Bunch J, Nelson B, Sainsbury P 1974 A hundred cases of suicide: clinical aspects. British Journal of Psychiatry 125: 355–373

British Medical Association and the Royal Pharmaceutical Society of Great Britain 1999 The British national formulary. BNF Number 38. British Medical Association and the Royal Pharmaceutical Society of Great Britain, London

Drug and Therapeutics Bulletin 1981 What should we tell patients about their medicines? Drugs and Therapeutics Bulletin 19: 73–74

Fara M, Davidson K G 1996 Definition and epidemiology of treatment-resistant depression. Psychiatric Clinics of North America 19: 179–195

Gostason R 1985 Psychiatric illness among the mentally retarded: a Swedish population study. Acta Psychiatrica Scandinavica 318(71): 1–117

Greenblatt M, Grosser G H, Wechler H 1962 A comparative study of selected antidepressant medications and ECT. American Journal of Psychiatry 119: 144–153

Greenblatt M, Grosser G H, Wechsler H 1964 Differential response of hospitalized depressed patients in somatic therapy. American Journal of Psychiatry 120: 935–943

Halmi K A, Eckert E, La Du T J, Cohen J 1986 Anorexia nervosa treatment efficacy of cyproheptadine and amitriptyline. Archives of General Psychiatry 43: 177–181

Helzer J C, Robins L N, McEvoy L 1987 Post-traumatic stress disorder in the general population: findings of the Epidemiological Catchment Area survey. New England Journal of Medicine 317: 1630–1634

Hojer J 1994 Management of benzodiazepine overdoses. CNS Drugs 2: 7–17

Jus K, Jus A, Gautier J et al 1974 Studies of the actions of certain pharmacological agents on tardive dyskinesia and on the rabbit syndrome. International Journal of Clinical Pharmacology, Therapeutics and Toxicology 9: 138–145

Kaplan H I, Sadock B J 1995 Comprehensive textbook of psychiatry, 6th edn. Williams and Wilkins, Baltimore

Kendell R E, Zealley A K 1993 Companion to psychiatric studies, 5th edn. Churchill Livingstone, Edinburgh

Klein D F, Gittelman R, Quitkin F H, Rifkin A 1980 Diagnosis and drug treatment of psychiatric disorders: adults and children. Williams and Wilkins, Baltimore

Kushlik A, Cox G R 1973 The epidimiology of mental handicap. Developmental Medicine and Child Neurology 15: 748–759

Lohr J B, Caligiuri M P 1996 A double-blind placebo controlled study of vitamin E treatment of tardive dyskinesia. Journal of Clinical Psychiatry 57: 167–173

Medical Research Council 1965 Chemical trial of the treatment of depressive illness. British Medical Journal i: 881–886

Ratey J J, Salzman C 1984 Recognizing and managing akathesia. Hospital and Community Psychiatry 35: 975–977

Regier D A, Boyd J H, Burke J D et al 1988 One-month prevalence of mental disorders in the United States, based on five Epidemiologic Catchment Area sites. Archives of General Psychiatry 45: 977–986

Robins E, Murphy G E, Wilkinson R H, Gassner S, Kayes J 1959 Some clinical considerations in the prevention of suicide based on a study of 134 successful suicides. American Journal of Public Health 49: 888–899

Schildkraut J J 1965 The catecholamine hypothesis of affective disorders: a review of supporting evidence. American Journal of Psychiatry 122: 509–522

Weschler H, Grosser G H, Greenblatt M 1965 Research evaluating antidepressant medication on hospitalization mental patients: a survey of published reports during a five year period. Journal of Nervous and Mental Disease 4: 231–239

Wing L 1971 Severely retarded children in a London area: prevalence and provision of services. Psychological Medicine 1: 405–415

World Health Organization 1992 International Classification of Mental and Behavioural Disorders ICD-10. WHO, Geneva

Resources

A number of contact points are identified that will provide additional information on various aspects of mental illnesses and their treatment. For example the Royal College of Psychiatrists provides a range of excellent fact sheets that are useful for both lay people and professional carers.

The Royal College of Psychiatrists
www.rcpsych.ac.uk
17 Belgrave Square
London, SW1 8PG
Tel: 0207 235 2351

British Institute of Learning Disabilities
www.bild.org.uk
Wolverhampton Road
Kidderminster
Worcs
Tel: 01562 850251

The Arc of the United States
http://Thearc.org/welcome.html
500 East Border Street
Suite 300
Arlington
Texas 76010
USA
Tel: 1 817 261 6003

American Association on Mental Retardation
http://www.aamr.org
444 North Capitol Street NW
Suite 846
Washington DC 20001-1512
USA
Tel: +1 202 387 1968

7 Gentle Teaching

Siobhan O'Rourke and Jane Wray

Key issues
- Gentle Teaching is an approach to working with people with learning disabilities that is based upon unconditional valuing of others and places relationships at the centre of learning and development
- The approach is based upon humanistic psychology and incorporates non-aversive strategies to promote client independence and mutually liberating relationships
- Values such as respect, equity and mutual change lie at the core of Gentle Teaching and the approach requires an explicit adherence to these values for change to occur
- Research into the effectiveness of Gentle Teaching remains equivocal, although services continue to advocate its use

Overview

Gentle Teaching is a therapeutic approach that was first developed working with people with learning disabilities. The approach is based on the unconditional valuing of others, and places relationships at the centre of learning and development. The chapter commences with an explanation of the philosophy and values underlying Gentle Teaching, and documents the development of this approach. The evolution of the approach from a non-aversive behavioural position to an emergent humanistic approach is also described. Using case illustrations, the practical application of the approach is demonstrated, and in particular, how the approach can be used to work with people who display behavioural distress. Finally, available research evidence is discussed and the relative strengths and weaknesses of the approach are explored.

Gentle Teaching

The approach is based on the unconditional valuing of others and it requires carers to question their own attitudes, behaviour and responses towards the people they care for. It incorporates a non-aversive strategy that aims to promote complex, meaningful relationships between client and carer, and in this respect it is considered to go beyond behavioural techniques (see Ch. 9), whose focus is often merely to eradicate unwanted behaviour. Gentle Teaching is considered a practical way of helping people to live meaningful and purposeful lives, and it uses specific techniques and procedures to achieve these objectives. Gentle Teaching seeks to reach out to people who are alienated from others and invites them to participate in relationships built on the safety and security of interdependence. One of the principle proponents of Gentle Teaching, John McGee, has described the approach (McGee et al 1987) as follows:

> *Gentle Teaching is based upon a posture that centers itself on the mutual liberation and humanisation of all persons, a posture that strives for human solidarity and one that leads care givers to teach bonding to those who attempt to distance themselves from meaningful human interactions. It is a pedagogical process that rejects cruel and cold practices and focuses on teaching the value inherent in human presence, human interactions and human reward.*

[p. 11]

Gentle Teaching's philosophy assumes that each person's value is inherent, that their value exists simply in being human. In Gentle Teaching, this philosophy is encapsulated in a new attitude or posture; carers work in partnership with people with learning disabilities. Gentle Teaching views people as social beings, and its definition of a person includes reference to the existence of others and the relationship that exists between people. People who are displaying behavioural distress and behavioural difficulties (challenging behaviour) are therefore approached within the context of their relationships. The success of an intervention based upon Gentle Teaching is determined by the extent to which parties involved in a relationship move towards a more functional form of interaction – that is, the extent to which they have ceased relating in maladaptive ways and are participating in life and living interdependently.

Gentle Teaching was first applied in the field of learning disabilities, and in particular with those clients who displayed behavioural distress. Gentle Teaching recognises that learning disabilities affect people's cognitive functioning, with consequences for the way in which they perceive the world and express themselves to the world. Also, people can be affected as much by the way the world sees them as they are by their actual disability. Supporting and empowering a person with learning disabilities can require additional understanding and skill on the part of carers. In the past it was not at all unusual for people with learning disabilities who experienced behavioural distress to have also experienced relationships that were both unfair and controlling. There are three common ways that this tendency towards control can be expressed within the 'practitioner' or 'carer' relationship. In Gentle Teaching these are called maladaptive postures (see Box 7.1).

The three maladaptive postures shown in Box 7.1 all lack the possibility of reciprocity and shared learning in a relationship. In Gentle Teaching, the practitioner assumes a 'posture of solidarity', and this is characterised by warmth, human presence, shared value and shared growth. It is a posture that enables people to accomplish in partnership things that cannot be accomplished individually. Gentle Teaching does, however, also encompass the adaptive elements of other postures: from authoritarianism it takes gentle leadership; from 'over-protectiveness' it takes safety and security; from coldness and distance it takes a sense of perspective. The central tenet of Gentle Teaching is that all human beings need to participate in reciprocal

Box 7.1
Maladaptive postures

> **The authoritarian posture**
> When a teacher relates to a distressed person from an authoritarian posture there is an underlying assumption that the practitioner knows best and that the only way positive change can occur is by the learner doing exactly what the teacher requires. This posture commonly involves the use of punishment and rewards. The availability of positive valuing is conditional upon the compliance of the learner.
>
> **The over-protective posture**
> Superficially this posture can appear to be very warm but the intention is to control the relationship and prevent the person from growing in ways that might destabilise the role of the practitioner as protector. The practitioner may stop asking the person to participate so as to avoid stimulating aggressive or self-injurious behaviour. This posture restricts growth and promotes dependence and vulnerability in the learner.
>
> **The cold and distant posture**
> Characterised by an apparent indifference to the well-being of the person, this posture assumes no real responsibility within the relationship and allows the person to discover the natural consequences of his or her actions. Where an agreed approach to supporting the person exists, this will be followed obediently without any concern for its effectiveness or fairness.

loving relationships and to participate with others in activities that comprise daily life. People who have difficulty with the former will often have difficulty with the latter and so activities are used as a tool to allow the relationship to unfold, and the relationship is used to support the development of participation.

It is not uncommon for texts on helping people who display behavioural distress to devote a chapter to the ethical issues that arise when offering support. Gentle Teaching does not separate ethics in this way. Gentle Teaching rests upon a humanistic philosophy, on which it builds a framework of values that seek to safeguard the dignity and humanity of all parties involved. The strategies and techniques are used within this framework of values. It is possible to encounter incompetence within any therapeutic approach, and Gentle Teaching is no exception. However, a practitioner who fails to value someone, who seeks to dominate, and who manipulates with rewards is not practising Gentle Teaching. It is possible (though not currently acceptable) to be a forceful or a controlling behaviour therapist without contravening the philosophy of behaviourism. It is not possible to do this and remain consistent with the approach of Gentle Teaching. Gentle Teaching developed as a moral reaction against unfair treatment, and therefore it stands as a check and balance for other systems whose internal logic does not embrace human relationships, their power dynamics and moral consequences.

The value system underlying Gentle Teaching

Values lie at the core of Gentle Teaching, and whilst its strategies share many similarities with other approaches (such as task analysis and the use of prompts and cues), it has an explicit and inherent commitment to positive values which is unusual.

Respect   Gentle Teaching understands respect to mean unconditional regard for the humanity of others. Respect is the awareness of other persons as self-conscious individuals who are 'complete' and 'whole' in themselves. This is in contrast to other approaches which focus on strengths, needs, skills and behaviours. Simply to be aware of being in the presence of another person whose humanity is exactly like yours is a profound and powerful introduction to new ways of reaching out to people in behavioural distress.

Equity   Gentle Teaching acknowledges that people have different needs and skills. Equality is therefore an ideal rarely attained or maintained in relationships. Equity, however, is an acknowledgement of the equal worth of the individual's contribution to a relationship, regardless of their skills or behaviour. A person who finds it difficult to trust others or to tolerate the presence of others may express a willingness to relate simply by remaining in the room, or by returning to the scene of an activity. This is of enormous value to the development of relationship, and needs to be noticed, acknowledged, welcomed and warmly praised.

Mutual change   When the focus of an intervention is on a relationship, it makes sense for both people to change. The distressed person may have spent years located in a spiral of isolation and hostility and is unlikely to initiate positive change. It is therefore up to a practitioner or teacher to begin this process. Some changes are 'changes of heart', that is, a shift in general attitude. Others can be very practical and specific, such as a change in the way the person is invited to participate, the practitioner learning to speak more gently or to express more enthusiasm. Every Gentle Teaching practitioner has his or her own individual style of self-expression: some are reserved, others gregarious, some very tactile, others less so. Within the range of our own natural expression we need to develop a sensitivity and responsiveness to the specific and changing needs of the individual. We cannot distort our own way of communicating; neither should we impose our style, disregarding the mood or personality of the other person.

The history and development of gentle teaching   The term 'gentle teaching' first appeared in professional journals in 1985 (McGee 1985a, 1985b, 1985c), but the ideas behind this approach can be traced to a paper by Menolascino & McGee (1983) that appeared in the *Journal of Psychiatric Treatment and Evaluation*. This paper suggested that the then current practice for dealing with severe behavioural problems for people with learning disabilities (psychoactive medication and applied behaviour analysis) was inadequate and inappropriate. The authors outlined a list of behavioural practices considered 'inhumane'; these included such techniques as the use of cattle prods, stun guns and ammonia spray.

When Gentle Teaching first appeared it rejected the then predominant homo-fabian model of mankind that stated that a person's value was seen in terms of deeds done (i.e. skills only). Gentle Teaching had much in common with other important contemporary developments that affected the lives of people with learning disabilities; these included the principles of 'normalisation' (Wolfenberger 1972) and the development of the disability rights and advocacy movements. Gentle Teaching responded to what Wolfenberger had highlighted as an important need in his development of social role valorisation (SRV): the formulation of a qualitative language (or posture) that attempted to prevent people with learning disabilities from being devalued and oppressed. Gentle Teaching also had much in common with humanistic psychology, and in particular the views of Rogers (1951) and Maslow (1954) and the fundamental right to self-actualisation for all people. A comparison of some aspects of psychodynamic, behavioural, humanistic and cognitive psychology can be found in Table 1.1 (Ch. 1).

Proponents of Gentle Teaching have argued that aversive procedures, typically, were ineffective, produced only temporary suppression of behaviour, were frequently associated with negative side-effects, were highly likely to be misused or abused, and lastly, were simply not necessary (Coe & Matson 1990). Gentle Teaching became clearly identified as part of the anti-aversive lobby and proclaimed its rejection of:

> *the hierarchical approach of traditional pedagogy and the authoritarian approach of behaviourism.*

[Stainton 1993, p. 29]

The use of aversive practices in the care and treatment of people with learning disabilities culminated in publicly debated court cases that centred upon inattention to human rights. The ethical concerns raised by the use of 'aversive' procedures led to several American states outlawing aversive behavioural interventions. Concern over the appropriateness of aversive techniques in the care and treatment of people with learning disabilities was at its peak when John McGee published his book *Gentle Teaching: A Non-Aversive Approach for Helping People with Mental Retardation* (McGee et al 1987).

Gentle Teaching was seen as representative of a larger movement that called for the abandonment of aversive procedures and a move towards a more humanistic perspective. Gentle Teaching questioned the behavioural approach for its focus upon behaviour and not the person, and its inattention to the rights of people with learning disabilities. Historically, behaviours considered challenging or difficult were modified and reduced using a range of behavioural strategies. Gentle Teaching gained increasing popularity with its novel approach to care:

> *The goal is not to eliminate the behaviour per se, but to instil in the client a new set of values that will result in mutually humanising and liberating interactions between the client and the caregiver.*

[Jones et al 1990, p. 216]

The practical application of Gentle Teaching

The primary focus of Gentle Teaching practice is the quality of people's relationships with others, and the quality of their daily life. Although some information gathering takes place before the work of Gentle Teaching commences, the emphasis is very much on beginning a gradual process of change. The Gentle Teaching practitioner seeks to develop a relationship with the person being helped. Defining the care-giving relationship is often extremely difficult as much debate goes on in care services about whether there is a distinction between care professionals and users. Gentle Teaching proposes a form of professionalism that includes genuine connection with people as opposed to detachment. Gentle Teaching holds that a relationship between care giver and service user can encompass warmth, genuine human connection and unconditional valuing, without in any way compromising the legitimate role of the care professional.

The next section of this chapter outlines the practical application of Gentle Teaching and focuses upon four key areas: gathering information, introducing participation through the use of activities, finding the 'entry point' and dealing with behavioural distress.

Gathering information

The Gentle Teaching practitioner will discover most about the other person through talking to him or her, rather than by prior analysis of information. Three important questions must be asked:

- How does the person participate?
- How does the person communicate?
- How does the person relate to others?

By asking these questions of the person's care givers, the practitioner gains powerful insights, not only into the life of the person, but also into the beliefs and attitudes of the care givers. Carers who support people with behavioural distress are often very focused on the harm caused by the behaviour, and forget to step back and look at the person's life. Frequently, in answering these simple questions, care givers may remember traumas the person has experienced, losses suffered and the lack of meaningful daily activity, as well as the paucity of human relationships in their lives.

By being with the person and noticing the person's posture, body language and facial expressions, a practitioner can gain a sense of 'who' the person is. When one concentrates on the deeds of a person, one risks neglecting the agent of these actions. Some simple human communication can originate from merely offering a warm human presence at a proximity and of a duration that feels safe for both parties. The practitioner can become aware of a person's anxiety, excitement, fear, distrust, pleasure or other emotion, and register a sense of how they are feeling. Participating with a person will also reveal much, especially about their skills, emotional state and tendency to communicate through behaviour that may be challenging.

It is common for people with learning difficulties and/or behavioural distress to have limited experience of life as it is ordinarily lived. This is even the case in small community settings, as well as in institutions. Knowing how people spend their time enables practitioners to understand them. Many people with learning disabilities are given detailed timetables listing a range of opportunities which are on offer. However, being offered an opportunity is not the same as actually taking part, and for many people the extent of the opportunities on offer does not reflect the actual quality of the participation. Most people referred for Gentle Teaching consultancy have the following experiences:

- They spend long periods of time being completely inactive.

- They are only willing to tolerate passive involvement.

- They prefer to be receptive rather than active, and select passive experiences (e.g. massage, listening to music) over interactive activities (e.g. playing football, washing the dishes).

- They participate exclusively on their terms ('it depends on his mood' or 'some days she'll get her own breakfast, other days she won't do a single thing for herself').

- They have limited experience of completing activities ('he can't concentrate on anything for long enough to finish it').

- They become stressed when asked to participate in an interactive activity.

The first case illustration ('John: gathering information to produce positive change') recounts the first named author's own experience with one individual who had limited experience of participating fully in life.

John: gathering information to produce positive change

John, a 19-year-old man, has lived in very different settings and had to leave all of them because of his self-injury and the extreme damage he has caused to property. By asking the three simple questions detailed opposite ('How does this person participate/communicate/relate to others?'), I was able to establish that John spent most of his day going for walks with staff. On further questioning it emerged that while he was on these walks he spent a lot of time collecting small pieces of 'rubbish' from the ground; they ranged from cigarette butts to leaves. When encouraged to drop the rubbish and move on he would bite his arm, sometimes causing the skin to break. John liked other activities including trampolining and cycling in the back garden. He liked to do these things according to his mood, and would cease doing them when he no longer felt like continuing. When encouraged to come in for a meal or move on to something new he often removed or tore his clothing and injured himself severely. Staff were trying, although with limited success, to teach a pictorial system of communication to John, who could not speak or use signs.

This profile suggested a young man who had very limited experience of interactive activity, whose life did not balance choice with responsibility, and who found transitions difficult. Because of the severity of his self-injury, and the staff's desire to make John feel safe and secure, staff very frequently followed John's lead and found themselves at a loss when he became frustrated and injured himself. As a Gentle Teaching practitioner, I focused on introducing simple daily activities to John in a structured, scheduled way while maintaining a warm, caring approach. (This Gentle Teaching response is explored in greater detail in 'Introducing participation', below.)

Sophisticated analyses of behaviour can often take months to reach a conclusion such as 'the function of this person's head-banging is to attract attention and to provide stimulation', or 'the function of this person's physical aggression is to avoid demanding activities'. For other approaches, the issue then revolves around satisfying that specific function, that is, providing attention or stimulation without reinforcing the behaviour. However, the gentle teaching approach suggests that it is much simpler, and feels more natural, to look compassionately at a person's life. Steps can then be taken to satisfy human need in ways that use structure, strategies and procedures in the service of those needs, rather than maintaining a focus on the behaviour.

Introducing participation through the use of activities

Ordinary activities form the major part of most people's lives, and it is through activities that our lives gain purpose, meaning and shape. Most people's lives are full of change and contrast. However, people with learning disabilities often have empty lives, one hour is much the same as another, morning is the same as evening, weekdays are no different from weekends. The absence of activities blocks the development of relationships, but a day filled with forced, meaningless activity can be just as futile as an inactive day. In order to interrupt destructive behaviour patterns, the practitioner has to initiate shared participation through the use of activities. Gentle Teaching sees activities as opportunities for bringing values into a person's life and chooses those activities that will provide the best opportunity for the Gentle Teaching process to take place. Usually, ordinary daily activities are chosen: examples of such activities include washing up, folding towels, filling the dishwasher, hanging out the washing, putting away the laundry and so on. Ideally, activities should be useful, interesting and age-appropriate, but where ordinary daily living activities are not available to the person, other activities can be adapted in order to help the person enjoy doing things with others. Box 7.2 outlines the key requirements of an activity that can be used to introduce Gentle Teaching.

Box 7.2
Choosing an activity

> The first activity should comprise the following elements:
> - Be simple
> - Be easily broken down into steps
> - Have a beginning, a middle and an end
> - Have repetitive sequences
> - Call for the use of materials
> - Be able to be done in a variety of places
> - Require active participation
> - Require two-way interaction
> - Have built in mini-breaks

Simple activities with sequences of repeated steps allow equal attention to be given to shared participation and to the relationship. Being too 'task centred' can make some people feel pressurised whilst, on the other hand, dwelling on relational aspects of interaction may feel too intense. The essential skill of Gentle Teaching is to introduce activities while at the same time generating opportunities for the expression of respect, equity and mutual change. Box 7.3 shows how the Gentle Teaching practitioner approaches the person in behavioural distress to commence an activity.

Box 7.3
Getting started with Gentle Teaching

> Before commencing an activity, the Gentle Teaching practitioner must remember to:
> - Approach the person with sensitivity and respect
> - Establish a positive rapport
> - Explain gently what is going to happen
> - Invite participation using materials as prompts
> - Demonstrate showing enjoyment and interest
> - Acknowledge and value the person's presence
> - Seek an entry point
> - Acknowledge and praise every sign of involvement
> - Balance shared valuing with shared participation

Complex activities may be well within a person's range of technical competence, but when introducing a new way of relating to someone in behavioural distress it is best to start with something simple that can easily be broken down into small steps. When an appropriate activity has been chosen by the practitioner, he or she then has to make both the environment and materials ready for the activity. The learner is not expected, or invited, to participate in this part of the work. The practitioner should estimate the approximate length of the activity (number of times/steps/turns) and communicate this clearly to the learner. It is important that an activity has a beginning, a middle and an end.

The beginning of the activity

When the activity is ready to commence, the learner is invited to become involved. The learner's involvement may be minimal at first (e.g. being present, watching, pointing) and should be warmly acknowledged ('it's lovely to have you here with me while I am doing [the activity]', or, 'I can see you watching – you know the next step in this activity don't you?').

The middle of an activity

As an activity progresses, the practitioner draws the learner's attention to the materials and says: 'We're halfway through now, only five steps more in this activity to go'. This helps the learner to gain a sense of how long the activity is going to last, and gives a sense of movement and progress by drawing attention to something that has already been accomplished. It also assures the learner that the end of the activity is approaching.

The end of the activity

It is sometimes common for care givers who are not using Gentle Teaching to try and motivate people by inviting them to do 'just one' step of an activity, and then ask them to do another, and another. In this situation, the person has no way of knowing how many steps they actually have to do, and as a result the individual may become very agitated and increasingly distressed. Consequently, the person learns to associate harmful behaviour with ending activities and gains little experience of completing a task successfully.

If the practitioner experiences difficulties during the activity, he or she may also find it useful to introduce 'mini-breaks', reduce demands or increase the amount of support given during the activity. Box 7.4 shows how support can be offered during an activity if the practitioner is experiencing difficulties introducing participation.

Box 7.4
During the activity

> If the practitioner is experiencing difficulties during an activity, he or she can use any or all of the following strategies:
> - Offer most to least support
> - Use mini-breaks
> - Reduce demands
> - Share valuing
> - Legitimise the behaviour
> - Shape the behaviour
> - Seek a fresh entry point
> - Redirect to scheduled activity

Mini-breaks are slight pauses of about 30 seconds when the teacher shifts the focus from the activity to the relationship in order to 'share values', have a rest, and take stock of shared progress. Mini-breaks help to prevent both the practitioner and the individual from 'rushing' or from being too 'task centred'. They can also reduce pressure, increase bonding and provide an opportunity to promote concentration and refocusing.

It is useful if a person expresses a preference for a particular activity. However, people in behavioural distress often do not know how to participate in any activity. The process of Gentle Teaching commences by interrupting the vicious circle of painful relationships, harmful behaviour and unfulfilled existence by introducing participation. Once a person is enjoying a single activity, a second or third activity can be introduced rapidly. In an environment that is reasonably well resourced, three or four activities can be scheduled to take place on a daily basis by the end of the first week. Each week, new activities can be added to the schedule, thus providing opportunities for choice, turn taking, responsibility, rest, leisure and socialising. As life gets busier, it becomes useful to plan and perhaps record participation. This also allows the person being helped to have information that is necessary to be part of that process. Some people benefit from augmented communication systems to plan and remember their routine. A pictorial timetable is a useful tool for promoting choice and responsibility.

People who display behavioural distress and who have learning disabilities often perceive interactive activities as a threat to their emotional security and safety. They may have experienced criticism, punishment and failure when participating in the past. This can result in reluctance to participate. Careful structuring of the activity will generate a feeling of safety and security, and greatly increase the likelihood of willing and enjoyable participation. It is important that the learner knows exactly what steps are involved and how long the activity is going to take. Trust and security depend upon clear information and a predictable, reliable sequence of steps. If the learner is having emotional or practical difficulty at any stage, the practitioner should give as much support as necessary, even completing entire steps for the learner to reduce anxiety and build trust. However, the person is invited to maintain some level of involvement (albeit intermittent or minimal) throughout the activity. When an activity is almost complete, the teacher points to the material and says: 'We are completely finished now. There is no more [of that activity] left to do.'

Finding the 'entry point'

Within each sequence of repeated steps in an activity, there is often one step which the person finds interesting or attractive. They may look up each time that step comes around. This is called the 'entry point'. A person who is reluctant to share participation is more likely to join in at the 'entry point' than at any other stage in an activity. Look at the case illustration entitled 'Max: finding the "entry point"', which shows how this point was identified for one young man.

Max: finding the 'entry point'

Max, aged 13, was very inactive and passive. He spent most of his home life sitting on the sofa and, apart from feeding himself, he was dependent on others for support. The gentle teaching practitioner looked for an appropriate activity in which to involve Max, and chose a pile of towels that needed folding. She brought the pile of unfolded towels and a laundry basket over to the sofa. After a few friendly words and a brief explanation the practitioner took a towel and slowly and deliberately folded it in half, smoothed it, folded it again, smoothed it again and, smiling, placed it in the basket. Max followed all her movements with cautious curiosity. Taking the next towel the practitioner repeated the process, placing the towel on Max's knee before lifting it and placing it in the basket. Max smiled at that part. This was his ENTRY POINT. Next time, the teacher placed greater emphasis on that part, making it Max's job. He anticipated the movement by holding his arms out to take the towel and put it carefully in the basket. Max smiled and gave a lot of eye contact during the second part of the activity and initiated a hug at the end.

Max's entry point was putting the towel in the basket; to direct him towards the folding during the first attempt would probably have alienated him. Every aspect of the practitioner's posture and behaviour has a bearing on the relationship with the person who is behaviourally distressed. The practitioner uses this consciously to promote a warm, safe and empowering relationship. Eye contact, facial expression, tone, pitch, volume, the pace at which one walks toward someone, how close one is and in what position one sits or stands, how one uses the language of touch – all of these can be an expression of commitment to relate in a fair and empowering way.

The Gentle Teaching response to behavioural distress

Relating to a person in a warm, equitable way and empowering the learner to participate in a balanced schedule of activities brings about significant changes in lifestyle, self-expression and personal relationships. However, patterns of extremely harmful behaviour can be very deeply entrenched, and may be a person's primary manner of making an impact on their external world. Consequently, this behaviour often continues even when an environment has changed.

Whilst Gentle Teaching does not focus on behaviour as such, it acknowledges that certain actions may adversely affect a person's quality of life and/or cause harm to themselves or others. Some of these behaviours may limit participation in daily life as well as damage relationships with others. Information about such behaviour emerges from the questions on participation and communication, but it is also essential for the practitioner to document a detailed description of any behaviours considered to be harmful. By examining the behaviours in the context of a person's life, any areas of need seen to underlie the behaviour can be immediately addressed. Behaviours which cause serious harm or disruption need to be described very accurately and in detail in order for any interventions aiming towards life change to be successful.

Difficulties with relationship can block participation, and problems with participation can interfere with the development of relationship. Emotions experienced within this vicious circle are often expressed through behaviours such as:

- Verbal aggression
- Physical aggression
- Inappropriate social behaviour (e.g. undressing in public)
- Inappropriate vocalisation (e.g. shouting and screaming)
- Self-injury
- Damage to property
- Compulsive behaviour
- Obsessive behaviour
- Extreme withdrawal.

Such behaviours are viewed as communicative messages through which a client indicates distress, discomfort or anger. Some people with learning disabilities are considered at risk of exhibiting such behaviours because their ability to communicate effectively is often hampered by a combination of psychological, sensory, neurological and physical difficulties. These behaviours also impede the development of relationships and participation in everyday life. It is important to distinguish between two 'types' of challenging behaviour: low intensity, high frequency behaviour, and high intensity, low frequency behaviour.

Low intensity, high frequency behaviour

An example of this type of behaviour is given in the case illustration 'Rajid'.

Rajid: an example of low intensity, high frequency behaviour

Rajid was always on the move, always up to mischief, knocking things over, grabbing people, spitting, kicking, scratching, biting, exposing himself. Periods when he was not thus engaged were rare. His behaviour had an adverse effect on his relationships and on his participation in life. He never caused serious harm to anyone, although the continued risk of broken skin and slight bruising from his self-injury was extremely difficult for his family and professional carers.

For people with low intensity, high frequency behaviour (as for John in the first case illustration), it is sufficient for the practitioner to note and remain aware of the behavioural precursor, that is, behaviours which, though harmless in themselves, indicate that the person is distressed and likely to behave in a challenging way (for example a person might have a pattern of pacing up and down before smashing the television). To work alongside Rajid one had to balance physical support and emotional warmth with the need to protect oneself from his scratching, kicking and biting. The key questions the practitioner supporting Rajid asked were:

- Does he scratch with both hands?
- Does he usually scratch a particular body part, for example hands, arms, face?
- Does he maintain the pressure or scratch and let go quickly?
- Will he approach a person in order to scratch them?
- If you move away when he is trying to scratch, will he follow?
- Does he kick when he is sitting and you are standing, or the other way around?
- Does he kick a person sitting beside/near him?
- Does he kick when you and he are both standing?
- Is it a single kick, a few kicks, or prolonged kicking?
- Does he kick particular body parts, for example groin? shinbone?

To interrupt this vicious circle the practitioner needed to introduce participation whilst developing a relationship. Knowledge of the behaviour enabled the practitioner to choose the best activity, the best place to sit or stand, where to position materials, and to work out a plan for redirecting Rajid from challenging behaviour to shared participation. For Rajid, the practitioner chose to work sitting on a sofa arm with Rajid sitting next to her on the sofa. The activity selected was dusting and polishing, an ordinary daily activity well within Rajid's capabilities. The materials (a duster and polish) were placed within the practitioner's reach but not Rajid's, and the practitioner encouraged Rajid by stroking his hand and placing the duster in it. Once Rajid was comfortable with this, the practitioner then concentrated upon moving his hand towards the table.

High intensity, low frequency behaviour

The case illustration entitled 'Stuart' provides an example of a young man who displays the type of challenging behaviour that can be described as high intensity, low frequency.

Stuart: an example of high intensity, low frequency behaviour

Stuart could go for weeks without challenging. When supported by skilled and valuing staff members he participated enthusiastically in a range of activities. However, if he experienced acute stress, uncertainty or insensitive attitudes from others he occasionally became extremely aggressive, causing serious harm (for example, he once broke a staff member's nose, and extensively damaged property). This behaviour was perceived by staff as being unprovoked, unpredictable, sudden and inexplicable.

When all other options have been exhausted, it is not uncommon for care givers to respond to high intensity, low frequency behaviour by using physical restraint, or the emergency administration of tranquillising medication. The adverse effects of such a response on the health and happiness of the person and on those close to them is immense. The distress, anxiety, fear, longing and desperation that is expressed in this way must be correspondingly painful. To move beyond a pattern of harm followed by control, a practitioner must empathise fully with the person, acknowledge their distress and skilfully and gently guide him or her to a relationship of shared valuing and shared participation. In order to maintain a posture of solidarity, a practitioner has to gain a thorough understanding of the behaviour itself. This is not necessarily an understanding of the specific causes of the behaviour, but an empirical description of the actual behaviour. This type of description allows the care giver to respond early on in a behavioural cycle.

High intensity, low frequency behaviour generally commences with harmless precursors (for example pacing, muttering, rocking, adjusting clothing, staring, avoiding eye contact), before building up to more intense behaviour (for example shouting, running back and forth, swearing, threatening gestures or words, pushing or shoving, picking at a sore spot). These more intense activities continue to intensify further until the harmful behaviour itself occurs (for example fast repeated biting of own arm causing bleeding, throwing and smashing of furniture, kicking, scratching and biting of another person causing severe lacerations and severe bruising). These behaviours may cease spontaneously but will sometimes continue until someone intervenes. The harmful behaviour is followed by a return to the person's usual state. Each stage of a person's behaviour needs to be described in clear, precise and factual detail. These descriptions should not include interpretation, judgement or recommendation.

The categories of 'low intensity, high frequency' and, 'high intensity, low frequency' behaviour provide a framework within which the practitioner can endeavour to understand the behaviour of the individual. These categories are, however, a simplification, and most people do not fit neatly into them. For example, some people can have a low intensity, high frequency behaviour which occasionally escalates into a high intensity behaviour. If this is the case they will need strategies to manage behaviour in the context of shared participation in activities and relationships, as well as gentle teaching response procedures. Strategies for preventing and responding to potentially harmful behaviour are developed in the context of doing activities together. People with the experiences described above often have very strong and entrenched ways of responding to any invitation to share participation. Therefore, very careful consideration must be given to the type of activity selected, with attention to its structure, how the person is invited to participate, the use of the practitioner's physical position and the prevention of, and response to, harmful behaviour. The challenges for a practitioner are to:

- Maintain a valuing relationship
- Minimise harm and damage
- Re-establish shared participation.

When managed with compassion and skill, a potentially risky situation can be transformed into an opportunity for showing a person that commitment to valuing them is not conditional upon 'good behaviour'. The 'defusion' response is used to provide emotional and physical safety whilst continuing to value the person. This response is outlined in Box 7.5.

Box 7.5
Defusion

By using the following steps (the 'defusion' response), emotional and physical safety can be provided whilst continuing the activity:
1. The teacher reduces or removes the demands being placed on the person: ('Don't worry, we'll have a little break and then *I'll* do the next part', or, 'Let's walk to the other side of the room, we don't have to finish that straight away').
2. If possible, the teacher legitimises the behaviour: ('That's OK, you can throw that T-shirt to me if you like', when the person's intention was to throw the T-shirt away, or, 'Fine, let me shake your hand, thank you', when the person was hitting out not trying to shake hands).
3. The teacher provides a breathing space to take stock and allow the person a little time to relax.
4. The teacher expresses value towards the person and acknowledges that the situation is new and difficult for the person: ('I know this is hard, everything is fine. I'm glad you're still here, you're trying really hard').
5. The teacher gradually and gently recommences the activity, seeking an entry point.
6. The teacher shifts the person's focus from the intensity of their emotions to the calm, predictable safety of the shared activity.
7. The teacher values and praises the person's presence and involvement while being mindful and respectful of the fragility of the person's participation.

As the distress abates and trust re-emerges, the person is again invited to share participation in the presented activity. Each of the steps outlined in Box 7.5 takes a minute or two, but they may need to be repeated or partly repeated a great number of times before trust and safety are established. Also, the steps do not always follow in the same order. Judgement and skill are needed to balance safety and growth, and where serious harm is a possibility care givers should consider training before using the strategy. The aims of a Gentle Teaching response procedure are to maintain a posture of solidarity, to maintain emotional and physical safety, and to facilitate growth and empowerment. The earlier in the course of a behaviour a care giver responds, the more they will be able to use defusion and redirection to whatever activity the person would normally be engaged in at that time. If the care giver misses the early indications, and a build-up occurs, the person can be directed towards a sequence of activities selected and structured to provide an absorbing alternative to the emotional intensity expressed by the behaviour. The sequence of activities should be:

- Attractive to the person
- Familiar to the person
- Readily accessible and practical at all times
- Unconditionally available to the person.

The first activity in the sequence should be the most attractive, that is, something the person is known to really enjoy doing, and this activity may be quite intense and vigorous (such as football, sweeping leaves, pulling clothes from washing machine). The second and third activities should place slightly greater demands on the person. The care giver can also rely upon a response procedure which prioritises emotional and physical safety. Such a response, though not as powerful as one involving a sequence of activities, is nonetheless very effective at maintaining respect and equity within a relationship. The caregiver's demeanour should always communicate:

- Gentle leadership
- Compassion
- Respect and equity
- Safety and warmth.

Organisational principles of Gentle Teaching

Gentle Teaching requires commitment from care givers, as well as commitment at an organisational level. Service providers who wish to embrace the philosophy of Gentle Teaching as part of their service culture will need to consider the factors identified in Box 7.6 to gain maximum benefit from gentle teaching.

Staff working within an organisation which does not have a positive and dynamic value base can still use Gentle Teaching as part of their philosophy, but change is likely to be slow and uneven. Staff in such an organisation will need to be strong and resourceful, and remain non-confrontational and non-judgmental of others within their organisation, if Gentle Teaching is to succeed.

Gentle Teaching training

Although the underlying principles of Gentle Teaching appear simple, translating them into practice requires skill and judgement. These are best developed with the support and guidance of a competent Gentle Teaching

Box 7.6
Organisational
considerations

Service providers who wish to embrace Gentle Teaching as part of their service culture will need to invest in the following:

- Adequate Gentle Teaching training, both theoretical and 'hands on'
- Access to ongoing support and guidance from a competent practitioner
- Effective systems of feedback between colleagues
- Effective methods of communication with and without the organisation
- Proactive management systems
- Regular and frequent supervision
- Adequate staffing levels
- Access to activities of daily living within the organisation itself, as well as the wider community
- Appropriate monitoring and inspection

practitioner or trainer. People supporting individuals showing only slight behavioural distress and/or participation problems may find a basic Gentle Teaching seminar sufficient to point them in the right direction. Staff teams with controlling postures will benefit more from intensive training, and those supporting people with deeply entrenched patterns of harmful behaviour will benefit most from a combination of seminar training, followed by hands-on support. Hands-on support is where a trainer introduces Gentle Teaching to a person and staff directly, and establishes a level of skills within the situation before withdrawing support. This has been found to be the safest way to introduce the approach in a high risk situation.

If a service wishes to purchase Gentle Teaching training, the following characteristics of the trainer and participants are worth considering:

1. The trainer

- The trainer has experience of working within services for people with learning disabilities before becoming a trainer.

- The trainer continues to practice hands-on Gentle Teaching.

- The trainer can provide hands-on training if appropriate.

- The trainer can provide references and test materials from people who have received training.

- The trainer is competent in managing conflict and other emotionally intense situations (this refers to the dynamics with staff groups as well as people being helped).

2. The participants

- The participants are offered opportunities to explore their existing attitudes and values without judgement or condemnation.

- The participants are clear that Gentle Teaching requires a commitment to positive values.

■ The participants are offered practical advice and guidance in relation to specific situations.

■ The participants are offered access to sources of theoretical/academic material.

Criticisms of Gentle Teaching

Many criticisms have been levelled against Gentle Teaching, including the following:

1. That it is ineffective at reducing behavioural difficulties and that this is proven by research
2. That it is potentially aversive
3. That the central tenets of gentle teaching are loose and not operationally defined, therefore making objective evaluation difficult
4. That Gentle Teaching uses behavioural techniques.

Each of these criticisms is now explored in more detail, and possible responses to the criticisms are discussed.

Gentle Teaching is ineffective at reducing behaviour difficulties and that this is proven by research

McGee (McGee et al 1987) has presented group data from 73 individuals treated for self-injurious behaviour (SIB) to demonstrate the therapeutic effect of Gentle Teaching. The vast majority of persons (86.3%) entered the programme with high intensity SIB, and none displayed this level upon discharge or up to 5 years later. Further papers by McGee confirmed these results: in a study of a sample of 40 people (McGee & Menolascino 1992), an average 78.8% reduction in self-injury and a 90.6% reduction in aggression was documented. These results were impressive and McGee et al (McGee et al 1987) have suggested that Gentle Teaching is universally effective, or at least as effective as alternative interventions. However, questions have been asked concerning the legitimacy of the data collection methods in these studies, including the sample selection, levels of learning disability, which types of self-injurious behaviours were changed, and medication levels (Mudford 1995).

Jordan et al (1989) found that visual screening and Gentle Teaching were more successful than task training and the no treatment condition in reducing rates of stereotyped behaviour. They also found that visual screening was more effective than Gentle Teaching, and that bonding did not occur more often under the Gentle Teaching condition than in the visual screening condition.

Jones et al (1990, 1991) reported that there were few clinically significant differences in terms of effectiveness between Gentle Teaching and visual screening, and this was true for the reduction of challenging behaviours and for bonding. They concluded that the two procedures were equally effective with one subject and ineffective with the other. More recently, Gates et al (1997) conducted a comparison between Gentle Teaching, behaviour therapy and a control group in the management of behavioural difficulties in children with learning disabilities. Parents were taught the techniques of one of the two interventions at workshops, and the child's behavioural difficulties were monitored for 12 months. They found that when measuring 'maladaptive' behaviour, in the majority of measures employed little statistical difference was found between Gentle Teaching and behaviour therapy. Only one area of statistical significance was found, and that was in the domain of social engagement: significant differences existed between both Gentle Teaching and the control (at 12 month follow-up), and between behaviour therapy and the control (at 3 and 6 month follow-up). This study indicated that Gentle Teaching had a therapeutic effect, and that this effect was comparable to behaviour therapy. However, further research in this area still needs to be undertaken.

The argument that Gentle Teaching is ineffective at dealing with behavioural difficulties is a misleading one. Proponents of Gentle Teaching claim that the approach is not a form of treatment, nor something one does to the another person to prevent the behavioural difficulties. The building of the relationship between client and carer remains the primary focus of the approach, and not a reduction in difficult behaviours. Gentle Teaching has never professed to be an alternative method of modifying behaviour. McGee (1992) stated that:

> *the initial purpose of care-giving is to establish a feeling of companionship between the caregiver and the individual with behavioural difficulties.*

[p. 869]

Any reduction in the behavioural difficulties of a person with learning disabilities that occurred as a natural consequence of this interaction was considered a bonus.

Research to date questions the claim made by McGee of the universal successfulness of Gentle Teaching. McCaughey & Jones (1992) have concluded that any future findings will confirm the findings of Jones et al (1990) that it was effective for some individuals and ineffective for others. The same conclusion could be made regarding most interventions, including applied behaviour analysis (Didden et al 1997). Within the field of learning disabilities there has been an increased acceptance of the need for alternative approaches, not just Gentle Teaching but for non-aversive practices in general (Crowhurst 1991).

Gentle Teaching as an approach can be considered to be in its infancy in terms of research, particularly in comparison to behaviour therapy. Behaviourism began its research with animals in the late 19th century and the first recorded incident of its successful use with people with learning disabilities was in 1949 (Fuller 1949), over half a century later. Gentle Teaching first appeared in 1983, a mere 15 years ago. The studies conducted in the 1980s and 1990s are insufficient to support many of the claims made for gentle teaching, but that does not mean that Gentle Teaching does not have a future as a therapeutic intervention. On the contrary, practitioners in the field of learning disability care provision in particular continue to advocate the use of Gentle Teaching as a positive way of working with people.

Evidently, there remains a continuing need for further research in this area. Given that independent investigations have been criticised by McGee, and his own work has been heavily criticised by proponents of behavioural interventions, it appears reasonable to consider whether research into Gentle Teaching can be conducted in such a way as to be acceptable to both schools of thought. Mudford (1995) suggested that there are five minimum requirements for future research:

1. All aspects of treatment to be supervised by a teacher or therapist approved by McGee.

2. Empirical evaluation should be supervised by behaviour analysts with considerable experience in direct observational measurement of human behaviour.

3. An initial study might employ the multiple baseline across-subjects experimental design.

4. Observations should be conducted when the participants are with the teachers to ensure that Gentle Teaching's independent variables can be described fully.

5. Observations should be conducted for no longer than 4–15 minutes, in 2 hour sessions, as reported by McGee and Gonzalez (1990), to assess maintenance and generalisation of effects.

In addition, Jones & McCaughy (1992) suggested that the research should be conducted over months rather than weeks.

Gentle Teaching is potentially aversive

Barrera & Teodoro (1990) found that self-injury did not decrease significantly with the use of Gentle Teaching, and that it was reduced to its lowest levels only when restraints, edible reinforcers and isolation between sessions were used in one of the experimental conditions. In this study variations of Gentle Teaching were employed with a client who had self-injurious behaviour. The client made no significant progress during treatment, and following consultation with John McGee himself, amendments to the procedures were made. Head hitting continued to increase past baseline levels and finally Gentle Teaching was discontinued. Barrera & Teodoro (1990) suggested that:

our participant's attempts to resist and terminate session, as well as to escape from the training area in most phases, suggest that this approach acquired undeniable aversive properties.

[p. 210]

This has led to some authors suggesting that in some contexts Gentle Teaching might be:

highly aversive to people whose self-injury is motivated by a desire to escape others.

[Emerson 1990, p. 94]

However, McGee himself has also suggested that, at the beginning of the process of Gentle Teaching, the person will display behaviours which obviously indicate that they do not want anything to do with a care giver, for example screaming, hitting, biting, kicking, scratching or avoiding (McGee 1985a). If a person has spent years expressing themselves through such behaviour it is likely that it will emerge again, even when the practitioner is providing a safe and secure environment. Trust in, and connection with, other people takes time to grow. The person exhibiting a particular kind of behavioural distress may feel a little suspicious of such positive regard. Also, if people have experienced maladaptive postures from care givers in the past, they may feel very uncertain about what is going to happen now and in the future. People who have been controlled or punished may be expecting more of the same to happen. Those who have been left to their own devices, or who are accustomed to having everything on their own terms (within the limits of what is usually available to people with learning difficulties and behavioural distress in our society) may feel rather threatened; this is often expressed by behaviour which is harmful.

The central tenets of Gentle Teaching are loose and not operationally defined therefore making objective evaluation difficult

Independent evaluations of Gentle Teaching have been limited because of the failure of Gentle Teaching practitioners to define independent and dependent variables in terms of observable behaviour (Bailey 1992, Cuvo 1992). McGee & Gonzalez (1990) designed the 'Caregiver Interactional Observation System' (CIOS) and the 'Person Interactional Observation System' (PIOS) with which to code the dyadic variables of interactional change. The CIOS and the PIOS have provided a measurement tool with which to systematically evaluate Gentle Teaching. However, authors who attempted to replicate the variables under research conditions (Barrera & Teodoro 1990; Jones et al 1990, 1991) failed to find any statistically significant differences in therapeutic effect between Gentle Teaching and other interventions. McGee (1992) has suggested that independent evaluations of Gentle Teaching have failed to analyse and measure interactional change and:

have deviated from the Gentle Teaching intervention in methodology and procedures.

[p. 870]

However, in the Barrera & Teodoro study (1990), McGee himself was consulted. For Gentle Teaching practitioners, the effectiveness of the approach can be measured in terms of outcomes, and these are outlined below.

Outcomes for gentle teaching

The approach is perceived as being successful when:

1. The person being helped welcomes, or seeks human presence.

2. The person expresses regard for others by behaviours such as offering a handshake, smiling or passing materials to the teacher (or other participant) as part of an activity.

3. The person begins to show an interest in functional activities such as play, housework or leisure by remaining in the room where the activity is taking place or by following the movements of the teacher with his or her eyes. Also, by entering or returning to the place where the activity is happening, handling materials appropriately as part of an activity, showing pleasure by smiling, laughing or producing a thumbs up sign when being involved.

4. The person participates in scheduled activities until each activity is completed and expresses satisfaction with this.

5. The person communicates functionally about the activities scheduled, as well as about other aspects of life.

6. The person exercises a range of choices in the schedule of activities as well as other aspects of life.

7. The person develops greater access to a range of socially valued relationships.

8. The person participates in life with less reliance on maladaptive forms of self-expression which are potentially harmful.

Gentle Teaching uses behavioural techniques

Much of the literature has debated whether Gentle Teaching can in fact be distinguished from (non-aversive) behavioural techniques. Critics have argued that Gentle Teaching was:

essentially no more than a set of behavioural principles packaged with a heavy dose of old-time patent-medicine showmanship.

[Linscheid et al 1990, p. 7]

An analysis of Gentle Teaching from the perspective of applied behaviour analysis (Jones & McCaughy 1992) has indicated that the two approaches need not be regarded as mutually exclusive. McGee (McGee et al 1987) has described Gentle Teaching as 'a non-aversive behavioural intervention strategy', and as 'an attempt to adapt a number of behavioural techniques'(McGee 1990, p. 86). McGee elucidated further by saying:

Gentle Teaching is distinct from applied behaviour analysis in its unconditional valuing, its focus on mutual change, its analysis and measurement of dyadic variables, and its underlying assumptions. It is congruent with applied behaviour analysis in that it uses several behaviour change techniques in its intervention procedure.

[McGee 1992, p. 871]

Gentle Teaching uses a range of therapeutic techniques that could be described as behavioural. According to McGee (1989), Gentle Teaching emphasises the need for co-participation with a person with learning disabilities and, amongst other techniques, makes use of dialogue to express unconditional valuing. Many of these procedures include well-established behaviour analytic techniques, however, they do not include aversive stimulation (McGee et al 1987) or contingent reinforcement (McGee & Menolascino 1991). Bailey (1992) has suggested that:

Gentle Teaching proposes to be a philosophy, a humane technology, and a insightful, politically correct view of behaviour problems.

[p. 879]

It appeared that the techniques used by both approaches were similar; however, the focus and purpose of Gentle Teaching and behaviour therapy were considered to be entirely different. The main differences between Gentle Teaching and behaviour therapy are outlined in Table 7.1.

Table 7.1

The differences between behaviour therapy and Gentle Teaching

Behaviour therapy	Difference	Gentle teaching
To change undesirable behaviour	Goal	To teach bonding
The identification and elimination of behaviour	Focus	Solidarity and interaction with the person
Contingent reward, aversive and non-aversive practice	Strategy	Non-contingent valuing, non-aversive practice. Using tasks as a vehicle to establish bonding
Change in behaviour, compliance	Outcomes	People learning the value of human relationships, mutual liberation

The debate regarding whether Gentle Teaching is 'behavioural' or not has been misleading. In fact it can be easily demonstrated that it does use behavioural techniques and consequently there must be a demonstrated therapeutic effect. Gentle Teaching evolved out of behaviourism and adopted those techniques considered useful, therapeutic and positive and abandoned the elements of the approach that were seen to be focused upon behaviour and aversive. Although the advocates of gentle teaching have been reluctant to associate themselves with their behavioural history, there is an inherent strength in this association. For Gentle Teaching, this association actually offers hard empirical evidence to support its claims to effectiveness. In addition, it has combined a well-evidenced approach with a more ethically acceptable – by contemporary standards – attitude to the care of people with learning disabilities. However, continual focus on the strategies themselves fail to accord significant attention to the crucial importance of the spirit behind Gentle Teaching – the genuine warmth, acceptance and empathy of the practitioner.

Conclusion

Gentle Teaching can be understood as a response to and comment upon behaviourism. Behaviourism has evolved and embraced a variety of different forms over the last 40 years, and has had little choice but to adapt as society and attitudes have changed. Gentle Teaching can be seen as one therapy among many that reflect these changes. The focus and purpose of the Gentle Teaching approach is quite different from behaviourism, concentrating upon the whole person and relationships rather than on specific behaviours. This focus helps care givers to cope with and accept the often seemingly intractable problems experienced by many of their clients. For Gentle Teaching practitioners, the question is not whether the approach is more effective at reducing challenging behaviour, but whether it is effective at helping and caring for people with learning disabilities who display behavioural distress.

Gentle Teaching evolved out of the current dominant paradigm of behaviourism but its starting point was a non-aversive behaviourist approach rather than simply a behavioural approach. Gentle Teaching has both encapsulated and fuelled the development of non-aversive approaches, and was part of a 'new attitude' which questioned the authority of behaviourism and rejected the behaviourist approach to human behaviour.

It could be argued that Gentle Teaching not only emerged out of, and away from, behaviourism, but that it has also influenced the direction that behaviourism has taken in the last 15 years. Within behaviourism itself there has been increasing emphasis placed on relationships, self-expression and emotional needs. Perhaps in the future, a gradual convergence will emerge between the two approaches as Gentle Teaching develops its own scientific credentials, and behaviourism becomes less dependant upon conditional valuing.

Further reading

McGee J J, Menolascino F J, Hobbs D C, Menousek P E 1987 Gentle Teaching: a non-aversive approach to helping people with mental retardation. Human Sciences Press, New York
This is the first book on gentle teaching published by McGee and colleagues, and outlines the main concepts and values underlying the approach as well as strategies that can be used by practitioners. The final section of the book also details McGee's seminal piece of research undertaken in the University of Nebraska during the early 1980s.

McGee J J, Menolascino F J 1991 Beyond Gentle Teaching: a non aversive approach to helping those in need. Plenum Press, New York
The second book by McGee (with Menolascino) explores further the concepts and values outlined in his first book. This book elaborates upon the approach, using case studies to illustrate the approach in action and is aimed at direct care workers.

Mudford O C 1995 Review of the Gentle Teaching data. American Journal on Mental Retardation. 99(4): 345–355
This paper provides a comprehensive overview of the research conducted to date into the efficacy of gentle teaching.

References

Bailey J S 1992 Trying to win friends and influence people with euphemism, metaphor, smoke and mirrors. Journal of Applied Behaviour Analysis 25(4): 879–883

Barrera F J, Teodoro G M 1990 Flash bonding or cold fusion? A case analysis of gentle teaching. In: Repp A C, Singh N N (eds) Perspectives on the use of non aversive and aversive interventions for persons with developmental disabilities. Sycamore Publishing, Sycamore, Illinois

Coe D A, Matson J L 1990 The empirical basis for using aversive and non aversive therapy. In: Repp A, Singh N N (eds) Perspectives on the use of non aversive and aversive interventions for persons with developmental disabilities. Sycamore Publishing, Sycamore, Illinois

Crowhurst G 1991 Work for non-aversive practise, not just gentle teaching. Community Living 5(2):20

Cuvo A J 1992 Gentle teaching: on the one hand . . . but on the other hand. Journal of Applied Behaviour Analysis 25(4): 873–877

Didden R, Duker P C, Korzilius H 1997 Meta-analytic study on treatment effectiveness for problem behaviours with individuals who have mental retardation. American Journal on Mental Retardation 101(4): 387–399

Emerson E 1990 Some challenges presented by severe self injurious behaviour. Mental Handicap 18: 92–98

Fuller P R 1949 Operant conditioning of a vegetative human organism. American Journal of Psychology 62: 587–590

Gates R, Newell R, Wray J 1997 Comparing the efficacy of two therapeutic interventions used in the management of children with learning disabilities who exhibit challenging behaviour (behaviour difficulties). Final Report to the Northern and Yorkshire Research and Development Directorate. East Yorkshire Learning Disability Institute, University of Hull

Jones R S P, McCaughey R E 1992 Gentle Teaching and applied behaviour analysis: a critical review. Journal of Applied Behaviour Analysis 25(4): 853–867

Jones L J, Singh N N, Kendall K A 1990 Effects of Gentle Teaching and alternative treatments on self-injury. In: Repp A C, Singh N N (eds) Perspectives on the use or non aversive and aversive interventions for persons with developmental disabilities. Sycamore Publishing, Sycamore, Illinois

Jones L J, Singh N N, Kendall K A 1991 Comparative effects of Gentle Teaching and visual screening on self-injurious behaviour. Journal of Mental Deficiency Research 35: 37-47

Jordan J, Singh N N, Repp A C 1989 An evaluation of Gentle Teaching and visual screening in the reduction of stereotypy. Journal of Applied Behaviour Analysis 22 (1): 9-22

Linscheid T R, Meinhold P M, Mulick J A 1990 Gentle teaching? Behaviour Therapist (letter) 13: 32

McCaughey R E, Jones R S P 1992 The effectiveness of gentle teaching. Mental Handicap 20: 7-14

McGee J J 1985a Gentle Teaching. Mental Handicap in New Zealand 9(3): 13-24

McGee J J 1985b Bonding as the goal of teaching. Mental Handicap in New Zealand 9(4): 5-10

McGee J J 1985c Examples of the use of Gentle Teaching. Mental Handicap in New Zealand 9(4): 11-20

McGee J J 1989 Being with others: toward a psychology of human interdependence. Creighton, Omaha, Nebraska

McGee J J 1990 Gentle Teaching: the basic tenet. Nursing Times 86 (2): 68-72

McGee J J 1992 Gentle Teaching's assumptions and paradigm. Journal of Applied Behaviour Analysis 25 (4): 869-872

McGee J J, Gonzalez L 1990 Gentle Teaching and the practise of human interdependence: a preliminary study of 15 persons with severe behavioural disorders and their caregivers. In: Repp A, Singh N N (eds) Perspectives on the use of non aversive and aversive interventions for persons with developmental disabilities. Sycamore Publishing, Sycamore, Illinois

McGee J J, Menolascino F J 1991 Beyond gentle Teaching: a non aversive approach to helping those in need. Plenum Press, New York

McGee J J, Menolascino F J 1992 Gentle Teaching: its assumptions, methodology and application. In: Stanback W, Stanback S (eds) Controversial issues confronting special education: divergent perspectives. Allyn and Bacon, Boston, pp 183-200

McGee J J, Menolascino F J, Hobbs D C, Menousek P E 1987 Gentle Teaching: a non-aversive approach to helping people with mental retardation. Human Sciences Press, New York

Maslow A H 1954 Motivation and personality. Harper, New York

Menolascino F J, McGee J J 1983 Persons with severe mental retardation and behavioural challenges: from disconnectedness to human engagement. Journal of Psychiatric Treatment and Evaluation 5: 187-193

Mudford O C 1995 Review of the Gentle Teaching data. American Journal on Mental Retardation. 99 (4): 345-355

Rogers C R 1951 Client centred therapy. Houghton Mifflin, Boston

Stainton T 1993 A philosophy of equal human worth. Community Living 6 (4): 29

Wolfenberger W 1972 Normalisation: the principle of normalisation in human services. National Institute of Mental Retardation, Toronto

Resources

Contact details for training services:

Siobhan O'Rourke
Positive Support Services
Highfields
Brynymor Road
Aberystwyth
Caredigion SY23 2HX
UK
Tel/Fax: 01970 627337

Dan Hobbs
19706 South 168 Street
Springfield
Nebraska 68059
USA
Tel/Fax: +101 402 2532941

Dan Hobbs is one of the leading proponents of Gentle Teaching in the USA. He is one of the authors, with John McGee, of the first book on Gentle Teaching (see Further Reading list, above). He runs workshops in the UK (through Hexagon Publishing) and can be contacted for information and advice about Gentle Teaching. (Remember that Nebraska, USA, is 6 hours behind the UK!)

For further information about Gentle Teaching workshops contact:

Hexagon Publishing
2 Whitehouse Cottages
Washford
Watchet
Somerset TA23 0JZ
UK

'Mutual Change' (Gentle Teaching training package) is also available from Hexagon Publishing. This pack is used to provide people with the resource to train others in Gentle Teaching. The pack contains video material and booklets, tutors' presentation notes, timetables, exercises, and handouts.

http://www.gentleteaching.com/

This is the website of Gentle Teaching International (GTI). It provides a resource for all those who wish to learn about and practice Gentle Teaching. On the site you will find information about GTI, conference details, articles, training news, a newsletter and connections to other sites.

Structured teaching

Owen Barr, David Sines, Ken Moore and Gillian Boyd

Key issues
- Structured teaching is one aspect of the programme developed with Division TEACCH for the treatment and education of people with a range of autistic spectrum disorders
- The approach is essentially a method of education that relies upon systematic routines provided by trained teachers and professional staff with parents acting as co-therapists
- The five major dimensions of structured teaching provide a structure for assessment, planning, implementation and evaluation of the curriculum
- Quantitative and qualitative evaluation of structured teaching has indicated that the approach can result in a reduction of the severity and incidence of inappropriate behaviours amongst clients and simultaneously enhance opportunities for skill development

Overview
This chapter discusses a technique developed for people who fall within the spectrum of autistic disorders. However, its methods are equally applicable to other people, including children and adults with learning disabilities, who may also have deficits in communication. This chapter focuses most attention on structured teaching, which is one aspect of the programme developed at the University of North Carolina within Division TEACCH. The acronym (although not a perfect match) stands for 'treatment and education of autistic and communication-handicapped children'. The chapter commences with a brief exploration of some of the characteristics of people within the range of autistic spectrum disorders that originally stimulated this approach, then offers a short history of its development followed by a detailed description of how the approach may be applied to practical situations. Two individual client histories are offered to illuminate the practical application. The chapter concludes with a discussion of the perceived limitations of its method.

The nature of the spectrum of autistic disorders

What is autism?

The diagnosis of autism has been an issue that has aroused considerable debate since Kanner first described it in 1943. A point of particular debate was whether 'classic' autism as described by Kanner (1943)(Box 8.1) was a specific identifiable condition, or whether it was one of a number of conditions with overlapping characteristics that were best viewed along a continuum of differing levels of ability and impairment (Wing 1988, Trevarthen et al 1998). A variety of conditions may be grouped together in what has loosely been described the 'autistic spectrum', and includes semantic pragmatic disorder, deafness, blindness, disintegrative disorder, elective mutism, Rett's syndrome, emotional deprivation and idiopathic learning disability. The term autistic spectrum disorder (ASD) will be used in this chapter to reflect the growing recognition of a range of conditions that have previously been loosely referred to as autism or autistic traits. Two key emerging areas of increasing research interest are, firstly, early diagnosis of ASD (Baron-Cohen et al 1996, Stone et al 1999). Secondly, much attention in recent years has been given to understanding more about the aetiology of the condition, and in particular the contribution of genetics (Rutter 1999, Rutter et al 1999).

Box 8.1
Classical characteristics of people with autism as described by Kanner (Trevarthen et al 1998)

- An inability to establish social relatedness
- A failure to use language 'normally' for the purpose of communication
- An obsessive desire for the maintenance of sameness
- A fascination for objects
- Good cognitive potential
- These characteristics appear in the child before the age of 30 months

It has also been noted that people with ASD have social interactions that are not reciprocal and often lack empathetic understanding. Another feature is resistance to change, with a key focus on repetitive activities and lack of creativity (Baron-Cohen & Bolton 1993).

The prevalence of ASD is influenced by the criteria used to diagnose it. The rates of autistic and autistic-like conditions have been reported to range between 4.9 in 10 000 (Wing & Gould 1979) and 11.6 in 10 000 (Gillberg et al 1991). More recently, Wing (1996) has suggested that the prevalence rates for ASD may be as high as 91 in 10 000. More males than females appear to present with autistic spectrum disorders by a ratio of 3 to 1 (Gillberg 1996). Data from the 1993 census indicated that there were some 26 200 people with ASD in the UK, of whom 7 000 were under 18 years old (Trevarthen et al 1998). However, it is important to note that prevalence rates of the number of this group of people can vary considerably across different countries, depending on criteria used to diagnose the condition. Because of this, caution should be exercised when comparing prevalence across different countries.

Wing (1996) regarded a child as falling within the autistic continuum if they presented with a 'triad' of social impairment in relationships, communication and imagination, associated with behaviour that was characterised by rigid repetitive patterns. Bishop (1989) has suggested that a continuum approach should be used and Happe (1994) has stated that ASD could have many different manifestations. This continuum comprises two extremes ranging from people with very low levels of ability – in particular poor social, communicative and imaginative functioning – and, at the other end, people with exceptionally high levels of functioning who have devised coping strategies that facilitate their personal adaptation to their unique individual circumstances. Several people with ASD are accomplished authors and have provided important insights into their world as they view it (Williams 1994, 1998, 1999; Grandin 1995; Miedzianik & Croskin 1997). Despite consensus on some of the key characteristics, it is essential to recognise that, as is the case in the general population, considerable individuality exists in the personal likes, dislikes and personalities of people within this spectrum. (For a detailed discussion about individual differences between people with ASD and their abilities and needs see Firth 1989, Baron-Cohen & Bolton 1993, Trevarthen et al 1998.)

The majority of people with ASD have a range of different symptoms and therefore they may be located at different points on the continuum previously outlined. The possible range of abilities and needs of children in this spectrum, together with a lack of certainty over absolute criteria for diagnosis, can make the process of obtaining a diagnosis very difficult for parents. Parents often seek clarification of their child's condition, but sometimes find that they have to visit a number of professionals, most of whom are reluctant to confirm the diagnosis of ASD (Moore et al 1999).

Communication and people with autistic spectrum disorder

Communication deficit is a major feature of the presence of ASD, consequently it needs to be a key focus within any strategy aiming to increase skills development and social interaction in individuals with any of these conditions. Rutter (1985) reflected this when he described a range of goals (Box 8.2) for intervention programmes designed to enhance skills and social functioning amongst people with ASD. The centrality of the need to increase communication ability was recognised by Howlin (1998) in a review of treatments.

Box 8.2
The range of goals for intervention programmes designed to enhance skills and social functioning of people with autism spectrum disorders (developed from Rutter 1985)

- Fostering social and communicative development
- Enhancing problem solving
- Reinforcing those responses that are appropriate to verbal instructions presented and increasing learning/access to opportunities for 'normal' experience
- Decreasing behaviours that interfere with learning and access to opportunities for 'normal' experience
- Shaping behaviours toward the achievement of appropriately targeted outcomes
- Programmes that include sequences designed to help the person reach objectives based on functional analysis, and involving systematic manipulation of stimulus conditions, consequences, instructional stimuli, and other variables

Apart from the importance of aiming to alter inappropriate behaviours, Mesibov et al (1994) have described the need to include instruction to enhance social skills for children, adolescents and adults with autistic spectrum disorders. The latter involves structured teaching sessions and social activities followed by an opportunity to practise skills in naturally occurring social situations. Within such structured sessions a range of approaches may be used to assist people in developing skills. Mesibov et al (1994, p. 194) have pointed out that:

> *social skills training follows a cognitive, social learning model; improving understanding of social expectations through specific teaching techniques such as role playing and behavioural rehearsal, participating in social activities in natural social settings, and understanding social expectations through discussions and group activities.*

They have also applauded the use of peers without learning disabilities as co-workers, having found that they were effective in teaching social behaviours to such individuals (see also Box 8.3).

Box 8.3
Key aspects of structured teaching

- Clear structure
- Respect for individuality
- Respect for the complexity and meaning within the world of people with autistic spectrum disorders
- Use of symbols and colour to assist teaching and learning of:
  — communication
  — socialisation
  — personal care skills
  — practical independence
- Family involvement
- Opportunities for activities with non-autistic children

Although the above goals of intervention programmes have been written specifically with people with ASD in mind, again it is important to emphasise that these goals are equally applicable to other people with learning disabilities who may have deficits in communication (Fitton 1994, Bradley 1998).

History of structured teaching

Origins of structured teaching

The TEACCH programme was first developed in 1972 at the University of North Carolina at Chapel Hill in the USA. It provides a comprehensive programme of support for people with ASD and related disorders. The programme was officially inaugurated by the North Carolina General Assembly who mandated the creation of Division TEACCH for the 'treatment and education of autistic and related communication handicapped children'. Division TEACCH is responsible for planning, delivering and assuring quality services to over 6000 people with autistic spectrum and related disorders in North Carolina and delivers its service through six regional centres geographically distributed throughout the state (Division TEACCH 1992). It relies on effective collaboration with key state agencies providing services for people with developmental disabilities, for example health and education. Its overall aim is to provide lifelong support for people with ASD and their families. Since inception the TEACCH programme has received international recognition as an effective model of intervention for working with this group of people.

Schopler et al (1979) have described the purpose of the programme as fourfold. Firstly, they viewed it as having a role in avoiding unnecessary use of residential care services for children; secondly, facilitating and improving adaptation for the child and family; thirdly, providing individualised special education for each child; and finally reducing the stresses of a child with disabilities on their family. Further to these broad aims, specific objectives have been outlined for localised structured teaching projects (Box 8.4).

Box 8.4
Specific objectives outlined for the TEACCH project in Northern Ireland (Sines 1996)

- Assessment of developmental delay and severity of autism spectrum disorders
- Individualised educational programmes to clients in four selected schools and one adult day service
- Support and advice to teachers and other professionals working with people with autistic spectrum disorders
- Advice on behaviour management at school/work and at home
- Examples of educational materials/tasks and schedules
- Monitoring of subject progress
- Education and training in the form of parent and professional workshops
- Home consultation (and consultation with other agencies)
- The facilitation and consolidation of an inter-professional team ethos to maximise the effectiveness of TEACCH methods
- Data to inform systematic monitoring, review and evaluation of the effectiveness of the TEACCH method

In pursuit of these aims and objectives, Division TEACCH provides a wide range of services to a broad section of people with ASD of all ages. The main features of the TEACCH programme are the provision of services to children and their families in their own home and in their school settings. These include aspects such as regional clinical and diagnostic evaluations, social skills training, home based intervention services, support and consultation to classrooms and residential services, behaviour management procedures and home based intervention services, as well as pre-school demonstration classrooms. Services are also provided to older people with ASD, including adolescent and adult support services and supported employment services. Finally, staff are involved in professional training and consultation services as well as research and dissemination of the work of the department (Division TEACCH 1992). (Regularly updated details of the nature and scale of the services provided by Division TEACCH can be obtained by visiting their website at www.unc.edu/depts/teacch.)

Watson et al (1989) have outlined specific considerations that should be taken into account when developing individualised structured teaching for people with autistic spectrum disorders or communication handicap. It is therefore necessary to distinguish between the TEACCH programme – that is, the overall service operated and managed by Division TEACCH (delivered in North Carolina) – and the development of individualised structured teaching strategies used with children with ASD. The former relates to the state-wide provision available only in North Carolina, USA, that includes a wide range of services. The latter relates specifically to the development of structured teaching when working with individuals. As already noted, the origins of this type of service can be traced back to the early 1970s in North Carolina. However, it is only during the past decade that this approach has gained widespread recognition within the UK as a valuable approach when working with people with ASD. Frequently, these 'structured teaching' services are called 'TEACCH classrooms/projects' to denote their original influence, but it is important to recognise that structured teaching is only one of a number of services provided by Division TEACCH.

The theoretical basis

An overview of the main approaches used in teaching new skills

A wide variety of approaches and their respective techniques have evolved from the interplay of clinical observation and research (Rutter 1999) in response to the challenges of teaching new skills, and responding to the behavioural distress among people with ASD (Howlin 1997, 1998). Historically, the predominant intervention used with this group of people appears to have been based on the behavioural approach. This approach has incorporated the use of teaching and learning in incremental steps. There has indeed been considerable success over a number of years in developing communication skills in people with learning disabilities through the use of behavioural techniques (Lovaas 1977, Yule & Carr 1987, Kazadin 1994). However, the limitations of such approaches have also been noted (Carr 1985; see also Chs. 9 and 10).

An important contribution has also been made by psycholinguistic approaches to enhancing the communication abilities of people with ASD. Within this approach an emphasis is placed on how children develop communication abilities, and how development in this area relates to development in other aspects of cognitive and social skills. The focus of interest has shifted over time from an initial interest in the development of language structure to an interest in the meaning of language and aspects of social communication, and the use of appropriate language in a range of school settings. Whilst having a different focus, in reality the psycholinguistic approach to language development uses behavioural techniques in the way in which the interventions are structured and implemented. In many ways this enhances the previous behavioural approach rather than replacing it.

Increasingly, the possible contributions of cognitive strategies are being highlighted in services for people with learning disabilities, and evidence of their effectiveness with people with ASD has been reported (Kroese et al 1997). As a result, within most current intervention strategies there is now a tendency to integrate previous approaches and less use of exclusively behavioural, psycholinguistic or cognitive approaches. All of the above approaches have influenced the development of structured teaching.

Structured teaching: an integrated approach

Schopler & Reichler (1971) were the first to describe a specific form of structured teaching by demonstrating that people with ASD processed visual information more easily than verbal information. As the result of other observations of children with ASD during the 1960s and 1970s, structured teaching was developed as a programme for working with them (Mesibov et al 1994). At a later stage the effectiveness of a model of psycho-educational intervention was found to be generalisable to people with ASD of all ages and levels of functioning, by organising their environments and providing:

‘clear, concrete and meaningful visual information.’

[Mesibov 1997]

The result was the development of the structured teaching programme that involved parents and people with ASD (and their instructors) as co-workers. This developed as a psycho-educational model that incorporated aspects of developmental, behavioural, cognitive and psycholinguistic theories.

This developmental approach to teaching communication skills stressed the need for an individualised diagnostic assessment. It also accepted the importance of parents and other family members as co-workers developing appropriate competence in the application of the teaching method, alongside professionals. The developmental aspects are evident in the staged approach to the development of new skills, which accepts that new skills are built upon existing skills and that some skills are needed as a prerequisite level of maturity.

Aspects of behavioural techniques are evident in the practical application of structured teaching. The behavioural techniques include a detailed comprehensive assessment of the communication process, and this process recognises the importance of family members as a source of relevant information. The completion of baseline measurement, the setting of clear objectives and the use of teaching strategies (including prompting, shaping, fading and a range of reinforcers and reinforcement schedules – see Ch. 9) are evidence of a behavioural influence on the structured teaching approach. However, the importance attached to learning and processing of cues in structured teaching has a cognitive basis. The psycholinguistic influence is also evident in the categorisation of an individual's communication across the main dimensions of structured teaching (Box 8.5).

Box 8.5
Five dimensions within structured teaching (after Watson et al 1989)

Functions/purposes of communication
General purposes in mind when communicating. These include: getting attention; requesting; rejecting or refusing; commenting; seeking information; expressing feelings

Context or situations of communication
Different situations in which people communicate, different situations requiring different skills

Semantic categories/meanings
This relates to the meaning of a word when used to communicate a concept. Such concepts include reference to actions (walk), objects acted on (pulled toy), person acting (dad pulled toy) and location (on floor, in cupboard), person feeling (sister happy)

Words, gestures, signs used in communicating
Words or other 'units of communication' used, such as gestures or signs

The form the communication takes
Includes reference to the method of communication (such as pulling a person to a place, pointing, picture boards, sign language or spoken word). Also relates to the level of complexity in the 'form' of communication used (single actions and words or a variety of appropriately arranged actions or words)

The five major dimensions of structured teaching provide a structure for assessment, planning, implementation and evaluation of the curriculum. In addition, there are practical aspects relating to the learning environment such as the provision of clear structure and the organisation of teaching materials to provide direction for the commencement and completion of a task. These specialised procedures and services are designed to build on existing abilities and meet the individual needs of people with ASD. (The application of these aspects of structured teaching is discussed in more detail below, under the heading 'The practical application of structured teaching'.)

The structured teaching programme therefore adopts an interdisciplinary approach to the delivery of services, focusing primary attention on the needs of children and adults (and of their families/carers) rather than on the needs of various support staff, professionals and agencies. Rather than untrained people attempting to implement some limited aspects, ideally only people who have been appropriately trained should implement structured teaching. All instructors were originally designated as psycho-educational therapists but in reality they worked as an inter-professional team. However, irrespective of their professional backgrounds they have provided a general TEACCH service to clients and their families/carers. All staff also require intensive training in the use of structured teaching methods in order to become experienced in the application of a broad range of interventions including behaviour management, language and social development, special education and family interaction/intervention approaches. Home teaching and behavioural management programmes are also envisaged as being an integral component of the structured teaching method. The services provided by TEACCH teams in North Carolina normally include the facilitation of diagnosis and assessment, the support of staff using TEACCH, the provision of workshops for parents and professionals and the implementation of a home based support service, in order to enable parents and carers to work as co-therapists.

The philosophical basis

The philosophy of approaches and strategies that are prominent in services are often a reflection of an overall guiding philosophy of service structures and systems. This has been evident in services for people with learning disabilities over the past few decades. Structures of services have tended to be segregated and have often failed to respect the individuality of people with learning disabilities. As the philosophy of services has altered to incorporate the influence of 'normalisation', previous group and depersonalised approaches to services have become less acceptable and an emphasis has been placed on the need to value people as individuals (Barr 1999). This has resulted in a wider consideration being given to the impact of environmental factors and of other people on the behaviour and lives of people with learning disabilities (Gates & Beacock 1996).

There has also been a shift away from the view that any difficulties presented by a person with learning disabilities were innate and that therefore it was the person with learning disabilities who needed to change. This continuing evolution of approach is noticeable in the growing prominence of the concept of 'inclusiveness', talk of citizenship and person-centred approaches (Sanderson 1998), and the need for evidence of effectiveness and quality in services (DHSS 1995, Mental Health Foundation 1996, Redworth & Redworth 1997). The principles of 'inclusion' and 'person centredness' underpin services delivered by Division TEACCH and the implementation of structured teaching.

Central to structured teaching is a recognition of individuality among people with ASD, along with their individual social circumstances. Further to recognising individuality, this individuality is respected and valued, as is evidenced in the development of flexible personal learning and development plans. Opportunities are presented to people with ASD to influence the nature of their activities, including the pace and direction of their individualised teaching plans. Mesibov (1998) emphasises the importance of:

cultivating strengths and interests rather than dwelling solely on deficits.

Consequently, a key aspect of structured teaching is building on the strengths of this group of people, and using these as a basis for developing new skills. It is argued that strategies that purposefully structure the physical environment, as well as developing schedules and work systems assisted by visual cues that provide clear directions, build on the abilities of people with ASD and fit with the 'culture of autistic spectrum disorder' more effectively than other approaches. This culture is characterised by: excessive focus on details with limited ability to prioritise the relevance of details; distractibility; concrete thinking; difficulty with combining or integrating ideas; difficulty with organisation and sequencing; difficulty with generalising; strong impulses; excessive anxiety; and sensory/perceptual abnormalities (Mesibov & Shea 1999).

Structured teaching recognises the positive contribution parents and other family members can make, as well as the difficulties they may encounter in assisting the person with ASD to develop increased independence. The importance of family members is evident in their integral involvement in the development and implementation of individualised teaching plans for their relative (Watson et al 1989). Care is taken to work at the pace of the individual, and as their social circumstances allow. This reduces the risk of exploitation of family members, or increasing pressure on the family circumstances. Such a focus is consistent with the importance now being attached to careful negotiation of care and interventions with family members (Dale 1996).

Whilst structured teaching services continue to be primarily focused on children with ASD and those with other communication handicaps, they strive to have a real world focus and an inclusive approach in their activities (Mesibov 1998). A key aim of structured teaching is to enable people with ASD and other communication handicaps to become more included in their local communities as their abilities of communication and other social skills develop. The use of local community facilities alongside an emphasis on individuality and 'inclusion' reflect the importance attached to citizenship evident within structured teaching and wider Division TEACCH services.

There is a long history of evaluating the effectiveness of the services provided for this group of people within Division TEACCH (Schopler & Reichler 1971, Mesibov et al 1994). This history reflects the need to be aware of the latest research about the nature of this group of people concerning aspects such as communication difficulties, teaching strategies, and the effectiveness of different types of service provision. The findings of ongoing research within Division TEACCH, their associated research projects and the wider research community form the basis for the refinement of the services provided by Division TEACCH and the implementation of structured teaching.

The practical application of structured teaching

Key concepts in structured teaching

Structured teaching is essentially a method of education that relies upon systematic routines provided by trained teachers/professional staff. Parents/carers act as co-therapists, thus emphasising the importance of the transfer of learning between the formal learning environment and the home setting. This model is characterised by the key concepts outlined in Box 8.6.

Box 8.6
Key concepts in the structured teaching model (after Watson et al 1989)

- Spontaneous communication is both the basis of assessment and the final goal
- Use of five dimensions for assessment and programme planning – namely, functions, forms, semantic categories (meanings), words and contexts
- The student is required to learn only one new skill in each dimension
- The need for flexibility in the curriculum to encourage a broader perspective on the integration of skills across dimensions
- 'Real world focus' relates to the need to communicate better in naturally occurring situations
- Collaboration with parents in assessment, goal settings, and the implementation of teaching activities

Structured teaching within Division TEACCH regards the characteristics of ASD as affecting the ability of people to learn effectively through conventional teaching methods. Communication, both receptive and expressive, is often impaired. As a consequence an individual may find difficulty both in understanding spoken language and instructions and in making themselves understood through the use of expressive language. These difficulties are likely to lead to some degree of challenge to the services. Social skills are often impaired, making it difficult to attend and work in groups and to find any reward in praise, or in pleasing people. Imaginative processes are restricted, which inhibits play and the generalisation of learned behaviours to new situations and creates a need for routine and sameness (Trevarthen et al 1998; Williams 1998, 1999).

Structured teaching seeks to provide an environment that can be understood by the child or adult with ASD. This is undertaken in pursuit of the primary aim of Division TEACCH, which seeks to enable this group of people to function meaningfully and independently within their communities (Mesibov 1998). Teaching approaches are structured, incorporating clear visual aspects with the aim of helping this group to predict, control and thus understand the world around them. As with other educational approaches the cyclical process of assessment, planning, implementation and evaluation is central to effective implementation of structured teaching.

Assessment

Division TEACCH originally developed the Psycho Educational Profile (PEP) assessment for use with children with ASD (Schopler & Reichler 1983a). A revised version of this (PEP-R), prepared by Schopler and colleagues, was published in 1988 (Schopler et al 1988). The PEP profile is a directly administered test that measures student achievement on a range of behavioural and developmental sub-scales. The behavioural sub-scale considers aspects such as relating and affect, play and interest in materials, sensory responses and language. The developmental sub-scale collects data on imitation, perception, fine motor skills, gross motor skills, eye–hand integration and cognitive and verbal performances. Sub-scale scores are totalled and a developmental score/age is calculated. The scales have been tested for both reliability and validity (Schopler et al 1979, Mesibov 1988) and are considered to provide an effective method for the objective measurement of behavioural and social/emotional gain for pupils/students. A variation – the Adolescent and Adult Educational Profile, or AAPEP – has been adapted and is used for the assessment of adolescents and adults. In the adult form, the assessment has been expanded to focus on vocational behaviours, work related socialisation, vocational skills, self help skills, independent work skills and leisure activities (Mesibov et al 1988a, 1989).

The manuals for the assessment instruments provide explicit instructions on how to present each task, together with guidance on the scoring format and criteria. The results are plotted on a master sheet providing a developmental profile that typically shows an uneven profile with functioning often being age appropriate in gross motor skills, but lower in cognitive and verbal skills. The PEP-R and AAPEP can be used in conjunction with other assessment scales such as the Bayley Scales of Infant Development, the Merrill-Palmer, the Wechsler intelligence tests, the Leiter International Performance Scale and the Childhood Autism Rating Scale (CARS). This last instrument assesses the level of abilities and needs of individuals by the use of questions about the responses and functioning level in sensory areas. Within the CARS instrument, parents of children select a response from a choice of five statements about their child's behaviour and the scores are added to give a total that is put against a scale of severity within the spectrum of autistic conditions (Schopler et al 1980).

An additional advantage of this assessment is that attempts at completing a task by the person being assessed can be recorded as an 'emerging skill'. Such attempts should demonstrate some understanding by the individual of what is required, so that it can be incorporated into the child's subsequent teaching programme. Staff carefully assess each individual and a strategy is decided upon which details the actions to be taken in respect of the pupil's immediate physical environment in the workplace, their individual daily timetable, the structure of each task and the type of instruction needed for each task.

Planning and implementation of structured teaching

A child's educational psychologist may have conducted some of the assessments and the teacher will undertake other aspects of the structured teaching assessment. Both sets of results will be available to the teacher and are of value in planning the child's individual educational programme (IEP). Typically the developmental profile will show peaks, indicating areas of achievement, and troughs, indicating areas of difficulty for the pupil. Strengths should be worked on to enhance the areas in which the child excels, and doing this will often increase the child's abilities within other areas of difficulty. For example, gross motor skills are often good, whilst cognitive and verbal skills may be poor. With a child who has such a profile, developing communication skills could be linked to enjoyable gross motor activities, such as encouraging the child to shout 'jump' before being assisted to jump into a swimming pool. Or, if the pupil has poor imitation skills, then strategies and exercises can be planned to strengthen these; if the child has good visual discrimination skills, then teaching methods would use visual instructions. The teacher will be able to observe the pupil's preferences for some tasks and perhaps dislike of others. This will enable the teacher to plan the order of tasks on the pupil's schedule with a less favoured task being followed by a preferred one, which can have the effect of increasing pupil motivation. The more it is possible for the child to be motivated by the intrinsic reward of understanding and completing the work task, the greater the potential learning.

Structured teaching emphasises that teaching goals should be selected against the criteria that:

- Meet the child's needs at home, in school and for the future
- Meet the parents' priorities and concerns
- Are realistic expectations for the pupil.

Further guidance on suggested teaching strategies and activities can be found in manuals produced by Division TEACCH. These provide advice for using assessments and on how to plan and write a learning plan for the child (Schopler & Reichler 1983b) as well as guidance on a range of detailed activities in ten function areas with suggestions on how to teach the activity (Schopler & Reichler 1983c). Following the identification and agreement of teaching goals with parents and, when possible, the pupil, it is necessary to develop an individualised plan for each child.

Structured classrooms are designed to provide children with individualised programmes that emphasise skills appropriate to the children's age and developmental level. Each child is provided with an individual workstation, work schedule and work system. Teaching methods rely on the use of symbols and colour codes to reduce reliance on verbal communication that can often be confusing for people with autistic spectrum disorders (Watson et al 1989). There is an emphasis on communication, socialisation, practical skills and fostering of independence. Classes usually serve no more than six pupils and have a minimum of two staff in attendance. Opportunities for integration in specific activities within school activities with other children are also provided. The individualised plan outlines what will occur within the teaching environment and provides guidance to staff and parents.

The individualised education plan will indicate the nature of the structured teaching environment and the manner in which the four main dimensions of the teaching environment will be individualised. The four key dimensions are:

- The structure of the immediate physical environment
- The structure of time through use of a timetable, known as the schedule
- The structure by a work system explaining the task and how to complete it
- The visual instruction and clarification.

Each of the four dimensions is now briefly described:

Structure of the immediate physical environment

The classroom or workplace should be structured in such a way as to provide a dedicated area for specific activities. This should be an uncluttered and clearly defined environment. Within the classroom there can be areas for play or leisure, individual work, group activities, eating and arts and crafts.

Each area is labelled if necessary, so that the pupils can understand what to do there. Areas can be separated using screens or cupboards and bookcases, but each part of the classroom should be easily visible to staff members (see Fig. 8.1, plate section between pp 112 and 113).

When using structured teaching it is necessary to provide a transition area. This is an area of the classroom where the pupils can gather when it is time to change activities during the day. The location and identification of this area requires to be clearly thought out in order to select the most appropriate area within the space available. The area should be central, easily accessible from all other areas of the room, and should be a calm and quiet place where students can come and look at their work schedules to see what they must do next. The area in which the work schedules are placed should be large enough to accommodate all the necessary work schedules when placed out flat for all the pupils in a group. The top of a cupboard or a round table can be used to place work schedules on, and these can become the location of the exchange of these schedules. This surface should be at the right height for both the children and the adults who have to use the work schedules.

Structure of time

The way in which time is structured depends on the level of ability and preference of the child or adult. The introduction of a photographic timetable can have a positive impact. The timetable will use photographic cues of points or activities that represent particular instructions. When possible, these cues should be selected from within the familiar environment of people with ASD. Work schedules or timetables are arranged from top to bottom, or left to right, in a prominent place were they can be easily seen. Single word labels can be attached to the photographs at an early stage, as some individuals have such good visual ability and memory that they learn these associated words in print very quickly. This is seen as a 'goal directed positive progression approach'. Makaton symbols can also be used and some people may find these easier to understand than a photograph that may have too much distracting detail. Alternatively a mixture of words, photographs and symbols of differing sizes and complexities may be used if that is what is needed; the most important consideration is that the person using the timetable understands it.

People with ASD may find it very difficult to understand the concept of time, including the fact that one activity is not going to last forever, the school day will eventually end, and that they will go home again. The timetable acts to help the individual understand the sequence of the day's events and, through use of a picture of the school bus or Mum's car at the bottom of the timetable, reassures them that they will be returning home. Providing such guidance (and reassurance) can have a very positive effect on the behaviour of this group of people.

The younger child, when first introduced to structured teaching, is provided with an individualised work schedule that stays in the transition area. The children can easily identify their own card by their name and by colour if necessary (see Fig. 8.2, plate section). The schedules have Velcro strips to which are attached cards of the activity that the children will be following. For example, the first card may relate to a task which will then be removed from the larger card by the child, and taken to the work area where it will be put in an envelope on the child's worktable. After the task is completed a card indicating a play activity could be taken to the play area and put in a container there.

Structure by work system

The work system is used to provide information about how much work, what to do, how to do it, when it is finished, where to put it, and a reward motivator to work towards. The allocated task and instructions for its completion are usually conveyed by having each task contained in separate boxes (see Fig. 8.3, plate section). For example, a workbox relating to number identification could contain work cards explaining the task of matching the numeral with a picture and a picture of the correct number of objects. The workboxes may be left next to the pupil's worktable or, as the child becomes more able, across the room so that he or she must walk over to collect them. The card can be coloured or numbered and the pupils will follow a work card telling them what order to do their work in and what to do when they have finished it.

The pupils must easily understand instructions in the workboxes, as they should be able to complete the work independently. To help the pupils to match up the correct components of the task, specially prepared templates may be used (see Fig. 8.4, plate section). A picture may then show the pupils how to put them together. If a pupil can read, written instructions are used; a picture dictionary can extend the child's vocabulary where needed. The workboxes may also contain more conventional work tasks such as written exercises or number work.

Visual instruction and clarification

The timetable is presented in a visual form as this can help pupils to predict what is going to happen during the day and bring order to it. Visual information can be revisited whenever students need to reassure themselves or in case they forget what is next. Staff do not demonstrate a task and then expect pupils to copy them, instead they provide visual instructions and/or physical prompting during the completion of the task. Pupils with ASD generally do not learn by exploration or by trial and error; they tend to continue to repeat the same actions, and the same mistakes, over and over again. Therefore it is important that pupils are taught to carry out a task correctly the first time that they attempt it (Trevarthen et al 1998).

Evaluation of progress

The evaluation of progress involves the collection of quantitative and qualitative data from parents, structured teaching staff and other professionals who work with pupils. Evaluation should review the frequency with which pupils have located their individual work schedules and the degree of prompting necessary. It is important to record the number of tasks pupils can complete from their work schedules, and the extent to which this has developed during the time they have been receiving structured teaching. Furthermore, any progress in the use of visual and object cues on the individualised work schedules should be accurately recorded. Such broad quantitative measures used to assess progress can be further validated by the 6-monthly analysis of PEP-R or AAPEP scores (see Figs 8.5 and 8.6, below).

These instruments measure aspects of performance in the relevant developmental sub-scales such as improving self-help skills; social skills; reduction of problem behaviours and reduction of obsessional behaviours; enhancement of coordination skills; improvement of fine and gross motor skills; enhancement of communication skills; and improved concentration. Comparisons can then be made with baseline data gathered from earlier psychometric assessment. This is further validated by the completion of a full PEP-R or AAPEP assessment each year, to

Fig. 8.5
PEP–R developmental scale profile for Michael (see case illustration) (reproduced with kind permission from PRO-ED. Inc.)

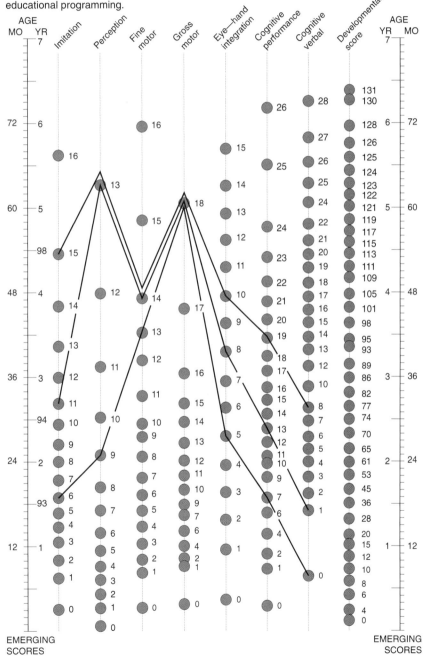

PEP–R DEVELOPMENTAL SCALE PROFILE

Name __Michael__   Case # _____

Date of test __1993—1998__ Date of Birth _____   Chronological Age _____

Mark the point on each scale that represents the number of Ps (passes) scored in that Developmental area. In the Developmental Score column, mark the point that represents the total number of Ps for all seven Developmental areas. (Where a number is missing in the scale, mark the next lowest point on the scale.) In the box at the bottom of each column, record the total E (emerging) scores for that Developmental area. These Emerging scores reflect the child's readiness to learn new skills and indicate appropriate starting points for educational programming.

EMERGING SCORES

Fig. 8.6

PEP-R developmental scale profile for Jonathan (see case illustration) (reproduced with kind permission from PRO-ED. Inc.)

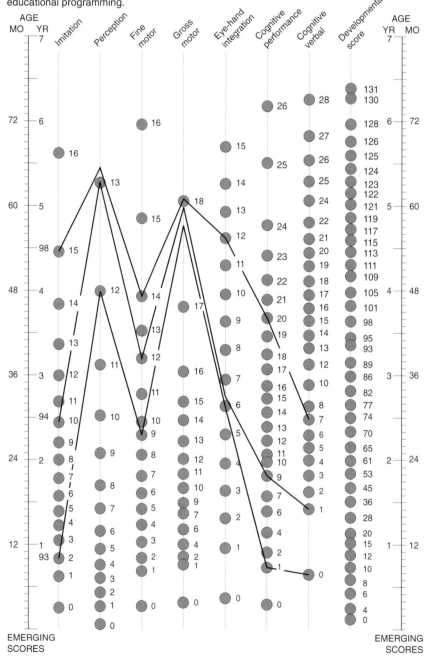

PEP–R DEVELOPMENTAL SCALE PROFILE

Name ___Jonathan_____ Case # _____

Date of test _1993—1998_ Date of Birth _____ Chronological Age _____

Mark the point on each scale that represents the number of Ps (passes) scored in that Developmental area. In the Developmental Score column, mark the point that represents the total number of Ps for all seven Developmental areas. (Where a number is missing in the scale, mark the next lowest point on the scale.) In the box at the bottom of each column, record the total E (emerging) scores for that Developmental area. These Emerging scores reflect the child's readiness to learn new skills and indicate appropriate starting points for educational programming.

illustrate how progress within the individual sub-scales influences the pupil's overall developmental profile. The conclusion from the above data can be complemented by the collection of qualitative measures that monitor improvements in progress in areas relating to quality of life, such as the development of new skills, maintenance of existing skills and interaction ability.

Evidence should be collected following personal observation of each class, self-reports from teachers and from an objective evaluation of the extent to which each structured classroom accords with recommended standards. The criteria outlined for enhancing quality within environments in which structured teaching is delivered provides an indication of the key aspects that should be evaluated (Box 8.7).

Box 8.7
Enhancing quality in structured teaching provision

Physical structure
■ Clear labelling indicating the functions of defined areas
■ Uncluttered floor, surfaces and walls
■ Safe and observable
■ Suitable fixtures and fittings in relation to type, age and colour

Classroom schedules and work systems
■ Visual
■ Clear
■ Consistent
■ Relevant to each pupil's level of understanding
■ Reviewed regularly and adjusted if necessary

Communication system
■ At each pupil's level
■ Portable
■ Everyone knows each child's method and uses it consistently

Individualised education programmes
■ Developed for each child
■ Each team member is familiar with them
■ Shared with parents
■ Developed and implemented in discussion with parents
■ Roles of all involved are clearly outlined

Behaviour management
■ Level and type of structure is individually tailored and suitable
■ Communication system in use for the pupil
■ Consistent approach by everyone
■ Clear communication and appropriate sharing of information between staff and family members

Parental involvement
■ Daily communication systems (e.g. diaries)
■ Parents have opportunities to work in the classroom
■ Parents' group established
■ Social activities within school to enhance support networks
■ Information and library facilities easily accessible
■ Established systems for two way exchange of information on the child

Case illustrations 'Michael' and 'Jonathan' provide details of two children who were involved in a structured teaching Programme. Figs 8.5 and 8.6 show a PEP-R Developmental Profile for each child. After looking at these, look at the activity that follows them (p. 204).

Michael

Michael was an attractive looking child, with large blue eyes and golden curls. He did not speak, nor had he any other form of vocal communication. He had a particular skill for spinning objects and was fascinated by reflected light and helicopters. His appearance, however, did not portray the challenges encountered by his mother and the school staff in living and working with Michael. He was at times an extremely difficult child to manage with frequent periods of distressed behaviour that could involve him shouting or screaming and waving his arms around excitedly. On top of this he would run away from his mother and other carers, if he had a chance, and seldom slept through the night. His mother could not take him into any shops or cafés because of his behaviour, and driving with him in the car had become dangerous, as he would strike out at his mother if she deviated from the route he had become accustomed to.

The constant demands of living with Michael resulted in his mother frequently asking for respite (short break) care in the evenings and over the weekend, often as things appeared to be approaching crisis situations. Michael did not like the disruption of his routine arising from the frequent use of respite care and consequently his behaviour became worse. This created a spiral of unhappiness that left Michael and his mother exhausted and trapped in an apparently unbreakable chain of events.

In school Michael joined a class in which a teacher who had undertaken additional training had set up a structured teaching environment. Michael was 6 years old and assessed on the PEP; following this, a highly structured individualised programme was prepared to respond to his identified abilities and needs. Michael settled into the structured teaching programme quite quickly and his behaviour began to improve slowly over the first year, followed by considerable progress in subsequent years. The class teacher talked with Michael's mum at length and often visited her at home to work on his programme and his timetable that used photographic cues for activities to be completed. His mother, schoolteacher and community nurse (learning disabilities) collaboratively established an acceptable behaviour management strategy. This included the scheduled use of respite care for one full week every month, as a focus on reducing the need for 'crisis' admissions. A plan was also worked out to respond to Michael's most disturbed behaviour at home. This involved his mother responding in a consistent and structured manner. The community nurse (learning disabilities) provided much needed support in this area. Within a short space of time Michael's behaviour began to improve, the periods of distressed behaviour became shorter and his sleeping began to improve at night.

In school Michael worked steadily, though not always willingly, through his programme. The teacher was pleasant but firm, teaching Michael new tasks on a one-to-one basis, and providing plenty of opportunities for these skills to be used both inside and outside of the school. The development of recognisable communication was a priority and frequent opportunities to prompt verbalisation were taken. The speech and language therapist who came to the school worked closely with the teacher and his mother on this, and gradually Michael's sounds became recognisable as the beginnings of words. Michael was encouraged to extend his language skills at home and in school through being understood and receiving high levels of praise.

After a year Michael was reassessed on PEP-R and showed improvements in all areas (Fig. 8.5), and this progress has continued consistently for several years, as is noted on his reassessment after 4 years. He is now on a school reading scheme, completing addition based mathematics, and shows considerable improvement in his communication skills. He speaks in sentences and can be understood by the people he speaks to. His understanding has improved to the extent that his mother can reason with him, and this has contributed significantly to managing his behaviour. His mother accepts that Michael will always have autism, however, at present he is well behaved most of the time and therefore less respite care is required. Both Michael and his mother enjoy life at present and whilst it was not always an easy path to follow at home or in school, the framework provided by structured teaching and the bringing together of the relevant professionals has resulted in considerable progress in Michael's independence and communication skills. He can now make much more use of facilities at home, at school and in his local community. He has made remarkable progress that will continue to be built upon by all involved.

Jonathan

Jonathan joined the structured teaching environment when he was 6 years old. He had a history of being a difficult child to manage, as he would not sit on a chair or near other children. His only vocal form of communication was to shout loudly. He was easily upset by too much noise or activity and would sometimes head-butt anyone near him if he was distressed. He would also run away from home or school if he had the opportunity.

On a more positive note, at 6 years old he was able to sequence the alphabet (backwards only) and was very interested in videos. The schoolteacher spoke at length with Jonathan's parents, who were concerned about him, about his abilities and needs. The structured teaching environment and programme that could be offered was explained to them and they viewed it as a worthwhile approach to pursue.

Jonathan required a work space with limited surrounding stimulation from the classroom, and this was achieved by placing screens on each side of his table. His individual education programme used a timetable with photographs (with words below) as cues. Initially two tasks (workboxes) were used during each work session. Jonathan made considerable progress and within a week five tasks were completed during each work session. Within 6 weeks Jonathan was working for up to an hour at a time. The schoolteacher incorporated activities into his programme that built upon his remarkable visual memory. She showed him how to use letter tiles to spell out some of his needs (e.g. 'biscuit' and 'drink'). Jonathan quickly extended his list of words and was able to use and develop his new skills further in his home.

The teacher worked closely with the speech and language therapist to help Jonathan master the use of a 'light writer'. This is a small 'qwerty' keyboard with a liquid crystal display. This made it easier to spell out his needs than using letter tiles. The schoolteacher made many visits to Jonathan's home and his mother was helped to implement a very structured environment for him at home. This appeared to considerably increase his level of independent functioning at home. Now, 5 years on, Jonathan has two work sessions each day and completes eight tasks during each session.

Baseline and follow-up PEP assessments were completed (Fig. 8.6) and it appears that Jonathan not only actively participates in his work sessions but also enjoys them, and they have a calming effect on him. He still gets upset if there is too much activity or noise near him, and he retreats to his workstation within the structured teaching environment. However, some progress has been made with his acceptance of noise and other people and he was willing and able to participate in the school's Christmas show. He is on a reading scheme and is completing the early stages of addition mathematics. He is now able to communicate very effectively using his 'light writer' at home, however he does not use it as effectively in school. He has acquired a vocabulary of over 300 words and with some prompting he can speak the first syllables of a limited number of words.

His behaviour has improved considerably and, at home, he enjoys using a computer, on which he takes turns with his brothers and sister. He understands most language used in the home and he is very much loved and valued as a family member. His mother feels that speech is not as crucial an issue for her as it used to be, as Jonathan can now communicate effectively with his light writer. She is very happy with the progress Jonathan continues to make.

Explanations

After studying the PEP-R Developmental Scales (Fig. 8.5 and Fig. 8.6) it can be seen that improvement has been made particularly during the period 1993–94. Other than the introduction of a structured teaching approach, can you think of other possible explanations for the progress made by the children? You may find it useful to discuss this with a group of your colleagues.

The empirical basis of structured teaching

In 1971, Schopler and colleagues confirmed the benefits that structured teaching had on learning processes for people with ASD and noted that a key determinant of success in learning depended on the instructor's ability to alter the degree of structure in a planned teaching programme for individual students. In their study the researchers defined a structured session as one in which the instructor determined what material the child would use, how long the child would work, and how the child would work. The results were encouraging and improvements were noted in the child's attention span, relatedness, affect and general behaviour. Other investigators have reported similar results over a number of years (Rutter et al 1967, Sines 1996).

Parents form an essential part of the TEACCH structured teaching application and in 1978 Marcus and colleagues demonstrated improved effectiveness in the parents' use of the structured teaching and learning approach (Marcus 1978). The outcome of the parent–child intervention sessions confirmed an increase in child cooperation as well as a general improvement in skills and well-being. Schopler & Reichler (1971) described the outcomes of a study designed to empower parents to act as co-therapists. They found that parental involvement was greater than they had originally anticipated. Parents attended instructional classes and reported that improvement in their children's functional ability was more noticeable when mothers became more involved in the extension of classroom based teaching to the home. Schopler & Reichler (1971) concluded that therapists should be encouraged to involve parents as co-therapists and thus recognise the valuable role that parents can play in 'solving' their child's problems.

Short (1984) examined the effects of the structured teaching programme by comparing pre- and post-test data with regard to the child's behaviour. Children (and parents) who had been trained and exposed to structured teaching methods showed a marked improvement in the incidence of appropriate behaviours and in the management of inappropriate behaviours. As with all Division TEACCH's work, investigations into the effectiveness of communication skills development is based on sound empirical research.

The curriculum is underpinned by behaviourist principles (Lovaas 1977) and advances in Division TEACCH's understanding of psycholinguistics (Tager-Flusberg 1985). The current model emphasises the meaning of communication and demonstrating its use in multiple situations (O'Neill & Lord 1982).

To demonstrate communication in varied situations, instructors relate learning experiences to the functional world, thus encouraging the association of learning experiences with everyday situations. Opportunistic teaching and ensuring that advantage is taken of every learning encounter (Carr 1985) further complement this approach. A third aspect of the TEACCH communication approach involves the use of a range of forms of communication (Mesibov 1997) that might, for example, include sign language, picture systems and written forms of communication (Layton & Watson 1995).

Division TEACCH have recommended that a series of outcome measures should be combined to provide a cumulative body of evidence to evaluate the effectiveness of structured teaching (Schopler et al 1982). Despite the many studies that have been published on the effectiveness of structured teaching, Schopler et al (1982, p.262) have concluded that:

> *The development of convincing evidence for treatment effectiveness with psychiatric and behavioural disorders is not a simple research task. Complex factors are involved with changes in symptoms and problem behaviours. Influences outside the specific treatment modality also affect every outcome. Control groups are not always available. Not only is the specific treatment difficult to measure, the question of outcome is further complicated over time in the distinction between short and long term effects. The financial cost of outcome research is another factor. However, the need of parents and professionals to identify the most effective treatment procedures for similar children maintains the pressure on all of us to know or find empirical bases for evaluating treatment.*

It is necessary to acknowledge that the challenges of investigating the effectiveness of interventions with people who fall within the spectrum of autistic disorders can be compounded by the complex nature of such disorders. Consequently such studies often require the use of multiple outcome criteria as the only reasonable approach to evaluating structured teaching interventions (Mesibov 1988).

Since the structured teaching programme includes complex components, several lines of evaluation data must be compiled and applied to any research study. These include the use of informal evidence and objective measurement of outcomes in the following domains:

- Social
- Cognitive
- Behavioural
- Self-help skills
- Parental/professional perceptions of treatment outcome effectiveness
- Changes in parent/staff skills.

Structured teaching has been evaluated throughout the world and Mesibov (1997) has advised that the 'most comprehensive' study was performed in Northern Ireland (Sines 1996) where five structured teaching programmes were systematically evaluated against the following outcome measurements:

1. Data provided by 19 parents, 11 project staff and 28 professionals in respect of their perceptions of the effectiveness of structured teaching for the 19 children and seven adults receiving the service (data collection was through questionnaires and personal parental interviews).

2. Independent rating of structured classroom provision against prescribed criteria.

3. Comparison of baseline and post-baseline measurement of pupil/student psycho-educational gain following implementation of structured teaching methods (the measurement tool used for this purpose is the Psychoeducational Profile (PEP or AAPEP)).

The severity of autistic spectrum disorder experienced by all children included in the study was assessed using the Childhood Autism Rating Scale (CARS) (Schopler et al 1986) as this has been reported as useful for children aged from 3–4 years onwards (Garfin et al 1989).

In the Northern Ireland structured teaching study, Sines found that 86% of the parents and professionals who responded to a postal questionnaire described structured teaching as effective, citing examples of improvements in self-help skills and social skills, and a reduction of 'inappropriate' behaviours. Improvements in communication, concentration and independence were also highlighted. Over 90% of participants claimed that this approach had enhanced improvements in social interaction and the quality of life for the children receiving the service. Evidence of effectiveness was noted in parents' reports of increased skills in self-help, social and communication skills. The majority of parents also reported improvements in mobility, coordination and concentration. Further to this, the majority of parents reported reductions in stereotypical, obsessional, aggressive and other 'problem' (as recorded by parents) behaviours. In conclusion, the majority of parents and professionals involved with the structured teaching project viewed it as making a 'great difference' to the quality of life for the children and adults in the project (Sines 1996).

The same study also documented the effectiveness of structured teaching training techniques through the provision of workshops to parents and professionals from the TEACCH project team. Evaluation of the experience of the participants in over 400 structured teaching workshops provided evidence of their effectiveness as a means of preparation to deliver structured teaching (Sines 1996).

Several other outcome studies have examined the effectiveness of structured teaching and the comprehensiveness of structured teaching intervention programmes. Bristol & Schopler (1983) have reported on the relationship between family stress and support networks. Parents reported that structured teaching was the most helpful strategy in reducing the stress. In a later study, Bristol et al (1993) found a decrease in depressive symptoms over time amongst a group of parents participating in the structured teaching programme. In contrast, mothers of developmentally disabled children without this intervention showed no change in depressive symptoms over time.

In conclusion, the available evidence suggests that structured teaching methods provide an effective service both to children and adults with ASD and to their carers. The emphasis within the programme on collaboration between parents and professionals has been described as being the 'potent force' in the provision of comprehensive services for people with ASD (Sines 1996, Mesibov 1997). The empirical and robust theoretical principles upon which structured teaching has been built evidences the success of the programme's dissemination throughout the Western world.

Limitations of the structured teaching approach

Division TEACCH places an important emphasis on the need to evaluate the achievements of the components of overall TEACCH services. It stresses the need to update and adapt practices on the basis of:

1. Research findings about the characteristics of people with ASD or other communication handicaps
2. The evidence about the effectiveness of individual teaching strategies
3. The overall organisation of services.

The above emphasis aims to ensure that services from Division TEACCH, including structured teaching, are as effective as possible on the basis of current knowledge. Despite this emphasis, a number of limitations relating to value for money, suitability for home, availability of community support and training requirements for implementation of structured teaching need to be considered (Sines 1996).

As noted earlier, the eligibility criteria for entrance into structured teaching services restricts the number of people who can access the services. Whilst this strategy may increase the likelihood of success among the pupils of such services, it also excludes other people who may benefit from considerable individual attention. Structured teaching is labour-intensive and the extent to which initial investment actually results in 'value for money' is therefore an area for further consideration. The successful implementation of structured teaching depends on the deployment of additional peripatetic professional staff to fulfil the home based interventions. Inadequate investment in this area may result in reduced effectiveness of interventions. Preliminary findings arising from Sines's study in 1996 have suggested that the provision of structured teaching results in a reduction in the incidence and severity of 'inappropriate' behaviours amongst clients, and enhances opportunities for skill development. In turn, overall service costs may be reduced as the need for long-term residential care is reduced. However, any such savings must be balanced against the initial and maintenance costs associated with the provision of structured teaching (Sines 1996).

Structured teaching requires a major investment of parents' time and energy. In addition, it impacts on other family members and activities within the home to varying degrees, depending on the flexibility within the home setting. The effective implementation of structured teaching in the home setting requires:

- Training opportunities for parents and other family members.

- That training opportunities and practical support services are provided at times that are suitable to the needs of the family.

■ That training opportunities should not be restricted to the working week, since this may not meet the needs of key members of the family and may result in an inconsistent application of structured teaching at home.

The following issues must also be considered:

■ Some parents and other family members may view structured teaching as a highly emotive issue.

■ Some carers may believe that the success of the interventions is dependent upon their own personal efforts in the home.

■ Parents and other family members who are unable to invest the time required to implement the method successfully (alongside the other demands of caring for both a family and the specific needs of a family member with a disability) could be burdened with additional feelings of guilt.

The following are essential to the successful implementation of structured teaching in the home setting:

■ It is essential that parents remain central in the assessment and planning stages of the process in order to match realistically the tasks to be undertaken with the resources available.

■ The availability of appropriately trained staff to both lead and implement structured teaching is a key factor in its successful implementation (Mesibov et al 1988b).

When considering training and staffing issues, the following must be taken into account:

■ This approach requires considerable investment in training of professionally qualified staff and other care staff, as it is often necessary to bring trainers from outside the local area (possibly from the USA).

■ Training requires the release of staff for several days to attend training workshops.

■ Due to the evolving nature of our understanding of people with ASD and of the most effective manner in which to provide support to them and their families, staff must also have access to regular updating and this clearly has ongoing cost and staffing implications.

Conclusion   Increasingly, the implementation of structured teaching is being recognised as providing a feasible way of supporting both children and adults with ASD within school, day centre and, to some degree, home settings. It does not have all the answers (nor does it claim to have) but it does provide a research based framework for increasing our understanding of the experiences of this group of people and the development of their skills. However, further research is required to validate the effectiveness of structured teaching, outside of the overall services provided by Division TEACCH. As the availability of structured teaching increases within the UK, its achievements need to be monitored and the transferability of this approach between the USA and the UK confirmed by research studies.

The availability of structured teaching is likely to expand within the UK and other European countries, and could become a valuable resource for people with ASD and their families. As the effectiveness of structured teaching becomes established and more widely available it is likely that the principles of structured teaching will become more widely used with other people with communication and learning disabilities, and not be confined largely to services for people with ASD. Sines (1996) has outlined a series of key measures that need consideration in order to facilitate the successful introduction of structured teaching into new settings (Box 8.8), and emphasises that the successful introduction of structured teaching into services will require investment and a long-term commitment to service development.

Box 8.8
Key considerations when introducing structured teaching into new settings (Sines 1996)

- Parents require adequate and comprehensive preparation prior to its introduction. This should include attendance at parent workshops
- Home based liaison services should be provided as a requisite, complementary service
- Training opportunities should be provided for both parents and staff prior to the implementation of structured teaching
- Parents and professionals require access to any information relating to the availability of services, delivery and evaluation of structured teaching. This should also include the provision of practical advice on how to structure programmes and to accommodate the rigorous demands that the method places on family life
- Parents need to know that effective methods of measuring the quality of structured teaching provision are well developed. This should include the quality of preparation for structured teaching and evaluation of follow-up services at home, school and work
- People with autistic spectrum disorders also need to be adequately prepared for the implementation of structured teaching at home, school and work. This should include preparatory home visits prior to its implementation
- It is important to ensure the provision of adequate follow-up visits and support for families. Parents also require access to systematic appraisal of their child's progress. This could be provided in the form of monthly written progress reports to encourage parents in the implementation of the method at home
- Investment should be made to ensure that all professionals (including doctors, nursery staff and respite/residential care providers) are 'trained' in respect of structured teaching principles to enhance effective coordination of structured teaching strategies
- Structured teaching should be implemented at the earliest possible opportunity in the child's life. Local services should plan delivery of structured teaching services as soon as possible after diagnosis of autistic spectrum disorders or non-specific communication handicap

Further reading

Attwood T 1998 Asperger's syndrome: a guide for parents and professionals. Jessica Kingsley, London

This book goes a long way to clarifying the nature of Asperger's syndrome and its relationship to autistic spectrum disorders. It focuses on information for parents, including practical explanations of the condition and suggestions for living with people with Asperger's syndrome.

Dale N 1996 Working with families of children with special needs: partnership and practice. Routledge, London

This excellent text considers the practicalities of developing partnerships with families and focuses on family units rather than parents or siblings. It provides clear guidelines for developing effective partnerships with families of children with special needs.

Trevarthen C, Aitken K, Papoudi D, Robarts J 1998 Children with autism: diagnosis and interventions to meet their needs, 2nd edn. Jessica Kingsley, London

This comprehensive text outlines a historical journey from the 'discovery' of autism through to current understanding and approaches to working with people with autistic spectrum disorders. It combines easy to read chapters with sections of detailed information for those readers interested in more complex information. As information in this area changes quickly it is as well to ensure that you refer to the latest edition.

Williams D 1994 Somebody somewhere. Doubleday, London

This is one of a series of books in which Donna Williams, a woman with autism, through her ability as a writer provides clear insights into the world of some people with autistic spectrum disorders. The content challenges readers to recognise and grasp the opportunities that exist to assist people with autistic spectrum disorders. (See also reference list for some other texts by D. Williams.)

References

Baron-Cohen S, Bolton P 1993 Autism – the facts. Oxford University Press, Oxford

Baron-Cohen S, Cox A, Baird G et al 1996 Psychological markers in the detection of autism in infancy in a large population. British Journal of Psychiatry 168: 158–163

Barr O 1999 Learning disabilities and mental health. In: Gormley K (ed) Social policy and health care. Churchill Livingstone, Edinburgh, pp 125–142

Bishop D V M 1989 Autism, Asperger's syndrome and semantic-pragmatic disorder: where are the boundaries? British Journal of Disorders of Communication 24: 107–121

Bradley H 1998 Assessing and developing successful communication. In: Lacey P, Ouvry C (eds) People with profound and multiple learning disabilities. David Fulton Publishers, London, pp 50–65

Bristol M, Schopler E 1983 Stress and coping in families of autistic adolescents. In: Schopler E, Mesibov G (eds) Autism in adolescents and adults. Plenum Press, New York

Bristol M, Gallagher J J, Holt K D 1993 Maternal depressive symptoms in autism: response to psychoeducational intervention. Rehabilitation Psychology 38: 3–10

Carr E G 1985 Behavioural approaches to language and communication. In: Schopler E, Mesibov G B (eds) Communication problems in autism. Plenum Press, New York

Dale N 1996 Working with families of children with special needs. Routledge, London

DHSS 1995 Review of policy for people with a learning disability. DHSS, Belfast

Division TEACCH 1992 TEACCH annual report (1991–1992). Department of Psychiatry, University of North Carolina at Chapel Hill, North Carolina

Firth U 1989 Autism: explaining the enigma. Basil Blackwell, Oxford

Fitton P 1994 Listen to me: communicating the needs of people with profound intellectual and multiple disabilities. Jessica Kingsley, London

Garfin D G, McCallon D, Cox R 1989 Validity of the Childhood Autism Rating Scale with autistic adolescents. Journal of Autism and Developmental Disorders 18 (3): 367–378

Gates B, Beacock C 1996 Dimensions of learning disabilities. Baillière Tindall, London

Gillberg C 1996 High functioning autism and Asperger syndrome. Blake-Marsh Lecture, Winter Meeting, Royal College of Psychiatrists, Stratford upon Avon

Gillberg C, Schaumann H, Steffenburg S 1991 Is autism more common now than 10 years ago? British Journal of Psychiatry 158: 403-409

Grandin T 1995 Thinking in pictures. Doubleday, New York

Happe F 1994 Autism. UCI Press, London

Howlin P 1997 Prognosis in autism: do specialist treatments affect outcome? European Child and Adolescent Psychiatry 6 (1): 55-72

Howlin P 1998 Practitioner review: psychological and educational treatments for autism. Journal of Child Psychology and Psychiatry 39(3): 307-322

Kanner L 1943 Autistic disturbances of affective contact. Nervous Child 2: 217-250

Kazadin A E 1994 Behaviour modification in applied settings, 5th edn. Brookes Coles, Pacific Grove, California

Kroese B S, Dagnan D, Loumidis K 1997 Cognitive-behaviour therapy for people with learning disabilities. Routledge, London

Layton T L, Watson L R 1995 Enhancing communication in nonverbal children with autism. In: Quill K A (ed) Teaching children with autism: strategies to enhance communication and socialisation. Delmar, New York

Lovaas O I 1977 The autistic child. Irvington, New York

Marcus L M, Lansing M, Andrews C E, Schopler E 1978 Improving of teaching effectiveness in parents of autistic children. Journal of American Academic Child Psychiatry. 17: 625-639

Mental Health Foundation 1996 Building expectations: opportunities and services for people with a learning disability. Mental Health Foundation, London

Mesibov G 1988 Diagnosis and assessment of autistic adolescents and adults. In: Schopler E, Mesibov G (eds) Diagnosis and assessment in autism. Plenum Press, New York

Mesibov G 1997 Formal and informal measures of the effectiveness of the TEACCH programme. International Journal of Research and Practice – Autism 1(1): 25-35

Mesibov G 1998 What is TEACCH? (online) Division TEACCH. University of North Carolina. Available from http://www.unc.edu/depts/teach/Whatis.htm

Mesibov G, Shea V 1999 From theoretical understanding to educational practice. Plenum Press, New York

Mesibov G, Schopler E, Schafer B, Landrus R 1988a Individualised assessment and treatment for autistic and developmentally disabled children: the Adolescent and Adult Psychoeducational Profile – AAPEP. Pro-Ed, Austin, Texas

Mesibov G, Toxler M, Boswell S 1988b Assessment in the classroom. In: Schopler E, Mesibov G (eds) Autism in adolescents and adults. Plenum Press, New York

Mesibov G, Schopler E, Caison W 1989 The Adolescent and Adult Psychoeducational Profile: assessment of adolescents and adults with severe developmental handicaps. Journal of Autism and Developmental Disorders 19(1): 33-40

Mesibov G, Schopler E, Hearsey K A 1994 Structured teaching. In: Schopler E, Mesibov G (eds) Behavioural issues in autism. Plenum Press, New York

Miedzianik D, Croskin S 1997 Autism: a life history approach. Journal of Learning Disabilities for Nursing, Health and Social Care 1(1): 4-9

Moore K, McConkey R, Sines D, Cassidy A 1999 Diagnostic scoping study: a study to investigate the provision of diagnostic services for people with autistic spectrum disorders in Northern Ireland. PAPA Northern Ireland/University of Ulster, Jordanstown

O'Neill P, Lord C 1982 A functional and semantic approach to language intervention with autistic children. Paper presented at the Symposium on Research in Child Language Disorders, Madison, Wisconsin

Redworth M, Redworth F 1997 Learning disability and citizenship: paradigms for inclusion. Journal of Learning Disabilities for Nursing, Health and Social Care 1(4): 181-185

Rutter M 1985 The treatment of autistic children. Journal of Child Psychology and Child Psychiatry 26 (2): 193-214

Rutter M 1999 The Emanuel Miller Memorial Lecture 1998. Autism: two-way interplay between research and clinical work. Journal of Child Psychology and Psychiatry 40(2): 169-188

Rutter M, Greenfield D, Lockyer L 1967 A five to fifteen year follow-up of infantile psychosis. II. British Journal of Psychiatry 113: 1187-1199

Rutter M, Silberg J, O'Connor T, Simonoff E 1999 Genetics and child psychiatry. II. Empirical research findings. Journal of Child Psychology and Psychiatry 40 (1): 19-55

Sanderson H 1998 Person centred planning. In: Lacey P, Ouvry C (eds) People with profound and multiple learning disabilities. David Fulton, London

Schopler E, Reichler R J 1971 Parents as co-therapists in the treatment of psychotic children. Journal of Child Schizophrenia 1: 87–102

Schopler E, Reichler R J 1983a Individualised assessment and treatment for autistic and developmentally disabled children, Vol 1. Psycho-Educational Profiles. University Park Press, Baltimore

Schopler E, Reichler R J 1983b Individualised assessment and treatment for autistic and developmentally disabled children, Vol 2. Teaching activities for autistic children. University Park Press, Baltimore

Schopler E, Reichler R J 1983c Individualised assessment and treatment for autistic and developmentally disabled children, Vol 3. Teaching strategies for parents and professionals. University Park Press, Baltimore

Schopler E, Mesibov G, DeVillis R F, Short A 1979 Treatment outcome for autistic children and their families. Unpublished International Conference paper presented to the 5th International Congress of the International Association for the Scientific Study of Mental Deficiency (IASSMD), Jerusalem, Israel, August 1–7

Schopler E, Reichler R J, DeVellis R F, Dally K 1980 Toward objective classification of childhood autism: Childhood Autism Rating Scale (CARS). Journal of Autism and Developmental Disorders 10: 91–103

Schopler E, Mesibov G, Baker A 1982 Evaluation of treatment for autistic children and their parents. Journal of Abnormal Child Psychiatry 21: 262–267

Schopler E, Reichler R J, Rebber B R 1986 The Childhood Autism Rating Scale (CARS). Irvington, New York

Schopler E, Reichler R, Bashford A, Lansing M, Marcus L 1988 Psychoeducational Profile revised. Division TEACCH, University of North Carolina, North Carolina

Short A B 1984 Short-term treatment outcome using patients as co-therapists for their own autistic children. Journal of Clinical Psychological Psychiatry 25 (3): 443–458

Sines D T 1996 A study to evaluate the effectiveness of the TEACCH project. University of Ulster, Jordanstown

Stone W L, Lee E B, Ashford L et al 1999 Can autism be diagnosed accurately in children under 3 years? Journal of Child Psychology and Psychiatry 40 (2): 219–226

Tager-Flusberg H 1985 On the nature of linguistic functioning in early infantile autism. Journal of Autism and Developmental Disorders 11: 45–56

Trevarthen C, Aitken K, Papoudi D, Robarts J 1998 Children with autism: diagnosis and interventions to meet their needs, 2nd edn. Jessica Kingsley, London

Watson L R, Lord C, Schaffer B, Schopler E 1989 Teaching spontaneous communication to autistic and developmentally handicapped children. Pro-Ed, Austin, Texas

Williams D 1994 Somebody somewhere. Doubleday, London

Williams D 1998 Autism and sensing: the lost instinct. Jessica Kingsley, London

Williams D 1999 Like colour to the blind: soul searching and soul finding. Jessica Kingsley, London

Wing L 1988 The continuum of autistic characteristics. In: Schopler E, Mesibov G (eds) Diagnosis and assessment in autism. Plenum Press, New York

Wing L 1996 Autistic spectrum disorders. British Medical Journal 312: 327–328

Wing L, Gould J 1979 Severe impairments of social interaction and associated disorders in children: epidemiology and classification. Journal of Autism and Childhood Schizophrenia 9: 11–29

Yule W, Carr J (eds) 1987 Behaviour modification for people with mental handicaps, 2nd edn. Chapman and Hall, London

Resources

Beyond the home site of Division TEACCH, the information provided below is a combination of addresses and Internet resources that will be of use if the reader wishes to further develop knowledge of autism specifically. This section does not aim to provide a definitive list of available resources as these are regularly updated as new information and resources become available. Rather, the list below represents a series of starting points from which to gain further information across the UK, Ireland, Europe and North America.

Division TEACCH
University of North Carolina
http://www.unc.edu/depts/teacch
This is the home site of Division TEACCH at the University of North Carolina. It provides extensive information in relation to Division TEACCH services and contains a large number of fact sheets and other related publications.

Autism Europe (AE)
http://www.autismeurope.arc.be/
This association coordinates the efforts of some 60 national and regional associations of parents of children with autism in 25 countries, including links to NAS and PAPA Northern Ireland. The site can be accessed in English or French and contact details of a large number of related groups across Europe are available from the site. Autism Europe is an association whose main objective is to advance the rights of people with autism and their families and help improve their lives and it plays a key role in disseminating information to raise awareness about the abilities and needs of people with ASD.

Autism Research Unit
School of Health Sciences
University of Sunderland
Sunderland SR2 7EE
Tel: 0191 510 8922
Fax: 0191 510 8922
http://www.osiris.sunderland.ac.uk/aut-sgi/
homepage
This research unit is supported by NAS and provides up-to-date information on current research relating to people with ASD. Examples include research about diets, vaccines, medical advances and ongoing research projects. Some previous conference proceedings, details of upcoming conferences and links to Autism Europe are also available.

Autism Resources
http://www.autism-resources.com
This American based website contains comprehensive information about people with ASD clearly organised within a framework of 'frequently asked questions'. It also provides details of a wide range of books and other related websites of interest, which include information on organisations, support groups and treatments available.

Irish Society for Autism (ISA)
Lower O'Connell Street
Dublin 1
Ireland
Tel: +35 3 874 4684
Provides a range of residential services in Ireland for adults with autistic spectrum disorders and also support for parents of young children. A network of local groups exists throughout Ireland and can be contacted via the ISA in Dublin. No website was available at the time of writing, but one is under preparation and it would be worth looking for on the Internet. ISA also regularly publishes information on autistic spectrum disorders and related topics.

National Autistic Society (NAS)
393 City Road
London EC1V 1NG
Tel: 0207 833 2299
Fax: 0207 833 9666
http://www.oneworld.org/autism_uk
The society provides clear information about the nature of autistic spectrum disorders for people with autism, families, professionals and other members of the general public. It has a network of groups across the UK, which provide a range of support services directly to people with autism and their families. Contains information on publications by people with autistic spectrum disorders.

Parents and Professionals and Autism – Northern
  Ireland (PAPA)
PAPA Resource Centre
Graham House
Knockbracken Healthcare Park
Saintfield Road
Belfast BT8 8BH
Northern Ireland
Tel: 02890 401729
Fax: 02890 403467
http://www.ulst.ac.uk/papa
*Information available on support groups, services
available (including structured teaching),
publications, research and other aspects across
health, social services and education in Northern
Ireland. A web homepage may be accessed
through the Autism Europe site.*

Scottish Society for Autistic Children (SSAC)
SSAC Headquarters
Hilton House
Alloa Business Park
Whins Road
Alloa FK10 3SA
Tel: 01259 720044
Fax: 01259 720051
http://www.autism-in-scotland.org.uk/
*SSAC has a network of support groups and a
range of other services for people with autistic
spectrum disorders and their families across
Scotland. The website provides details of contacts
and the publications available.*

9 Behavioural interventions

Michael McCue

Key issues
- The roots of behavioural analysis can be found in the classical and operant learning theories developed in the behavioural school of psychology
- Modern behaviourism has resulted in the development of assessment technology based upon multiple aetiological sources that include biological, personal, social and environmental factors
- The management of behavioural distress involves the reduction of significant inappropriate behaviours as well as improvement in social and adaptive skills in other areas of functioning
- There is considerable research evidence to support the effectiveness of behavioural approaches for dealing with behavioural distress

Overview

This chapter outlines and discusses ways in which behavioural approaches may assist in the identification, understanding and management of behavioural difficulties and distress, either as an individual or conjunctive component of therapy. The text presents the historical, philosophical and theoretical bases that underpin the behavioural approach, before considering practical applications in assessment, therapy and evaluation of behavioural interventions. Additionally, both general and context-specific limitations in the use of behaviourally based interventions are addressed, and prospective developments in therapy and service responsiveness are discussed. A subject-specific annotated further reading list, a comprehensive reference section, and a list of useful websites and other resources are appended to provide the reader with an opportunity to consolidate and develop knowledge about behavioural interventions.

Introduction

The last decade has witnessed considerable change in emphasis from a person-oriented causal focus of behavioural difficulties towards a wider 'systems analysis' of factors contributing to, and maintaining, distress. Additionally, there appears to have been a move from a preoccupation with the socially disruptive outcomes of behaviour towards a greater sensitivity to the effects and longer-term consequences of difficulties for the individual.

215

Despite this understanding, however, effective service responses to, for example, the needs, rights and wishes of people with learning disabilities who may experience behavioural distress remain sporadic, inconsistent and inadequate. This chapter outlines and discusses ways in which behavioural approaches can be used to alleviate behavioural distress.

The author uses the term 'behavioural difficulties' in preference to 'challenging behaviours' (a more commonly used and preferred term found in the language of learning disability professionals). This is because, although all behaviours properly classified as 'challenging' are likely to be distressing, not all behaviour difficulties can be termed 'challenging'. Yet, arguably, the majority of these will at some time be precipitated by and/or result in some form of distress for the individual and/or others.

The successful application of behavioural approaches in the assessment and treatment of behavioural difficulties is well documented, both for the amelioration of problems and for the promotion of individual skills and competencies (Matson 1990, Emerson 1995). This chapter is presented within the context of what is known as the 'non-aversive' approach to behavioural change and considers assessment and treatment based upon constructing the least restrictive and socially acceptable criteria.

The behavioural approach

Historical development

The roots of behavioural analysis and intervention are to be found largely in the classical and operant learning theories developed by the behavioural school of psychology. These theories, as outlined in Chapter 1, challenged predominantly medical and psychoanalytic perspectives on behavioural difficulties which concentrated exhaustively on 'within person' causal factors. In the 1920s, American psychologist John Watson began to experiment with response conditioning to support his belief that observable, readily defined and measurable behaviour was largely determined by external, environmental factors (Watson & Raynor 1920). At roughly the same time, the Russian psychologist Ivan Pavlov was conducting experimental research on the conditioning of involuntary reflexes with dogs (Pavlov 1927). These experiments demonstrated that by 'pairing' a neutral stimulus (food) with an unconditioned stimulus (bell ring), an unconditioned response (salivation) was produced. When the bell ring stimulus was later presented on its own, salivation was still induced – thus the bell ring had now become a conditioned stimulus producing a now conditioned response. This theory may be applied, sometimes even unknowingly, in clinical practice. Consider a client who is comfortable with and responds very well to a particular carer. In order to introduce a new carer to the client and establish the same functional relationship, we may 'pair' the two carers interactions with the client in order that the 'new' carer becomes associated with the positive values initially held in respect of the 'old' carer.

The use of this and similarly applied procedures help to 'desensitise' clients to potentially unsettling changes in personnel and routine. In the late 1950s, in his work with post-war traumatised individuals, a South African, Joseph Wolpe, extended the classical learning theories of Watson and Pavlov and introduced the concept of 'mutual exclusivity' between certain behavioural states, for example relaxation and anxiety (Wolpe 1958). This work was seminal to the development and later refinement of graded exposure and systematic desensitisation techniques.

The beginning of operant conditioning theory developed in the late 19th century, through the work of Edward Thorndike and his 'trial and error' learning experiments with cats (Thorndike 1898). Thorndike developed the 'law of effect', a precursor to reinforcement principles, which demonstrated that positive outcomes at the end of a series of activities rendered the cats more likely to repeat these behaviours. Arguably, the work of B. F. Skinner in the 1940s and 1950s resulted in the dominant theory of operant conditioning – that is, behaviour is functional and is stimulated and maintained by environmental conditions. The early focus on the environmental influences on behaviour was predominantly consequence orientated, and Skinner developed the scientific and behavioural definitions of reinforcement (response strengthening), negative reinforcement and punishment (both response weakening) contingencies. Skinner's (1953) three-term contingency relationship of occasion-response-consequences has evolved, with slight variation, into the ABC – antecedent-behaviour–consequence – triad which has formed the basis of behavioural analysis for the last 30 years.

Theories of classical and operant conditioning are based upon observable experimental behaviours, whereas social learning theory reported on by Albert Bandura (1977) was pivotal to the understanding of behaviour determined by 'indirect' non-experimental processes such as observational and vicarious learning. In addition to providing the foundations for development of invaluable teaching methods such as modelling and role play, social learning theory stimulated greater recognition of the roles of emotion, perception and cognition in the learning process (factors not denied, merely not recorded by operant theories). Over the last three decades, behavioural learning theory precepts have been significantly influential in both informing and directing assessment and intervention practices applied not only to the amelioration of undesirable behaviours, but also to functional improvements in the development of adaptive skills and competencies (Barker 1982, Emerson 1995). However, advances in the application of behavioural technology have not gone unchallenged, on theoretical, moral and social acceptability grounds. (These issues are dealt with later in this chapter.)

In 1968, with the launch of the Journal of Applied Behaviour Analysis, Baerx Wolf & Risley (1968) presented their seminal paper 'Some current dimensions of applied behaviour analysis'. Affirming their position some years later, the same authors contested that the process of applied behaviour analysis should be, amongst other things:

- *Applied*: studied behaviours should be socially significant
- *Behavioural*: studies should be concerned with what people actually do
- *Analytic*: studies should demonstrate that behavioural changes are substantially linked to the environmental events and/or manipulations put forward.

It has been argued (Oliver 1993) that a major reason for the seemingly reduced acceptance of behavioural approaches in the UK lies in the historical tendency to apply these techniques divorced from a fundamental and continuous process of research and theoretical legitimacy. In relation to this controversy, Lovett (1996, p. 5) has argued that:

the problem is not behaviourism, but the way practitioners have chosen to apply it.

Theoretical bases for behavioural interventions

In the past, behaviour therapy has been seen as cold, mechanistic, coercive and controlling. Lovett (1996, p. 63) has contested that:

❲Behaviourism gave people skills with one hand, but withheld their dignity with the other.❳

More recently, the focus of behavioural analysis has widened to consider a system versus person causal attribution towards behavioural distress. This has resulted in development of assessment technology based upon multiple aetiological sources that include biological, personal, social and environmental factors (Gardner & Graeber 1994). Additionally, there has been a growth in sensitivity and responsiveness to the distressing and debilitating effects of behavioural difficulties within individual contexts, as opposed to preoccupation with system based consequences. The significance of these developments has been advancement in interventions based upon changing systems, culture and environment (rather than merely changing individuals), in order to both reduce distressing behaviours and promote skills. Secondly, there has been a shift from the perceived requirement for 'quick-fix' technologies towards a more 'functional' orientation of assessment and treatment that has taken therapy beyond the treatment of behavioural symptomatology towards a greater analysis and understanding of causation.

The use of behavioural labels such as 'attention-seeking' and 'non-compliant' can be seen to be cursorily dismissive of the real reasons for such behaviour. Carer responses to an individual's behavioural distress can be influenced by their personal beliefs, values and attitudes with respect to both the cause and effects of that behaviour (see Hastings et al 1997, Morgan & Hastings 1998).

If carers respond to symptoms in the absence of an understanding and appreciation of the cause and function of the behaviour, the outcomes can be damaging. Consider, for example, an individual with communication difficulties who is experiencing physiological pain due to toothache. In order to communicate his or her discomfort and distress, the person begins to scream. A carer who believes that this screaming behaviour is 'attention-seeking' is likely to ignore it in order to avoid reinforcing that behaviour. The carer may also advise other carers and prospective contacts with that individual to do likewise. A potential outcome may be that an individual remains unable to communicate significant and untreated discomfort due to carer withdrawal and avoidance of contact. If this discomfort persists, without opportunity for remediation, the individual is likely to become even more distressed and present more severe screaming behaviour, or to substitute aggression or destruction. This example illustrates both the reciprocity of influence between client and carer behaviour and the potential for exchanges in 'antecedent, behaviour and consequence'. In this illustration client screaming (behaviour) has resulted in carer withdrawal (consequence). This consequence, however, may then become a setting event (antecedent) for continued screaming, or for another form of behavioural distress.

A further development in both the analysis and treatment of behavioural difficulties has been the appreciation of their communicative function (Durand 1990, Murphy 1994). Thus, an appreciation of both the potential relevance of and continuous interaction between biological, behavioural and ecological models has moved analysis and intervention towards a more integrated, compatible and therapeutic fusion of ideologies. Lastly, recognition of the importance of a need for interventions to have social validity is being addressed. Acceptability of methodologies being employed and the requirement of therapy to result in socially relevant and enduring outcomes for both the individual and others are being taken into account (Kazdin & Matson 1981, Schwartz & Baer 1991). Criteria such as personal development, growth in self-esteem and self-control, satisfaction, increased choice and greater social integration are being used as indicators of desirable outcomes that are systematically contributing to what are broadly but crucially being defined as 'quality of life' criteria. Although there has been a hiatus of dissatisfaction, disillusionment and even dismissal of behavioural technology, this approach to the management of behavioural distress appears to be experiencing a renaissance (Oliver 1993). The behavioural approach appears to be maturing with a greater sensitivity and responsiveness to the personal context of behavioural distress than it has had in the past.

The principal tenet of behavioural theory is that behaviour is functional for the individual, and is both shaped and maintained by personal and environmental stimuli and consequences. These stimuli and consequences are determined by personal, historical and situational contexts which anticipate the development of positive (desirable) or negative (undesirable) outcomes. Within these contexts are sets of broad and specific setting events and discriminate stimuli. These events and stimuli facilitate an individual's differentiation between situations in which desirable or undesirable outcomes of behaviour are more or less likely. The learning, shaping and maintenance of behaviour are at least in part mediated through the presentation or removal of desirable or undesirable outcomes.

Historically, this has been described as the processes of positive and negative reinforcement, which are outlined below:

1. Presentation of positive (desirable) outcomes is referred to as positive reinforcement, and this has the effect of strengthening (reinforcing) behaviour by making its repetition more likely.

2. Presentation of negative (undesirable) outcomes is called punishment, since this tends to result in the weakening of behaviour, making its repetition less likely due to the aversive consequences presented. The premeditated application of punitive consequences has been referred to as aversive therapy – a technique that has stimulated more heat than light in the ongoing controversy with respect to its acceptability and necessity.

3. Removal of positive (desirable) outcomes also produces a punitive effect in behavioural terms since this also aims to result in the weakening of behaviour, not through the *presentation* of aversive consequences but through the *removal* of desirables. This procedure may involve the techniques of time-out and response cost (similar to a fining procedure) (described and discussed later in this chapter).

4. Removal of negative (undesirable) outcomes is referred to as negative reinforcement (arguably the most confusing procedure of the four), since this results in reinforcement (strengthening of behaviour) not by presentation of desirables for example money, food, tangibles, but by the removal or avoidance of undesirable consequences.

The following example illustrates this fourth process, referred to as negative reinforcement:

A man's wife has observed that the lawn needs to be cut. Given a temporary lapse in her usual generous and sensitive disposition, she has decided not to induce her husband to perform this task with the promise of 'payment' in the form of liquid refreshment (positive reinforcement). Rather she chooses to nag him with unbearable venom and intensity, until he escapes from this oppression by cutting the grass. Thus, grass-cutting behaviour is strengthened by removal of the particularly aversive nature of the wife's harassment. Additionally, if, sometime later, the same man observes that the lawn requires mowing again, he may be more likely to cut the grass in anticipation of his wife's badgering – thus avoiding a repetition of unpleasantness. Negative reinforcement, therefore, is often referred to as escape and avoidance behaviour.

Reinforcement, it might be said, is like beauty; it lies in the eye of the beholder. What is reinforcing (pleasing) to one person may be largely uninteresting or significantly unpleasant to another. Consider the pleasure or displeasure of human touch to different people. Similarly what may appear to be undesirable to us may be rewarding to others, for example verbal disapproval or moderate degrees of pain. Additionally, reinforcement potency is dependent upon such things as context, cultural preference, historical significance and transient preferences. The prospective value of food and drink will depend upon whether an individual is hungry or thirsty.

Although the focus of behavioural analysis is primarily on the function of behaviour in terms of its environmental stimuli and effect, the topography or form of behaviour is also important. Both similar and different presentations of behaviour may serve similar and different functions across situations, persons, context and time. Behaviours which produce the same, or very similar, personal and environmental outcomes are referred to as belonging to the same response class. These behaviours may be topographically similar, that is, they present in a similar form (for example finger sucking and hand biting) or dissimilar (for example head banging and kicking).

If these behaviours were performed successfully to produce the desired outcomes for their user, for example to obtain carer attention (positive reinforcement) or to escape/avoid carer contact (negative reinforcement), then they could be described as being in the same response class – they produced the same outcomes despite being of similar or dissimilar form.

In order to emphasise the constant dynamic and complex nature of interaction and of the multiple factors which may prospectively influence behaviour, it is important to be aware of the (not exclusive) considerations given in Box 9.1.

The issue of reciprocal influence between client and carer behaviour has already been discussed, and the reader is referred to McGill et al (1996) for illustration of more sophisticated models of client behaviour and carer response contexts. Additionally, some care staff may become 'habituated' to some forms of behavioural distress, and as an inadvertent consequence, both elicit and reinforce more distressing forms of behaviour. Research reported by Gelfand et al (1967) has demonstrated the unscheduled carer reinforcement of client's behavioural problems.

The development of behavioural change techniques has witnessed a radical decline in the use of punitive techniques to eradicate undesirable behaviour (Gardner & Graeber 1994), and has widely embraced a

Box 9.1
Interaction and its relationship to influences of behaviour

1. Behaviours belonging to the same response class may elicit the same or highly similar outcomes across persons, settings, contexts and time
2. Topographically similar and dissimilar behaviours may serve both the same and different functions across persons, settings, contexts and time
3. Causal and maintaining factors may differ between individuals
4. Maintaining factors may vary from causal factors across time. Self-injurious behaviour, for example, may have originally developed as a self-stimulating behaviour (causal) then later is maintained by contingent attention and/or escape/avoidance of carer interaction
5. Both causal and maintaining factors may vary across different forms of behaviour within the same person. For example, different forms of self-injurious behaviour, hand biting and head banging, may have developed as self-stimulating behaviour and attention demanding behaviour respectively. However, functional analysis may now reveal that the maintaining factor for the former behaviour is now task/demand escape/avoidance whilst the latter now appears to be maintained by self-stimulatory reinforcement
6. The same behaviour may serve different functions across settings. For example stereotypic hand waving behaviour may be self-stimulating at home but eliciting of carer attention within the day service setting
7. Some behaviours may be under multiple influences which may be a combination of both internal (for example biological) and external (for example environmental) factors (Murphy 1994)

constructional orientation (Goldiamond 1974). Constructional orientation is concerned with supplanting behavioural difficulties with skills and competencies to replace distressing behaviour formerly elicited by particular situations and contexts. Establishing functionally alternative and less distressing behaviour helps to avoid substitution of other behaviours and the 'negativity' resultant from 'control and counter-control' described in the earlier example of client screaming behaviour. The key elements of positive behavioural support are presented in Box 9.2.

Box 9.2
The key elements of positive behavioural support

- Consideration that behavioural difficulties can be functional for the individual
- Consideration of the multi-function and multi-context significance of behaviour
- Detailed functional assessment and analysis should always precede intervention
- Approaches to intervention should be constructional in their orientation, and utilise functional alternatives to replace behavioural difficulties
- Approaches should seek to change 'systems' rather than just the individual
- Outcomes should produce qualitative life changes for the individual, and not merely the reduction or elimination of undesirable behaviours

Practical applications

Assessment strategies

Having outlined the history, nature and theory bases that have underpinned the development of the behavioural approach, this section explores its application to assessment.

There are numerous examples of, and guides to, behavioural assessment (Durand 1990, O'Neill et al 1990, Zarkowska & Clements 1994, Gardner & Graeber 1994). Box 9.3 represents some of the main objectives sought by this process.

Box 9.3
The purpose of behavioural assessment

- The identification of behavioural difficulties based upon their 'impact' on the individual and others, that is, the personal, social and environmental impact of behaviour, including stress, physical damage to property, injury and exclusion from services
- The definition of the form of specific behaviours, as many behaviours are referred to in broad classifications, such as aggression, destruction and self-injury. There is a need to provide a specific definition related to the topography of discrete behaviours within these groupings, for example striking others with fists (aggression) or pulling hair from own head (self-injury)
- The functional relationship of each form of behaviour and biological, psychological, physiological, social and environmental factors require to be assessed. An essential first step is to eliminate any organic and/or physiological factors which might both ethically and functionally exclude a behaviourally oriented intervention strategy
- The assessment and refinement of function of different behavioural forms
- The generation of hypotheses through safe, sensitive and ethically sound methods
- The assessment of risk to the individual and others in terms of risk factors both without and in light of proposed intervention strategies – that is, in terms of the comparative risks of intervening or not
- The detailed analysis of the prospective disadvantages and advantages for the individual and others – such as a cost-benefit analysis of intervention (Barker 1982)
- The identification of socially valid outcomes for the individual and others – for example quality of life issues
- The identification of potential equivalent behaviour(s) which may be included in order to replace difficult behaviour (consistent with a constructional orientation towards behaviour change)

The following section addresses the main approaches used in behavioural assessment.

Behavioural assessment

There are largely three main strategies of behavioural assessment:

1. The use of interview methodologies with significant informants, particularly the individual, if possible.

2. The use of structured and semi-structured observational techniques both informing and informed by 'refined' information obtained by interview.

3. The development of individually based experimental analysis by the manipulation of identified setting events for, and contingencies of, behavioural difficulties.

Each of these approaches is now discussed in greater detail.

Interview strategies   There are many structured and semi-structured interview formats and schedules designed specifically to elicit information from those informants best placed to provide it (McBrien & Felce 1994, Zarkowska & Clements 1994). O'Neill et al's guide *Functional Analysis of Problem Behaviour* (O'Neill et al 1990) includes a number of well structured and very useful pro-formas to obtain relevant information. The Functional Analysis Interview Form identifies information included in Box 9.4.

Box 9.4
Criteria of importance in functional analysis

- The nature and presentation of behavioural difficulties, that is, their form
- Behavioural dimensions, including frequency, duration and impact of behavioural difficulties
- Broad setting events for behavioural difficulties such as physiological problems, lack of sleep, activity scheduling, crowding/lack of personal space and noise levels
- Specific situations predisposing behavioural difficulties such as time of day, situation and specific activity
- Perceived function of behaviour – for example, what are the consequences of same?
- Behavioural 'efficiency' in terms of physical effort, response ratio and response delay
- Communicative strategies including verbal, gestural and symbolic
- Reinforcing events, actions and objects
- Existing functionally alternative/socially appropriate skills/ behaviours
- Problem history and outcomes of previous intervention strategies
- Informant based strategies should consider issues relating to intervention priorities in terms of:
  — behaviour(s) presenting greatest danger to the individual and/or others
  — which behaviour(s) appear to preclude the development of appropriate skills or competencies
  — which behaviour(s) could replace or 'inhibit' behavioural difficulties
  — which behaviour(s) if changed, would best meet the needs and wishes of the individual
- Resource availability (material, carer time, etc.), and its prospective influence on behavioural difficulties
- Service organisation and culture and prospective influences on behavioural difficulties
- Carer beliefs about attitudes and responses towards the individual's behavioural difficulties
- The benefit of using individual self-recording methods, rating scales and questionnaires to inform the assessment process

Rating scales

Durand & Crimmins' (1992) Motivational Assessment Scale is an example of a questionnaire-formatted, 16-item, 7-point rating scale intended to establish/identify the motivational bases for behavioural difficulties. The scale seeks to identify the influence of sensory-social-tangible and negative social reinforcement upon the development and maintenance of these difficulties. Gardner & Graeber's (1994) Multimodal Diagnostic and Intervention Model provides an assessment structure and methodology which focuses on the potentially wide and complex range of physiological, psychological, social and environmental factors which may be instrumental in the cultivation and preservation of behavioural and emotional distress. This model serves to analyse both *internal* (individual) and *external* (socio-environmental) characteristics and variables which may function as setting events for the presentation of behavioural difficulties (see Fig. 9.1). It is suggested that a critical combination of the factors identified in this figure may serve to precipitate behavioural difficulties. Clearly this will be dependent upon the intensity of the variables and the vulnerability and/or sensitivity of the individual, conditions and characteristics which may vary considerably across situations, contexts and time.

It is useful to analyse the potential setting events for behavioural difficulties across a temporal continuum. Consider, for example, the myriad of individual experiences that might influence subsequent behaviour, including: the volume and quality of sleep the previous night; waking in

Fig. 9.1
Internal and external variables, a combination of which may precipitate behavioural difficulties

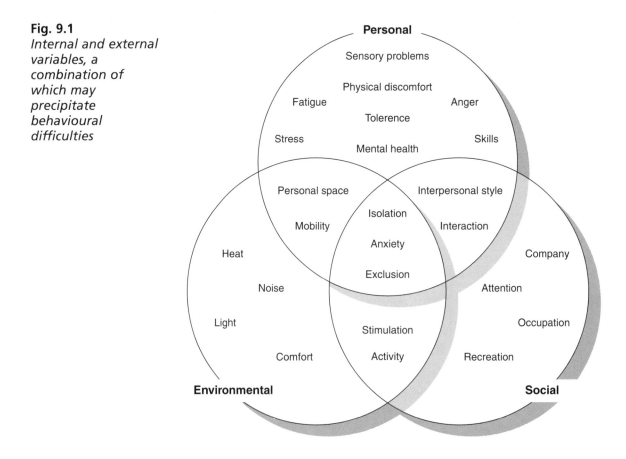

plenty of time to allow the usual routines that precede work; travel conditions en route to work; returning to work following leave; volume and type of work to be performed on arrival and throughout that day; pressure of deadlines and staff shortages; physical well-being and relationships with fellow workers. Consideration should also be given to the number of individuals, each with their own multiplicity of experiences and sensitivities, with whom interactions will take place. This complexity partly explains how difficult it may be to identify, far less analyse, the comparative significance and influence of a range of factors upon an individual's behaviour.

With respect to the prospective influence of skills based deficits on behavioural difficulties, Evans & Meyer (1985) have advised considering a 'discrepancy analysis' both to identify and to quantify those individual skill deficits associated with behavioural difficulties. This analysis typically involves comparing an individual's responses in problematic situations with those of a non-learning disabled peer in order to identify specific difficulties in need of redress, and prospective strategies to deal with them. (For other 'setting event' oriented checklists see Gardner et al 1986, Groden 1989, Van Houten & Rolinder 1989.) To address the subjectivity of informant based information, it is frequently necessary to consult with a significant 'width' of informants, to obtain more reliable, objective and valid assessment data.

Observational strategies

Recording formats

Although the assessment strategies discussed above rely on retrospective based observations of informants, it is useful to conduct progressively more structured and detailed observational and functional based analyses of the individual's behavioural difficulties. Figure 9.2 provides an example of a typical antecedent-behaviour-consequence (ABC) record format based on the three-term contingency theory of Skinner (1953) that an antecedent (or stimulus) sets the occasion for a behaviour (or response) to occur and in turn this behaviour produces a consequence (or outcome) which takes place sometime after the behaviour is displayed.

Analysis by this means enables consideration of the locational, situational, social and environmental antecedents to, and consequence of, behaviour. Although ABC records offer a significant range of information in an easily documented and compact format, disadvantages include the possibility of forgotten or unreliable information due to the retrospective nature of recording. The record can also be limited with regard to the predominant accounting of largely proximal antecedents and consequences. Typically, this method of recording does not yield information pertaining to either temporally or physically distant antecedents and consequences, including details of potentially significant happenings occurring some time before or after a 'target' behaviour, and the inclusion in records of possibly significant others or activities at some distance from the geographical proximity of that behaviour. If distal factors are considered to be significant, however, a follow-up interview with the relevant personnel may provide that information (O'Neill et al 1990 and Pyles & Bailey 1990 provide examples of three-term contingency based recording formats.)

Figure 9.3 presents a scatter plot assessment of an individual's behaviour (Touchette et al 1985). The shaded area represents a single occurrence of behaviour within 15 minute segments. More than a single occurrence of the behaviour may be recorded by numerical frequency in an unshaded

Fig. 9.2
An example of an ABC (antecedent-behaviour-consequence) record

	Antecedents		Behaviour	Consequences	
Date/time	Where was the subject before the incident ?	What was the subject doing before the incident ?	What actually happened ? Give a clear account of the details of the incident !	What happened after the incident ?	Sig

segment, or by using shading in different colours. By such graphical representation of observational data, behavioural 'density' may be highlighted across time. Similarly, and just as importantly, the lack of incidence of behavioural distress may be identified.

Fig. 9.3
Scatter plot analysis of behavioural difficulties (Touchette et al 1985)

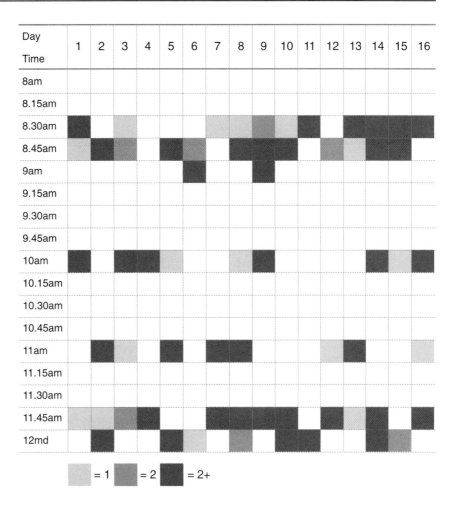

Subsequently, incidence or non-incidence can be analysed across contexts and settings, relative to time, which may be predictive of performance or non-performance of behaviour. In the illustration provided (Fig. 9.3) there appears to be a fairly consistent concentration of recorded incidents around times associated with periods of unstructured activity for this individual, those being arrival at the workplace, between activities, and prior to lunch.

Completion of a scatter plot format may be made using a transcript of salient information from ABC or other incident charts or through the use of direct observations of behaviour.

The case study entitled 'Peter' provides an example of how the use of a scatter plot analysis helped the identification, understanding and subsequent management of a young man's behavioural distress.

Peter

The need
Peter, a 27-year-old man, attends a local day service. This placement was in danger of breaking down due to an increased frequency of behavioural difficulties that were particularly aggressive and destructive. The implications of a placement breakdown were potentially traumatic for Peter and for his family, who would struggle to cope with

managing him at home without a structured schedule for occupying his week.

Approach
Problem incident assessment via ABC records and scatter plot analysis revealed that behavioural difficulties occurred most frequently at times of unstructured activity, such as arriving at and leaving the day service and in between scheduled occupation. Activities were preference ranked by Peter and then re-scheduled to take place immediately upon arrival and following lunch, to help motivate his attendance of these and reduce his capacity for delaying activities by wandering around the service complex. An activity diary was introduced in order to focus Peter's attention on his chosen schedule, and facilitate his self-cueing of attendance at the scheduled events. This also assisted carers by allowing them to prompt Peter to his next activity through consulting his diary.

Carers were trained to use an interactional style with Peter which was demonstrated to be sensitive to his needs and effective in attracting his attention and cooperation. Carers also became more aware of Peter's sensitivity to lack of structure, and were able to interact with him at other times as well as at programmed events to reduce the propensity for behavioural difficulties. Peter also became involved in a lunch-time service development group involving both clients and carers. This not only allowed him to contribute to the ongoing improvement of service delivery, but also reduced his capacity for unstructured activity during lunch.

Outcomes
Frequency of behavioural difficulties reduced significantly and the threat of placement breakdown was removed. There was improvement in Peter's co-operation within the service and his self-management skills. He now has greater choice regarding both the nature and scheduling of his activities. More 'out-of-service' activities have been arranged due to reduced management difficulties, increased confidence, and improved relationships with other service users and carers.

Direct (structured) observations

The use of direct participant based observational methods to assess behaviour is generally more time-consuming than non-participant based recording. Information obtained through interview or ABC records highlighting particular time or setting events predictive of behaviour will help inform and direct the nature and scheduling of direct observations; these in turn may facilitate the generation and testing of functional hypotheses. Conducting direct observations of behavioural distress is problematic. Consider, for example, the ethical implications of observing behaviour that may be potentially harmful to the individual and/or others. In such cases carers must consider, consult and attempt to reach a consensus concerning a range of issues that includes: prospective costs and benefits; informed consent; least restrictive alternatives; and safe and sensitive written protocols regarding contingency management of undesirable outcomes. In the case of potentially harmful behaviour, a retrospective analysis of behavioural context, dimensions and perceived functions may be indicated. Aside from developing an understanding of the 'functional setting events' for and consequences of behaviour, both participant and non-participant based observational recording allows the establishment of a baseline assessment of individual behaviour against which any intervention strategies may be evaluated. However, as previously stated, both quantitative (data based) and qualitative (positive life outcome based) therapeutic goals of intervention should be set and evaluated. It is possible to use computer technology to improve the accuracy and reliability of the recording and analysis of observational and statistical data. In addition, advances in both hardware and software and their increased availability have also contributed significantly to the process of behavioural and functional analysis (Repp & Felce 1990, Hall & Oliver 1992). A more sophisticated technique of behavioural assessment is described and evaluated by Emerson et al (1996). This approach is known as 'time based lag sequential analysis' and considers the predictability ('conditional possibility') of the onset, occurrence of termination of one event ('the conditional variable') across time, relative to the onset or termination of a second event ('the base variable').

Generating and testing functional hypotheses

The combination of information obtained through structured interview and behavioural assessment should help generate hypotheses regarding the causal and maintaining factors of specific behavioural difficulties. In turn, these hypotheses may direct the process of experimental analysis of behavioural function. The process of assessment of behaviour, therefore, follows a continuum of increasing specificity and contiguity: from what may be a distal/systemic oriented ecological analysis towards a proximal/person focused functional (experimental) analysis. Thus an individual's behaviour may be determined by a number of developing factors, for example: the amount of sleep from a previous night; familial harmony prior to departure for work; comfort of working conditions; physiological well-being and quality of interpersonal relationships throughout the day. Additionally, given the influence of others' experiences within these contexts upon both their own behaviour and that of those they come into contact with, the complexity of behavioural analysis may be even greater. It may not always be necessary or desirable to test generated hypotheses experimentally, for example if behavioural function is well established and defined prior to this stage, but testing and clear understanding may be necessary to satisfy ethical considerations of intervention strategies. The generation of functional hypotheses involves analysis of the often complex relationships between behavioural forms, causality processes and the contextual 'control' of these processes. From these, a number of hypotheses may be developed by analysis of relevant setting events and these relate to the bio-physiological and socio-environmental factors that are next briefly outlined.

Bio-physiological and socio-environmental factors

Bio-physiological factors include: hormonal changes, fatigue, pain, seizure activity. Socio-environmental factors include: carer interaction, peer taunts, instruction, crowding, noise, choice over activities, level of background stimulation such as music (Durand & Mapstone 1998).

Table 9.1 provides a framework for the consideration of functional hypotheses based on the process of positive, negative and automatic reinforcement. Note that with automatic reinforcement behavioural difficulties may occur in response to conditions of either deprived or intense stimulation and/or arousal, thus generating a functional hypothesis based upon behavioural difficulties serving either to compensate for levels of under-stimulation, or to suppress an unpleasant state of over-arousal (Horner 1980, Murphy 1982). It is potentially useful, at the stage when hypotheses are generated, to consider the functional relationships of behavioural difficulties presented in multiple forms. Where possible, these forms may be hypothesised and subsequently 'tested' as response class behaviours, that is those that result in the same or similar outcomes. The strategy most commonly used to conduct experimental analyses of behaviour from established hypotheses is analogue study (Sturmey et al 1988, Iwata et al 1994a). Analogue studies (also referred to as alternating treatment designs) involve the sensitive and systematic manipulation of environmental conditions, based on generated hypotheses, in order to establish the functional relationships of behavioural difficulties. These studies are potentially very powerful, concise and practical since:

- They may require only brief temporary changes to natural environments
- They can provide a very effective means of testing ideas regarding the motivational bases of behaviour
- They can introduce hypothesised 'setting events' which may only infrequently, even rarely, occur in the individual's natural environment
- They can be fairly easily replicated or repeated by others in different settings and contexts over time
- They afford the testing of setting conditions within the context of 'natural' environments.

Table 9.1

Generating functional hypotheses – some clues. Hypotheses as to behavioural function

Positive reinforcement	Negative reinforcement	Automatic reinforcement
↑ In behavioural difficulties when lacking direct contact/attention	↑ In behavioural difficulties when approached by carer	↑ In behavioural difficulties when understimulating OR overstimulating conditions (see text)
↑ In behavioural difficulties when people are 'around' but not in direct contact with the individual	↑ In behavioural difficulties when presented with task/activity request	↑ In behavioural difficulties when individual is alone
↓ In behavioural difficulties when people are interacting with the individual	↓ In behavioural difficulties when carer withdraws	↓ In behavioural difficulties when stimulation conditions are altered
↓ In behavioural difficulties when people are 'around' the individual, and contact is likely	↓ In behavioural difficulties when task/activity request is withdrawn	↓ In behavioural difficulties when individual is with others

Examples of experimental conditions that may be based upon generated functional hypotheses include:

- *Alone conditions*: individual alone with no peers or carers present and with or without available materials.

- *Continuous or contingent attention conditions*: carer gives attention continuously to the individual, or does so only in response to defined contingencies.

- *Task demand or instructional conditions*: presentation of task demands, perhaps with graded difficulty and level of prompting in order to test effects on behavioural dimensions.

- *Carer presence with no interaction*: carer is present but does not interact with the individual irrespective of behaviour.

- *'Control' condition*: to test the introduction of new stimuli and contingencies, for example carer attention/interaction or raised/lowered levels of background stimulation contingent on non-performance of difficult behaviour.

By evaluating the variation in behavioural dimensions as a consequence of environmental manipulation, hypotheses as to behavioural function may be further developed and refined. The following considerations should be satisfied prior to experimental analyses of behavioural function:

- The relevance, importance and requirement for this form of analysis with respect to the individual and others
- The requirement to conduct a detailed assessment of risk and analysis of prospective costs and benefits of performing such analyses
- The requirement for carefully planned ethical safeguards, risk reduction strategies and sensitive contingency protocols
- The consensus review of, and consent for, the application of these analyses by the individual and significant others
- The securing of sufficient resources to conduct the analyses, satisfy ethical safeguards and expedite protective contingency plans
- The methodology of evaluating and reporting on outcomes and their prospective influence on proposed intervention strategies.

The reader might wish to refer to Emerson et al (1990) for a comprehensive rationale and methods for the application of analogue studies. Figure 9.4 illustrates the results of a typical analogue study of an individual's screaming behaviour across four setting conditions. As can be seen, the frequency of the undesirable behaviour was greatest during the second setting condition (the

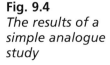

Fig. 9.4
The results of a simple analogue study

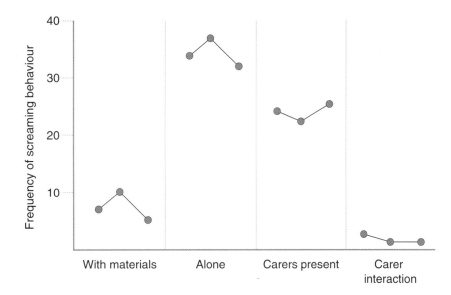

alone condition). Screaming behaviour was observed to be at relatively low frequency during the first (client with preferred materials) and fourth (client engaged in carer interaction) setting conditions. The third condition (carers present but not engaged with client) elicited a relatively frequent, but not most frequent performance of screaming behaviour. From these results, a preliminary hypothesis of a positive reinforcement-gaining function for screaming behaviour might be generated.

Figure 9.5 illustrates a more complex form of analogue study, or alternating treatment design. Readers may use this illustration to develop their own hypotheses as to the possible setting events and functions of the subject's behaviour prior to comparing these with the considerations offered in Box 9.5. There are a number of limitations in the application of behavioural approaches to assessment and these will be discussed later in this chapter. However, specific difficulties in the use of analogue studies include the capacity of experimental conditions to replicate 'natural' environments or conditions and the possibility of insufficient attention being given to the strategic ordering/scheduling of these conditions. Consider, for example, the relative satiable effects of scheduling a 'carer continuous attention' condition following a naturally arranged social event with the same carer; or the relative deprivation effects of scheduling an 'alone' condition following the same natural event, or following an experimental 'carer continuous attention' condition. Both examples are likely to produce a potentially distorted quantification of conditional influences on behaviour. The reader is advised that the use of such scales is extremely exacting, and a suitably qualified behaviour therapist must be consulted prior to

Fig. 9.5
A complex analogue study

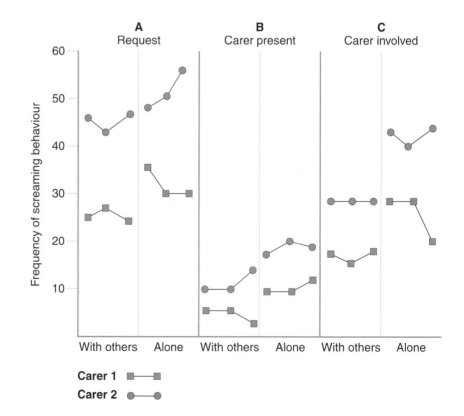

consideration of the use of analogue studies as a functional analysis of behaviour (see also further reading section at the end of the chapter).

Box 9.5
Preliminary hypotheses as to behavioural function (see Fig. 9.5)

Setting conditions
Frequency of screaming behaviour is consistently greater when the subject is alone rather than with others. A preliminary hypothesis based on this finding may be that the subject enjoys being alone, and that actual or perceived carer contact is aversive to them.

Experimental conditions
Frequency of screaming behaviour is highest under the request condition, followed by the carer involved condition. A relatively low frequency of screaming is experienced under the carer present condition. Again, a preliminary hypothesis may be that the subject finds carer requests and interaction to be unpleasant. Additionally, the performance of screaming behaviour during the carer present but not involved condition (albeit at comparatively low rate) may be due to the subject's perception of imminent carer request and/or interaction – especially when the subject is alone with a carer and may anticipate a greater likelihood of this outcome than when with others. The greater frequency of screaming behaviour when alone with carer(s) present, but not involved, would appear to support this hypothesis. Further, the finding that screaming behaviour is at a lower frequency during carer involved versus carer request conditions may be due to the relative acceptability to the subject of the nature of some forms of interaction over that of carer requests, including perhaps: method of presentation and/or interaction; difficulty of activity for the subject; level of carer assistance/encouragement; and duration of activity. Functional hypotheses, therefore, may be refined by subsequent analysis of these possible factors.

Carer comparison
Frequency of screaming behaviour is observed to be consistently lower across both setting and experimental conditions with carer 1. A preliminary hypothesis from this finding may be that the subject has a more comfortable relationship with carer 1, or that carer 1 uses a more positive style of interaction than carer 2. Additional considerations may include the respective gender, size, experience, communication skills and length of relationship with the subject of each carer. Again, further analysis of these and other factors would assist in the development and refinement of functional assessment.

Planning interventions

A number of strategies have been discussed that are helpful in identifying, quantifying and giving us a better understanding of behavioural difficulties and distress. The following section addresses the application of assessment outcomes to the planning and implementation of behavioural interventions. Important prerequisites for the development of both a rationale for and the approach to behavioural intervention should include:

■ A systematic orientation to the assessment of bio-psycho-socio-environmental factors which may serve to predispose and/or maintain behavioural difficulties

- A thorough assessment of the individual's attributes, strengths, skills and competencies
- Consideration of those skills and competency deficits which may be selected as constructional targets for intervention, and may serve as functional alternatives to behavioural difficulties
- The identification of individually based reinforcers which may be used to both establish and maintain new repertoires of behaviour
- The identification and evaluation of the prospective risks, costs and benefits of behavioural intervention
- A prospective analysis of proposed intervention in terms of ethical compatibility, social validity and quality of life enhancement.

Additionally, detailed consideration of any biological, psychological or physiological factors linked to behavioural difficulties should assist in defining the prospective legitimacy of behaviourally based interventions either as the main or as a conjunctive component of therapy. As previously discussed, detailed analysis of social and/or environmental setting events of behavioural difficulties may indicate the value of intervention strategies with a greater culture/systems focus. Assessment of an individual's skills and competencies is helpful in devising a constructional orientation of therapy and it also enables the use of established strengths to redress identified deficits. There are a number of skills assessment and checklists available (Hogg & Raynes 1986, Nihira et al 1993, Zarkowsa & Clements 1994). Over the last 10 years, particular attention has been directed towards the interpersonal and communicative context of behavioural difficulties. This has resulted in interventions being based on the establishment of augmentative (Beukelman & Mirenda 1992) or functionally alternative communication responses (Durand & Carr 1991, Thurman 1997). Additionally, skill deficits associated with setting events for behavioural difficulties may become targets for constructional intervention.

It is often the case that carers working with people with learning disabilities, for example, harbour unrealistic expectations of, or make unrealistic assumptions about, the ability of clients to demonstrate and transfer skills across a range of settings and situations that may not be accommodating of (or are even oppositional to) performance. Assumptions can be made regarding the individual's 'real' ability to exercise or use skills against choosing not to do so. This can result in a presumed motivational deficit to perform or 'behave'. Conversely, underestimation of an individual's abilities and strengths may also lead to false assumptions, with the potential of an illegitimate perception resulting in lowered expectation of a person. Some individuals may observe the competencies of other disabled or non-disabled peers and feel discontent, anger and frustration due to their own skill deficits. Such feelings may lead to behavioural difficulties.

Reinforcement

The identification of potential reinforcers that may be required in order to establish and maintain appropriate alternative behaviours is an important prerequisite to therapy. Reinforcement is the prime component in behavioural intervention strategies and has proved particularly useful in the case of people with learning disabilities who also have behavioural difficulties. The use of individually potent extrinsic reinforcement is particularly powerful in instances where the intellectual difficulties of a person may preclude the use of more 'natural' or intrinsically based motivators. Although researchers have observed the compromising effects of extrinsic reinforcement on intrinsic motivation (Carton & Nowicki 1998), when used sensitively and systematically, extrinsic reinforcement can provide a temporary but pivotal bridge towards the natural contingencies which maintain socially acceptable behaviours. Potentially effective reinforcers may be identified by consultation with the individual and/or appropriately knowledgeable informants. This may be achieved by using individual and/or informant based responses to structured reinforcement inventories (Willis et al 1993), and by testing reinforcement potency via sampling (Parsons & Reid 1990, Sigafoos & Dempsey 1992).

Risk analysis

The rationale for any behavioural intervention should reflect assessment of the prospective outcomes of therapy in terms of risk, costs and benefits to both the individual and others (See Ch.3). It may appear to be an obvious statement that the anticipated benefits of intervention should significantly outweigh any perceived costs, but it is a critical one. It should take account of the rights of the individual within the context of that individual's freedom of choice (Bannerman et al 1990). Identification of prospective risk factors is similarly crucial, in order both to avoid taking unacceptable risks and to make defensible evaluations of risk that are informed by carefully planned risk reduction and risk management strategies. It may often appear safer, and simpler, not to take risks at all, but at what cost to the well-being of the individual? The potential 'burden' of risk may be functionally quantified, managed, embraced and accepted by informed individual and multidisciplinary involvement. Emerson (1995) has provided an outline of some of the potential costs, benefits and risks of behavioural interventions that may be used in assessing their impact (Emerson 1995, pp. 114–115).

Outcomes analysis

Earlier in this chapter it was stated that behavioural intervention strategies should be socially and ethically acceptable and produce therapeutic outcomes which improve the quality of life for the individual and others. Increasingly, the outcomes of behavioural interventions are being evaluated from both quantitative and qualitative perspectives, that is, reductions in the dimensions of behavioural difficulty and distress, as well as advances in the wider aspects of life quality and personal well-being that may have been compromised by the behavioural distress (Meyer & Evans 1993, Felce & Emerson 1996).

Approaches to behavioural change

Once functional hypotheses for behavioural difficulties have been carefully developed, and relevant and valid behaviours have been identified as targets for intervention, the least restrictive methodologies for behavioural change should be considered. This section of the chapter aims to provide an outline and analysis of interventions aimed at reducing behavioural distress and producing desired behavioural change. Emphasis is placed on non-aversive technology of behaviour change, within a framework based upon the traditional ABC model:

1. *Antecedent based approaches*: the preventative/proactive approach to behavioural change, changing the context of behaviour and the modification of setting events.

2. *Behaviour based approaches*: the constructional approach to behavioural change, teaching new skills; 'establishing functional alternatives to behavioural difficulties by differential reinforcement of alternative or incompatible behaviours.

3. *Consequence based approaches*: the contingency approach to behavioural change, changing the consequences of behaviour; manipulating contingencies; methods of behavioural reduction.

Antecedent based approaches

By applying the traditional ABC model, behavioural intervention strategies may be employed within a range of contexts. Behavioural change methods based upon antecedent manipulation may assume a proactive orientation: they may prevent or reduce behavioural difficulties and distress by the alteration or removal of setting events identified as eliciting specific behaviours. The alteration or removal of setting events and specific stimuli can be used both to construct desirable behaviours and to reduce or eliminate undesirable behaviours.

Lovett (1996) provides an illustration of a lady who had spent many years in a large institution. One day she went out for lunch to a local restaurant. When the lady refused to leave the restaurant after a couple of hours, the owner alerted the police to resolve the situation. The lesson learned was that after many years of 'conditioning' to group eating – where everyone leaves the dining area together – this lady was merely waiting for other people in the restaurant to finish eating before 'cueing' her own departure. Similarly, a client was experiencing difficulties in using a shower after many years of using a bath. It appeared that this gentleman was uncomfortable about using a shower, and this became a problem when he moved to a residential facility that temporarily had only showering facilities. Someone from his care group mentioned that he enjoyed swimming very much, and since a 'natural' precondition of using the local pool was to shower, maybe this would be motivation enough. Subsequently, the gentleman used the shower, realised it was not so distressing after all, and overcame his temporary difficulty. The case study entitled 'Peter' (p. 227) contains a number of antecedent-control components to intervention that include interpersonal style profiling, environmental manipulation, and the provision of functional stimulus cues. The sections below provide further examples of setting event and stimulus change methods.

Interactional or interpersonal styles

Research studies have demonstrated that developing individually focused profiles of interactional or interpersonal styles can be very useful in both promoting adaptive behaviours and reducing or eliminating behavioural distress (McDonnell & Sturmey 1993, Yoder et al 1994). The development of an interpersonal style profile that responds to the needs of individuals requires a number of things. These include the use of eye contact, type and tone of voice, use of signs/symbols as communicative aids, the importance of personal space, distance, posture and touch, as well as the functional use of activities preparation, completion and scheduling.

Activities scheduling/ re-scheduling

Scheduling activities that are compatible with one another is important to instil motivation, preparedness, confidence and competence. For example, would any of us choose, or have it chosen for us, to bathe or do our laundry during our favourite television programme? Dunlap et al (1994) reported on how choice of preferred activities was used to increase engagement and reduce challenging behaviour. Case study 'Peter' (p. 227) provides an example of the therapeutic re-scheduling of activities at identified times of difficult behaviour for a young man working at a local resource centre. By affording him the opportunity to engage in favoured activities at stressful times, disruptive, destructive and aggressive behaviours were significantly reduced and participation and cooperation were greatly enhanced. Less preferred activities were then both sensitively and systematically introduced without recurrence of behavioural difficulties.

Introducing individual choice into the scheduling of activities is both motivating and empowering. Following such a strategy an individual's self-determination and control may be promoted and maintained and simultaneously developmental opportunities and goals may be realised (Foster-Johnson et al 1994). Further examples of activities based manipulations used to encourage desired behavioural change include the use of natural prompting (Ager & Reading 1992); matching tasks to abilities (Stubbings & Martin 1998); and using neutralising routines to reduce the likelihood of behavioural difficulties in identified high-risk situations (Horner et al 1997).

Changing setting events

Setting events alterations include: methods for changing strategies to control poor sleep patterns (Brylewski & Wiggs 1998); the use of non-contingent reinforcement (Fischer et al 1997, Hanley et al 1997) and response interruption and redirection (Duker & Schaapveld 1996). The latter procedure is similar to the interruption of response chains (Emerson 1995). An example of this can be provided from the workplace setting where the author of this chapter practices. At this setting a team of practitioners are working with a young man who has ASD and behavioural difficulties. We have identified a response chain pattern that, if left uninterrupted, frequently results in physically aggressive behaviours. Subsequently our intervention has been aimed at recognising and responding to behaviours that occur early in the chain, in order to alleviate the build-up of negative arousal leading to an aggressive response. (The reader may find it useful to compare this intervention with the structured teaching approach of Division TEACCH described in Ch. 8.)

Changing the setting events and contexts for behavioural difficulties provides a causal focus for intervention that may be preventative and proactive, rather than merely addressing symptoms. Changing setting events also places emphasis on systems and culture change versus a direct focus on person change only, and there is less likelihood of substitution of other difficult behaviours if the requirement for the target behaviour is removed. Additionally, alteration of setting events may be relatively easy to achieve and maintain, and relatively quick and durable desired behavioural change may be realised. Disadvantages and limitations include the difficulty, impossibility or undesirability of altering setting events which may be pivotal to the physical, emotional and/or developmental well-being of the client and/or others. Additionally, some setting event alterations (such as environmental enrichment and increased stimulation) may have the paradoxical and unintentional effect of producing over-arousal, withdrawal and reduced performance (Duker & Rasing 1989).

Behaviour based approaches

Behaviour based approaches are largely based upon the establishment of functional alternatives to the behavioural difficulty itself, whereby selection and reinforcement of a behaviour aims to satisfy the motivational purpose of the difficulty it seeks to displace (see Fig. 9.6). Further, the reduction or

Fig. 9.6
'Displacement' model
of behavioural
change and the
'traditional' ABC
model of behavioural
maintenance

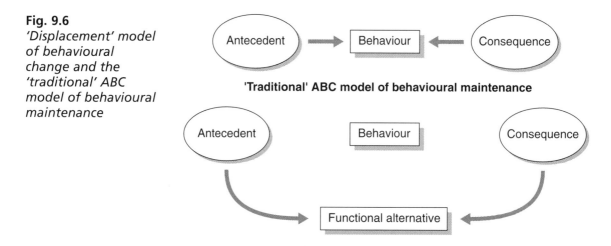

'Traditional' ABC model of behavioural maintenance

'Displacement' model of behavioural change

elimination of behavioural difficulties results from a systematic increase in frequency and duration of other appropriate behaviours. The second case study, 'Donald', describes the establishment of functionally alternative behaviour used to displace self-injury.

Donald

The need
Donald, a 50-year-old man with a diagnosis of profound learning disability and left-sided hemiplegia, had no verbal communication, and his comprehension skills were thought to be limited. At the time of intervention, Donald was living in a 12-bedded group home in the south of Glasgow. His presenting difficulties were high frequency self-injurious behaviour, and particularly severe hand biting and head hitting, causing significant tissue damage. This behaviour was very distressing for Donald, his fellow residents and carers.

Approach
Behavioural assessment was mainly by carer interview and analysis of incident records. Outcomes highlighted a relatively high frequency of self-injury when Donald was alone, and when carers and fellow residents were nearby but not interacting with him. A number of carers reported a higher incidence of self-injury when they and/or others were having conversations near him but that did not involve him.

Referral to, and subsequent input from, speech and language therapy revealed that Donald's comprehension skills were considerably more advanced than had been assumed and that the extent of his learning disability had been overestimated. Preliminary hypothesis of behavioural function was that it was communicative, and consideration was given to the selection of a suitable functional alternative behaviour which might displace self-injury.

After some discussion and consultation with Donald through the use of both verbal communication to him, and symbolic communication to and from him, it was decided to use a very small bell in order that Donald might cue the desire to communicate his needs. Donald kept this nearby, and would initiate interactions with others by ringing it gently. Advantages of this form of functional alternative included its capacity to trigger attention through aural as well as visual means. Carers were educated to the need to respond as soon as possible and enthusiastically to the functionally alternative behaviour and the input from speech and language therapy helped them devise a 'needs menu' for Donald; at first this consisted of broad needs categories such as food, drinks, activities, toilet and discomfort but later developed quite sophisticated and comprehensive sub-menus based on Donald's identified preferred needs and individual sensitivities. Other residents became aware of the function of Donald's 'ringing' and adapted their responses to facilitate appropriate action.

Outcomes
The incidence of self-injury stopped completely. Donald developed a greater capacity for communication through increased interaction, recognition of his intellectual capacity, and the technology supplied by the speech and language therapist. He now lives in his own tenancy with 24-hour carer support, and is employed on a part-time basis (at his request) in an administrative capacity with a well-established organisation which provides services to people with learning disabilities. He also now 'speaks' through his writing and communication aids.

There are number of factors that need to be considered in the selection and establishment of functional alternatives. Firstly, assessment should establish the motivation for specified behavioural difficulties across settings, situations and contexts. It is important that an existing appropriate behaviour, or a new behaviour of the same response class serving the same function, should be introduced in order to assume the same functional contingencies and displace the behavioural difficulty. It is also important that an appropriate and relevant response modality should be selected, whether verbal, gestural or symbolic (see Durand 1990). Alternative responses may be shaped if they are not in an individual's repertoire of behaviour already. Also, the natural antecedents to and consequences for the functionally alternative behaviour should be arranged. It is vital to consider whether a chosen appropriate behaviour may have been used naturally, given the ability, opportunity and encouragement. It is necessary to arrange meaningful outcomes for the alternative behaviour given the disproportionate attention given previously to the difficult behaviour.

In practice one should choose a response form for the alternative behaviour which is easy to use – and preferably less complex than the difficult behaviour – and ensure that the chosen alternative is understandable, relevant and able to be generalised across settings, situations and contexts in order to elicit the desired response. It is of paramount importance to establish a schedule of reinforcement for the alternative behaviour that is as potent, varied, sufficient and immediate as that obtained by the performance of the behavioural difficulty. Ideally, these properties should be intensified (at least in the short term), in order to establish the functional displacement of the undesired behaviour.

A common difficulty in pursuing schedules of reinforcement is ensuring consistency in response across people in order to strengthen the desired alternative behaviour. The importance of consistency cannot be overstated. Woods & Blewitt (1993) have referred to the problem of 'procedural decay' in reference to the possible deterioration in response efficiency and consistency. It may be useful to instigate trials of functionally alternative

response efficiency. The trials can be used in the short term to enhance initial effects. 'Distributed practice' (i.e. training throughout the day) may be introduced to promote generalisation of the desired behaviour. Across time, training may be systematically and sensitively phased to natural stimulus conditions within natural environments (see Durand 1990). The attitudes and conditioning of others and their responses to behavioural difficulties are also important (Hastings 1995, Hastings et al 1997). In addition to promoting a modified and strengthened response to functionally alternative behaviour, attitudes and conditioned responses to behavioural difficulties may require to be neutralised in order to consolidate reductive influences. Finally, increasing opportunities and setting events for functionally alternative behaviours, whilst simultaneously reducing or eliminating those for undesirable behaviours, is also most important. To be successful the alternative behaviour introduced must be of genuine functional equivalence to the behaviour being eliminated. Additionally, the alternative behaviour must demonstrate greater efficiency for the individual, relative to the behaviour they currently engage in.

Donnellan et al (1988) have discussed the use of alternative responses that are topographically similar to the behaviour being exhibited – by which it is meant that they must have similar response features (for example hitting others as opposed to touching others softly) – and those that are topographically dissimilar (for example biting one's own fingers as opposed to undertaking needlework). Additionally consideration should be given to topographical compatibility as opposed to topographical incompatibility. In the previous example finger biting and needlework would be topographically incompatible (the individual cannot physically perform both behaviours simultaneously). An example of topographically compatible behaviour might be shouting or swearing and watching television (the individual can perform these behaviours at the same time). These considerations are discussed further in the context of differential reinforcement.

The successful use of functional alternatives has been demonstrated in a number of studies (Durand 1990, Sprague & Horner 1992, Fisher et al 1993, Day et al 1994). Intervention through functional displacement has a number of difficulties. The process can be complex and resource intensive to initiate. Additionally, the legitimacy of providing functional alternatives for behaviours that serve to either access consequences which may be potentially harmful to the well-being of the individual or others, or to escape or avoid situations and or activities crucial to that well-being, is highly questionable. Given these examples, more ethically sensitive and constructive interventions would seek to reduce or eliminate the potentially harmful consequences in the former situation, and reduce or eliminate the individual's sensitivity to developmentally pivotal situations or activities in the latter.

Self-management approaches

Over the past decade, the use of interventions based upon self-control and self-regulation of behavioural difficulties has increased. Despite the significant therapeutic outcomes reported through the application of self-management procedures with people with learning disabilities in particular, their use remains relatively under-employed or under-reported. Since the use of self-management typically involves the combination of both behavioural and cognitive based components (for example self-monitoring, problem solving and self-evaluation), reported applications have tended to be with people who have a mild or moderate learning disability. It is not within the remit of this chapter to provide a detailed account of cognitive based approaches to reducing behavioural difficulties, as this will be comprehensively dealt with in the chapter that follows (Ch. 10). However, as Beck & Freeman (1990) have observed:

we must keep in mind that no techniques are purely cognitive or behavioral. Further, cognitive strategies can produce behavioral change, and behavioral methods generally instigate some cognitive restructuring.

Despite a more cognitive orientation, self-management interventions have produced favourable results using visual or symbolic cueing and feedback components in order to facilitate communication and comprehension (Cole et al 1985). Typically, self-management training will involve the use of the following procedures:

- *Self-monitoring*: the recognition and analysis of the nature and extent of the individual's own behavioural difficulties. Use of this procedure may in itself have the reactive effect of reducing behavioural difficulties (Ziegob et al 1978, Reese et al 1984).

- *Self-instruction*: the manipulation and self-determination of situational, behavioural and cognitive setting events for undesirable behaviour by the use of positive self-prompting and self-coping statements.

- *Self-evaluation*: the self-determination of behavioural performance against the desired or predetermined criteria. Functional use of this procedure requires both honest and accurate self-analysis and evaluation.

- *Self-consequation*: the self-determined application of consequences to behavioural performance dependent on the outcomes of self-evaluation – for example, self-delivery or self-denial of reinforcing contingencies.

Other, more behaviourally based constituents facilitative of self-management include relaxation, modelling, role play, prompting, self-recruited feedback and reinforcement by others.

Advantages of self-management approaches include:

- Demonstrable utility across a variety of behavioural difficulties
- Potential to realise the generalisation, maintenance and durability of desired behaviour change
- A self-regulatory orientation – promoting of independence and self-esteem
- Intrinsic motivational influences of self-determination, self-reliance and responsibility
- Reduced dependence on the external regulation and control of behaviour.

(See further reading with respect to both the application and outcomes of self-management based interventions for behavioural difficulties.)

Increasing other appropriate behaviours: differential reinforcement

Differential reinforcement procedures aim to reduce or eliminate behavioural difficulties via the systematic strengthening of other, alternative or incompatible behaviours. Differential reinforcement of other (DRO) behaviour is a non-constructional approach that is based upon the reinforcement of non-performance of behavioural difficulties. Since this procedure is used to deliver reinforcement contingent on non-performance of 'target' behaviour, it does not generally specify which 'other' behaviours should be rewarded. Subsequently, in using this procedure, there may be a danger that other problem behaviours may be inadvertently reinforced. This difficulty might be avoided to some extent by listing those undesirable behaviours the non-performance of which might be reinforced. Reinforcement scheduling is generally based on fixed or variable time intervals. These are determined largely by the frequency of the target behaviour, and the capacity of an individual to understand the relationship between non-performance of undesirable behaviour and subsequent delivery of reward.

It is best to pair tangible reinforcement with more 'natural' forms; these may subsequently be used to sustain the desired outcomes as tangible reinforcement is systematically phased out. Additionally, selected reinforcement should be outside the normal routine of the individual to enhance reinforcement potency. Donnellan et al (1988) have suggested the application of the 'Goldilocks rule' of reinforcement scheduling – not too large and not too small. This author's preference is to set initial reinforcement latency in response to the shortest time observed between episodes of behavioural distress. For example, if the shortest time between episodes was 12 minutes, then one would set the initial reinforcement schedule at 10 minutes, since this appears to be a realistic time to allow non-performance of undesirable behaviour. Reinforcement intervals may then be both sensitively and systematically phased to increase the time scheduling of reinforcement delivery. Should performance of undesirable behaviour occur between times scheduled for delivery of reinforcement, a reset procedure may be used in order to reduce the likelihood of unintentional rewarding of behavioural difficulties. For example, a reinforcement schedule which was fixed at half hourly intervals would reset reinforcement delivery to half an hour following undesirable behaviour which occurred between set times for reinforcement. Subsequent reinforcement intervals would then be set to correspond to the reset schedule. Although DRO has largely been applied to behaviours of relatively high frequency, Whitaker (1996) has discussed its efficacy in reducing behavioural problems occurring as infrequently as twice monthly. Variations in differential reinforcement approaches include:

Differential reinforcement of alternative behaviours

Differential reinforcement of alternative behaviours (DRA) refers to the differential reinforcement of specified alternative behaviours that may be used to displace undesirable behaviour(s). As the establishment of functional alternatives is one form of DRA, similar requirements should apply with respect to the increased rate, potency, immediacy and variety of the selected/chosen reinforcement. Donnellan et al (1988) considered the main advantages of DRA to be its potential to produce lasting results, its constructive orientation and its social validity.

Differential reinforcement of incompatible behaviours

Differential reinforcement of incompatible behaviours (DRI) refers to the differential reinforcement of appropriate behaviours that are physically incompatible with the undesirable behaviour. Donnellan et al (1988) assert that by satisfying the 100% rule, the differential reinforcement schedule will address only undesirable and directly incompatible behaviour. An example of this is non-compliance versus compliance: any increase in incompatible behaviour automatically guarantees a reduction in undesirable behaviour.

Advantages in using differential reinforcement approaches include:

- Speed of effect across a number of behavioural problems
- Few negative side-effects
- Good generalisation of positive outcomes
- Relative ease of use
- Recognised social validity

Disadvantages include:

- The non-constructive orientation of DRO (which may be best used in conjunction with constructive approaches)
- The potential for the inadvertent reinforcement of non-targeted undesirable behaviour
- Possible satiation to reinforcement
- Difficulty in the phasing out of reinforcement to 'natural' contingencies
- The prospective problem of procedural decay.

With respect to the latter phenomenon, some years ago a young woman who had difficulty wearing clothing underwent a differential reinforcement schedule to promote and encourage both clothes selection and wearing. This proved to be very successful, until the care team became rather relaxed with respect to the (by that stage) twice daily delivery of reinforcement (social praise, encouragement and interaction with the individual). Subsequently, the motivation for this young lady to continue to wear clothing decreased and the behavioural problem re-emerged. Additionally, the reinstatement of the management plan proved significantly less effective (in the initial stages) in producing the desired outcomes due to the individual's previous learning experience. (For further information on differential reinforcement procedures see Deitz et al 1976, Luiselli & Slocumb 1983, Jones & Baker 1990, Jones 1991, Whitaker 1996.)

Consequence based approaches

The removal of reinforcing contingencies: punishment 1

These are generally reactive interventions that aim to reduce or eliminate behavioural difficulties by the systematic manipulation or altering of the contingencies maintaining them. Since these approaches are the most restrictive strategies for behavioural change they should always be used as a last resort, in conjunction with constructionally based interventions and in line with ethical considerations.

Response interruption

This procedure attempts to delay or prevent the reinforcing consequences of undesirable behaviour by interrupting that behaviour, usually by prompting or reintroducing the individual to more acceptable behaviour, preferably towards responses incompatible with the difficult behaviour (Duker & Schaapveld 1996). An earlier example referred to the potentially therapeutic interruption of undesirable 'response chains'.

Extinction

This approach involves the removal of the consequences maintaining undesirable behaviour, for example by withdrawing attention to attention based responding or denying escape from interaction when that is the function of problem behaviour (Iwata et al 1990, 1994b; Zarcone et al 1994).

Sensory extinction

This procedure is used to alter or remove the stimulatory sensory based feedback that maintains undesirable behaviour (Rincover et al 1979, Rincover & Devany 1982, Iwata et al 1994b). The use of medication such as naltrexone (see Ch. 6) has proved to be effective in reducing self-injurious behaviour by blocking sensory-euphoric effects produced by stimulation of natural endorphins (Barrett et al 1989, Thompson et al 1994, Garcia & Smith 1999). It is important to acknowledge the ethical considerations of the use of extinction based procedures. These are considerable, since 'extinction bursts' (sudden increases in the frequency of undesirable behaviour) are common, due to exposure to conditions previously eliciting desired consequences, for example by the delivery of attention or escape from the 'aversiveness' of instruction or interaction. Unless the approach is consistent, the target behaviour and/or new undesirable behaviours may increase and emerge both within and outside the treatment setting. Additionally, there is a risk of symptom substitution, since the procedure does not address the construction of more appropriate alternative behaviours. The use of extinction based approaches may present unacceptable risks to the individual and/or others, due to the prospective escalation in severe behavioural difficulties.

Time-out   This approach involves the temporary removal of the opportunity to access positive reinforcement contingent on performance of problem behaviour. Typically, the procedure has two orientations:

Exclusionary time-out
This procedure involves the brief removal of the individual from a reinforcing situation to a less stimulating environment for a predetermined period of time (Mace et al 1986). Return to the reinforcing situation would normally be made dependent upon non-performance of the undesirable behaviour at time of reintroduction.

Non-exclusionary time-out
This approach involves the removal of reinforcing interactions, activities and/or materials from the individual – again for a set period of time and with reintroduction to reinforcement made contingent on the cessation of undesirable behaviour at that time (McKeegan et al 1984). A variation of this procedure involves removal of the opportunity to access or 'earn' reinforcement for a predetermined amount of time as a result of performance of undesirable behaviour.

Although the use of time-out based interventions has been observed to produce relatively quick and successful reduction in undesirable behaviour, the procedure has been found unintentionally to increase the frequency of behaviour whose function is escape motivated (Solnick et al 1977). This finding demonstrates again the need first to conduct a thorough functional analysis in order to determine the motivational bases for behaviour. Again, since it is a reactive and non-constructional approach, the use of time-out should be considered only in conjunction with more positive approaches when alternative, less restrictive, intervention strategies have been thoroughly exhausted without producing meaningful outcomes.

Response cost
This is a procedure similar to 'fining' that involves the permanent removal of a predetermined 'volume' of positive reinforcement as a consequence of performance of undesirable behaviour. The approach should only be used where a formally organised reinforcement system is in place, and should never compromise the everyday rights and lifestyle of an individual.

Visual/facial screening

Visual screening is a behavioural oriented procedure that involves occluding any visual reinforcement from the environment by using a piece of material or similar item as an immediate consequence of an undesired behaviour. This procedure has been successfully used to reduce undesirable behaviours related to visual reinforcement (Barmann & Vitali 1982, Jordan et al 1989, Jones et al 1991).

The presentation of punitive consequences: punishment 2

In behavioural terms, 'punishment' refers to any consequence of a behaviour that renders the probability of that behaviour less likely. As with reinforcement, there is danger in assuming the reductive capacity of punitive consequences outside the context of individual aversiveness. Consider, for example, unintentional reinforcement of undesirable behaviour through the implementation of time-out or social disapproval procedures. Additionally (as previously referred to), physical pain may act as reinforcement, and externally applied restraint and self-restraint procedures have been observed to function as both positive and negatively reinforcing contingencies (Favell et al 1981, Smith et al 1992, Powell et al 1996). Despite fairly widespread consideration of the successful application of punishment based approaches to the reduction of behavioural difficulties (Van Houten et al 1988, Matson & Taras 1989), the heated debate surrounding the acceptability, desirability and utility of such techniques continues. Over the last decade, the 'technicians' of behavioural interventions that seek to reduce behavioural problems experienced by people with learning disabilities have been embroiled in intense (and largely unresolved) deliberation over the application of restrictive procedures (see Sturmey et al 1993). Given the apparent increase in the social unacceptability for punishment based approaches (arguably in line with the advancement in constructional, non-aversive alternatives to behaviour change) and the negative outcomes associated with such invasive procedures, the legitimacy for and the application of these interventions must be analysed very carefully. They should only be used when less restrictive approaches have been *consistently* and *thoroughly* applied without achieving the desired therapeutic outcomes.

The implications of not intervening within a punitive context may be significantly harmful, even life-threatening, for the individual and/or others. In such situations, these approaches should only be considered in tandem with constructional interventions, with continuous and thorough evaluation, for very brief amounts of time, and with the minimum volume of intensity to bring about the desired therapeutic outcomes.

The limitations of behavioural approaches

The legitimacy, applicability and prospective effectiveness of behavioural approaches are limited or unclear when the underlying cause of that distress is not behavioural, but due to other factors (e.g. organic dysfunction). However, the process of assessing and isolating the relevant causal factors is often extremely difficult and complex. There are clear ethical implications in applying behavioural approaches to the management of difficulties that have an organic aetiology.

Assessment

The usefulness of methods of behavioural assessment are limited by their sensitivity in being able to identify desired information and their capacity to produce a reliable, accurate and broad enough analysis of behaviour. Additionally, there may be practical and organisational limitations because of the relative complexity and intensity of some assessment techniques. They may demand exhaustive commitment of time, training and resources. Accurate assessment is dependent on the competence, honesty, reliability and meticulous recording and provision of relevant information by others; insufficiencies or inconsistencies in these respects may understandably limit or preclude the effective application of assessment technology (Gates 1996). There may also be ethical requirements that could limit assessment outcomes, such as dependence on retrospective information (which may be incomplete and unreliable), should the 'real-time' analysis of self-injurious or aggressive behaviour be contraindicated in respect of the well-being of the client and/or others.

Reinforcement

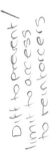

Limitations in the use of reinforcement include difficulties in the identification of sufficiently potent and easily delivered reinforcers. Some reinforcers may prove more vulnerable to satiation effects, and these can be limiting if only relatively few reinforcers can be identified. It can also be difficult to prevent or limit access to selected reinforcement outside the context of the treatment setting, which again may limit effectiveness. It is also important to note that the use of non-contingent (unconditional) reinforcement as the only component of intervention is not constructionally oriented; it will not, in isolation, establish new skills or facilitate the self-determination of access to reinforcement by the client, since availability is unconditional. Given the historical limitations imposed on the ability of people with learning disabilities (for example to exercise control), this procedure used in isolation may result in further disenfranchisement. The phasing out of reinforcement scheduling whilst maintaining desired results may also prove difficult, and the time-scale for this may be limited by the requirement to maintain therapeutic outcomes throughout such a sensitive and systematic process.

Ethical limitations concerning the use of reinforcement include the requirement to pair reinforcers such as consumables, special activities, tokens or points with the more natural contingencies of social praise, congratulation and encouragement. Additionally, these 'artificial' reinforcers should only be used for as little time as is necessary to substitute their function to more natural and intrinsic forms of reinforcement. Again, however, the relative ease of this process may be limited by the capacity of substitute reinforcers to maintain durable therapeutic outcomes. Another ethical concern arising from the use of reinforcement may be its propensity to compromise the physical and emotional well-being of the client. Consider, for example, the use of preferred foods or drinks as reinforcement for someone whose dietary intake requirements were compromised by the calorific, chemical or additive content of these consumables. Selected reinforcers may need to be limited to those outside routine access by the client, so that any withholding of these as a contingency of behaviour does not compromise the rights and integrity of an individual.

Intervention

Many behavioural approaches require the intensive use of resources and training of carers to be effective. Additionally, carers are required to be committed, motivated, consistent and sensitive in the application of behavioural techniques. Any limitations in these prerequisites may restrict the desired outcomes for the client. Approaches may also be limited by their potential or actual effect on others – for example environmental or

used gradual goals

setting event manipulations that may produce positive outcomes for one individual, but may compromise the well-being of another or others. The effectiveness of behavioural interventions may also appear to be limited due to the high expectations of the client and/or others. Both client and carers may expect the desired change to be rapid and dramatic, therefore failure to establish realistic time-scales and expectations could limit prospective outcomes. Some behavioural difficulties will endure a substantial amount of time and effort before any progress is observed. In such cases the more moderate expectation of gradual change in due course may preserve the motivation and commitment of both client and carer.

Ethical issues

The application of behavioural approaches to the assessment and management of behavioural difficulties is suffused with ethical considerations, a number of which have been identified and discussed throughout this chapter. The issue of maintaining informed client consent throughout therapy is a consideration that merits repetition. One must be sensitive to a consideration of the possible limitations imposed by an individual's capacity to make informed decisions regarding his or her treatment. The reader is referred to Morris et al (1993) and Arscott (1997) for further consideration of this issue, to Yule & Carr (1987), Presland (1989) and Emerson (1995), for further information on ethical issues relative to the application of behavioural approaches to the management of behavioural difficulties experienced by people with learning disabilities, and to Bicknell (1997) for more general information regarding ethical issues and people with learning disabilities.

Conclusion

This section summarises the main issues and challenges facing the development of behavioural assessment and intervention techniques.

As Owens & MacKinnon (1997, p.225) have stressed:

> *the basic process of functional analysis is itself still fraught with conceptual and theoretical problems.*

Behavioural assessment and analysis requires more sensitivity to the frequently changing and complex motivations that stimulate and maintain behavioural difficulties and distress. This may be assisted by recognising the limited validity and predictability of functional analysis, and greater awareness of the broad range of biological, physiological, environmental, social and behavioural factors involved in the genesis and maintenance of behavioural difficulties. Additionally, methods of analysis may require to become more sophisticated (Vollmer 1995) and individually tailored in their application (Toogood & Timlin 1996). A greater understanding of, and sensitivity to, the communicative function of behavioural difficulties is also necessary (Stansfield & Cheseldine 1994, Bolt et al 1997, Thurman 1997). The need to take into account the influence and effects of carers' attitudes, beliefs, interactions and reactions to behaviour is well documented, and this demands more detailed analysis (Bromley & Emerson 1995, Morgan & Hastings 1998).

Accurate and informed assessment is heavily dependent upon prerequisite competencies and adequate training in listening as well as observational and data collecting skills. A multidisciplinary approach to the assessment of risk, costs and benefits of the application of behavioural approaches may provide a process of analysis that is facilitative rather than compromising of the liberties of the client. Sensitivity to the risk of clients' well-being, as well as to the risk of the well-being of others, is also a key issue. Additionally, multidisciplinary approaches may facilitate continuous processes of informed consent to assessment and therapy in cases where a client's capacity to provide consent is either temporarily or persistently compromised. There is also a need for greater sensitivity to the early detection of factors known to precipitate behavioural difficulties, as well as to the early identification of the onset of these difficulties themselves (Murphy et al 1999). The process of planning both the application of behavioural approaches and the delivery of services to people exhibiting and/or experiencing behavioural distress requires the active involvement of clients, although working in genuine partnerships with clients may appear to be fallacious where there is a persistence of inequality in the balance of power within service cultures. Behavioural interventions and service responses should therefore promote client autonomy in safe and sensitive ways, and develop explicit policies and protocols for client involvement, choice and decision making in the design, delivery and development of services.

Services should also be both planned and evaluated in terms of quality of life outcomes for clients in order that interventions realise positive benefits as well as the reduction or elimination of distress (Felce & Emerson 1996). Service systems require the capacity to facilitate behavioural interventions by supporting carers and providing the training and resources necessary for the therapeutic application of these approaches. The early detection of factors known to precipitate behavioural difficulties, or the onset of these difficulties, affords opportunities for prevention or early intervention (Oliver 1995). Research has demonstrated the proactivity and effectiveness of early intervention, and both prevention and early intervention provide major therapeutic goals for the ongoing and future development of responsive behavioural management approaches (Emerson 1996, Felce & Emerson 1996).

There is also a need for the dissemination of information regarding the often complex and frequently changing motivational bases for behavioural difficulties, and both clients and carers require education to develop understanding of their sometimes unwitting contribution towards behavioural difficulties. Emphasis needs to continue to be placed on the importance of the provision of suitable recreational and occupational opportunities for clients, and the implications of such provision for the management of behavioural difficulties (Stevens & Martin 1999). Intervention strategies for behavioural difficulties that prove more durable and resistant to change need to be effective without compromising ethical considerations and quality outcomes. In evaluating the effectiveness of behavioural approaches there is clearly a requirement to develop greater sensitivity to the multi-factorial and multi-process context of behaviour in order to respond proactively, and produce strategies for modifying identified setting events. Well organised client and carer debriefing strategies provide not only much needed support and counselling, but also facilitate the development of approaches which may realise desired environmental, attitudinal, cultural or behavioural change. Evaluation, therefore, is not merely about outcome analysis, but is also about developing more effective and responsive services.

Further reading

Analogue studies

Iwata B A, Dorsey M F, Slifer K J, Bauman K E, Richman G S 1982 Toward a functional analysis of self-injury. Analysis and Intervention in Developmental Disabilities 2:1–20

This seminal text on the origins and rationale for the use of alternating treatment studies has stood the test of time as essential reading for those planning to use this approach to functional analysis.

Sturmey P 1995 Analog baselines: a critical review of the methodology. Research in Developmental Disabilities 16(4):269–284

As the title implies, this paper offers a detailed analysis of the contribution of analogue baseline studies to the analysis and treatment of behavioural difficulties, whilst providing a number of constructive criticisms with respect to potential limitations in their use. The text additionally points to further avenues of research with respect to the refinement and development of this method of functional analysis.

Self-management approaches

Gardner W I, Cole C L 1989 Self-management approaches. In: Cipiani E (ed) The treatment of severe behaviour disorders: applied behaviour analytic approaches. American Association on Mental Retardation, Washington DC, pp 19–35

This text provides a comprehensive introduction to the incorporation of self-control and self-determined management strategies in the assessment and treatment of behavioural difficulties. The chapter will provide the reader with an understanding of the development and advantages of self-management approaches from traditionally externally mediated and heavily behaviourally based interventions.

Rossiter R, Hunnislett E, Pulsford M 1998 Anger management training and people with moderate to severe learning disabilities. British Journal of Learning Disabilities 26(2):67–74

This paper presents a contemporary example of the therapeutic application of a cognitive/behavioural approach to the management of anger. The text appears to reflect a logical and legitimate advancement in intervention strategies for behavioural difficulties towards the incorporation of cognitively based treatment components wherever these appear appropriate and responsive to the needs of individuals and their behavioural difficulties.

Restrictive procedures

Butterfield E C 1990) The compassion of distinguishing punishing behavioural treatment from aversive treatment. American Journal on Mental Retardation 95(2): 137–141

This article provides a much-needed respite from the oppressive confusion and intense heat of the aversive debate by offering a passionate, but composed and sensitive plea for the application of enlightening and analytic thinking towards the prospective cost–benefit evaluation of the use, or not, of restrictive behavioural treatment.

Sturmey P, Rickets R W, Goza A 1997 A review of the aversives debate: an American perspective. In: Jones R S P, Eayrs C B (eds) Challenging behaviour and intellectual disability: a psychological perspective. BILD Publications, Kidderminster, pp 99–120

This chapter offers the reader an in-depth awareness and analysis of the aetiology and development of the aversive debate. Although the examination of the ideological and empirical bases for this are presented entirely from an American standpoint, it is suggested that the issues are applicable and relevant to the UK context, and this text is strongly recommended to the reader.

References

Ager A, Reading J C 1992 Teaching skills through the enhancement of natural antecedents. Journal of Intellectual Disability Research 36 (2): 157–169

Arscott K 1997) Assessing the capacity of people with learning disabilities to make decisions about treatment. Tizard Learning Disability Review l.2(2): 17–28

Baer D M, Wolf M M, Risley T R 1968 Some current dimensions of applied behavior analysis. Journal of Applied Behaviour Analysis 1: 313–327

Bandura A 1977 Social learning theory. Prentice Hall, Englewood Cliffs, New Jersey

Bannerman D J, Sheldon J B, Sherman J A, Harchik A E 1990 Balancing the right to habilitation with the right to personal liberties: the rights of people with developmental disabilities to eat too many doughnuts and take a nap. Journal of Applied Behaviour Analysis 23: 79–89

Barker P J 1982 Behaviour therapy nursing. Croom Helm, London

Barmann B C, Vitali D L 1982 Facial screening to eliminate trichotillomania in developmentally disabled persons. Behaviour Therapy 13: 735–742

Barrett R P, Feinstein C, Hole W T 1989 Effects of naloxone and naltrexone on self-injury: a double-blind placebo-controlled analysis. American Journal on Mental Retardation 93(6): 644–651

Beck A T, Freeman A 1990 Cognitive therapy of personality disorders. Guilford Press, New York

Beukelman D R, Mirenda P 1992 Augmentative and alternative communication: management of severe communication disorders in children and adults. Paul H Brookes, Baltimore

Bicknell J 1997 Philosophical and ethical issues. In: Russell O (ed) The psychiatry of learning disabilities. Royal College of Psychiatrists/Gaskell, London, pp 190–204

Bolt C, Farmer R, Rohde J 1997 Behaviour problems associated with lack of speech in people with learning disabilities. Journal of Intellectual Disability Research 41: 3–7

Bromley J, Emerson E 1995 Beliefs and emotional reactions of care staff working with people with challenging behaviour. Journal of Intellectual Disability Research 39: 341–352

Brylewski J E, Wiggs L 1998 A questionnaire survey of sleep and night-time behaviour in a community based sample of adults with intellectual disabilities. Journal of Intellectual Disability Research 42: 154–162

Carton J S, Nowicki S 1998 Should behaviour therapists stop using reinforcement? A re-examination of the undermining effect of reinforcement on intrinsic motivation. Behaviour Therapy 29 (1): 65–86

Cole C L, Gardner W I, Karan O C 1985 Self-management training of mentally retarded adults presenting severe conduct difficulties. Applied Research in Mental Retardation 6: 337–347

Day R M, Horner R H O, Neill R E 1994 Multiple functions of problem behaviours: assessment and intervention. Journal of Applied Behaviour Analysis 27: 279–289

Deitz S M, Repp A C, Deitz D E D 1976 Reducing inappropriate classroom behaviour of retarded students through three procedures of differential reinforcement. Journal of Mental Deficiency Research 20: 155–170

Donnellan A M, LaVigna G W, Negri-Shoultz N, Fassbender L L 1988 Progress without punishment: effective approaches for learners with behaviour problems. Teachers College Press, New York

Duker P C, Rasing E 1989 Effects of re-designing the physical environment on self-stimulation and on-task behaviour in three autistic-type developmentally disabled individuals. Journal of Autism and Developmental Disorders 19: 449–460

Duker P C, Schaapveld M 1996 Increasing on-task behaviour through interruption-prompting. Journal of Intellectual Disability Research 40: 291–297

Dunlap G, dePerczel M, Clarke S et al 1994 Choice making to promote adaptive behaviour for students with emotional and behavioural challenges. Journal of Applied Behaviour Analysis 27: 505–518

Durand V M 1990 Severe behavior problems: a functional communication approach. Guilford Press, New York

Durand V M, Carr E G 1991 Functional communication training to reduce challenging behaviour: maintenance and application in new settings. Journal of Applied Behaviour Analysis 24: 251–264

Durand V M, Crimmins D B 1992 The Motivation Assessment Scale. Monaco Associates, Topeka, Kansas

Durand V M, Mapstone E 1998 Influence of mood-inducing music on challenging behaviour. American Journal on Mental Retardation 102 (4): 367–378

Emerson E 1995 Challenging behaviour: analysis and intervention in people with learning difficulties. Cambridge University Press, Cambridge.

Emerson E 1996 Early interventions autism and challenging behaviour. Tizard Learning Disability Review 1(1): 36–38

Emerson E, Barrett S, Cummings R 1990 Using analogue assessments. South East Thames Regional Health Authority, Bexhill-on-Sea

Emerson E, Reeves D, Thompson S, Henderson D, Robertson J, Howard D 1996 Time-based lag sequential analysis and the functional assessment of challenging behaviour. Journal of Intellectual Disability Research 40(3): 260-274

Evans I M, Meyer L 1985 An educative approach to behavior problems. Paul H Brookes, Baltimore

Favell J E, McGimsey J F, Jones M L, Cannon P R 1981 Physical restraint as positive reinforcement. American Journal of Mental Deficiency 85: 425-432

Felce S, Emerson E 1996 Realities and challenges. Journal of Applied Research in Intellectual Disabilities 9 (3): 284-288

Fischer S M, Iwata B A, Mazaleski J L 1997 Non-contingent delivery of arbitrary reinforcers in treatment for SIB. Journal of Applied Behaviour Analysis 30 (2): 239-249

Fisher W W, Piazza C C, Cataldo M, Harrell R, Jefferson G, Conner R 1993 Functional communication training with and without extinction and punishment. Journal of Applied Behaviour Analysis 26: 23-36

Foster-Johnson L, Ferro J, Dunlap G 1994 Preferred curricular activities and reduced problem behaviours in students with intellectual disabilities. Journal of Applied Behaviour Analysis 27: 493-504

Garcia D, Smith R G 1999 Using analog baselines to assess the effects of naltrexone on self-injurious behavior. Research in Developmental Disabilities 20 (1): 1-21

Gardner W I, Graeber J L 1994 Use of behavioural therapies to enhance personal competency: a multimodal diagnostic and intervention model. In: Bouras N (ed) Mental health in mental retardation: recent advances and practices. Cambridge University Press, Cambridge, pp 205-223

Gardner W I, Cole C L, Davidson D P, Karan O C 1986 Reducing aggression in individuals with developmental disabilities: an expanded stimulus control assessment and intervention model. Education and Training of the Mentally Retarded 21: 3-12

Gates R 1996 Issues of reliability and validity in the measurement of challenging behavioural difficulties: a discussion of implications for nursing research and practice. Journal of Clinical Nursing 5 (1): 7-12

Gelfand D, Gelfand S, Dobson W R 1967 Unprogrammed reinforcement of patients'

behaviour in a mental hospital. Behaviour Research and Therapy 5: 201-207

Goldiamond I 1974 Toward a constructional approach to social problems: ethical and constitutional issues raised by applied behaviour analysis. Behaviorism 2: 1-84

Groden G 1989 A guide for conducting a comprehensive behavioral analysis of a target behavior. Journal of Behavior Therapy and Experimental Psychiatry 20: 163-169

Hall S, Oliver C 1992 Differential effects of severe self-injurious behaviour on the behaviour of others. Behavioural Psychotherapy 20 (4): 355-365

Hanley G P, Piazza C C, Fisher W W 1997 Non-contingent presentation of attention and alternative stimuli in the treatment of attention-maintained destructive behavior. Journal of Applied Behavior Analysis 30(2): 229-238

Hastings R P 1995 Understanding factors that influence staff responses to challenging behaviour. Mental Handicap Research 8(4): 296-320

Hastings R P, Reed T S, Watts M J 1997 Community staff causal attributes about challenging behaviour in people with intellectual disabilities. Journal of Applied Research in Intellectual Disabilities 10 (3): 238-249

Hogg J, Raynes N 1986 Assessment in mental handicap. Croom Helm, London

Horner R H 1980 The effects of an environmental enrichment program on the behavior of institutionalised profoundly retarded children. Journal of Applied Behavior Analysis 13: 473-491

Horner R H, Day H M, Day J R 1997 Using neutralising routines to reduce problem behaviors. Journal of Applied Behavior Analysis 30 (4): 601-614

Iwata B A, Pace G M, Kalsher M J, Cowdery G E, Cataldo M F 1990 Experimental analysis and extinction of self-injurious escape behavior. Journal of Applied Behavior Analysis 23: 11-27

Iwata B A, Pace G M, Dorsey M F et al 1994a The functions of self-injurious behavior: an experimental-epidemiological study. Journal of Applied Behavior Analysis 27: 215-240

Iwata B A, Pace G M, Cowdery G E, Miltenberger R G 1994b What makes extinction work: an analysis of procedural form and function. Journal of Applied Behaviour Analysis 27: 131-144

Jones L J, Singh N N, Kendall K A 1991 Comparative effects of gentle teaching and visual screening on self-injurious behaviour. Journal of Mental Deficiency Research 35(1): 37–47

Jones R S P 1991 Reducing inappropriate behaviour using non-aversive procedures: evaluating differential reinforcement schedules. In: Remington B (ed) The challenge of severe mental handicap: a behaviour analytic approach. Wiley, Chichester

Jones R S P, Baker L J V 1990 Differential reinforcement and challenging behaviour: a critical review of the DRI schedule. Behavioural Psychotherapy 18(1): 35–47

Jordan J, Singh N N, Repp A 1989 An evaluation of gentle teaching and visual screening in the reduction of stereotypy. Journal of Applied Behaviour Analysis 22 (1): 9–22

Kazdin A E, Matson J L 1981 Social validation in mental retardation. Applied Research in Mental Retardation 2: 39–53

Lovett H 1996 Learning to listen: positive approaches and people with difficult behaviour. Jessica Kingsley, London

Luiselli J K, Slocumb P R 1983 Management of multiple aggressive behaviors by differential reinforcement. Journal of Behavior Therapy and Experimental Psychiatry 14 (4): 343–347

McBrien J, Felce D 1994 Working with people who have severe learning difficulty and challenging behaviour. BILD Publications, Clevedon

McDonnell A, Sturmey P 1993 Managing violent and aggressive behaviour: towards better practice. In: Jones R S P, Eayrs C B (eds) Challenging behaviour and intellectual disability: a psychological perspective. BILD Publications, Clevedon, pp 148–172

McGill P, Clare I, Murphy G 1996 Understanding and responding to challenging behaviour: from theory to practice. Tizard Learning Disability Review 1(1): 9–17

McKeegan G F, Estill K, Campbell B 1984 Use of non-exclusionary time-out for the elimination of a stereotyped behavior. Journal of Behavior Therapy and Experimental Psychiatry 18 (3): 261–264

Mace F C, Page T J, Ivancic M T O, Brien S 1986 Analysis of environmental determinants of aggression and disruption in mentally retarded children. Applied Research in Mental Retardation 7: 203–221

Matson J L 1990 Handbook of behavior modification with the mentally retarded. Plenum Press, New York

Matson J L, Taras M E 1989 A 20 year review of punishment and alternative methods to treat problem behaviors in developmentally delayed persons. Research in Developmental Disabilities 10: 85–104

Meyer L H, Evans I M 1993 Science and practice in behavioral intervention: meaningful outcomes research validity and usable knowledge. Journal of the Association for Persons with Severe Handicaps 18: 224–234

Morgan G M, Hastings R P 1998 Special educators' understanding of challenging behaviours in children with learning disabilities: sensitivity to information about behavioural function. Behavioural and Cognitive Psychotherapy 26 (1): 43–52

Morris C D, Niederbuhl J M, Mahr J M 1993 Determining the capability of individuals with mental retardation to give informed consent. American Journal on Mental Retardation 98 (2): 263–272

Murphy G 1982 Sensory reinforcement in the mentally handicapped and autistic child: a review. Journal of Autism and Developmental Disorders 1(1): 36–38

Murphy G 1994 Understanding challenging behaviour. In: Emerson E, McGill P, Mansell J (eds) Severe learning disabilities and challenging behaviours: designing high quality services. Chapman and Hall, London, pp 37–68

Murphy G, Hall S, Oliver C, Kissi-Debra R 1999 Identification of early self-injurious behaviour in young children with intellectual disability. Journal of Intellectual Disability Research 43(3): 149–163

Nihira K, Leland H, Lambert N 1993 Adaptive behavior scale – residential and community, 2nd edn. Pro-Ed, Austin, Texas

Oliver C 1993 Self-injurious behaviour from response to strategy. In: Kiernan C (ed) Research to practice? Implications of research on the challenging behaviour of people with learning disability. BILD Publications, Clevedon, pp 135–188

Oliver C 1995 Self-injurious behaviour in children with learning disabilities: recent advances in assessment and intervention. Journal of Child Psychology and Psychiatry 30: 909–927

O'Neill R E, Horner R H, Albin R W, Storey K, Sprague J R 1990 Functional analysis of problem behavior: a practical assessment guide. Sycamore Publishing Company, Sycamore, Illinois

Owens RG, MacKinnon S 1993. The functional analysis of challenging bahaviours: some conceptual and theoretical problems. In: Jones R S P, Eayrs C B (eds) Challenging behaviour and intellectual disability: a psychological perspective. BILD Publications, Clevedon, pp 224–239

Parsons M B, Reid D H 1990 Assessing food preferences among persons with profound mental retardation. Journal of Applied Behaviour Analysis 23: 183–195

Pavlov I P 1927 Conditioned reflexes. Oxford University Press, London

Powell S B, Bodfish J W, Parker D, Crawford T W, Lewis M H 1996 Self-restraint and self-injury: occurrence and motivational significance. American Journal on Mental Retardation 101(1): 41–48

Presland J L 1989 Overcoming difficult behaviour. BILD Publications, Clevedon

Pyles D A M, Bailey J S 1990 Diagnosing severe behavior problems. In: Repp A C Singh N N (eds) Perspectives on the use of non-aversive and aversive interventions for persons with developmental disabilities. Sycamore Publishing Company, Sycamore, Illinois

Reese R M, Sherman J A, Sheldon J 1984 Reducing agitated-disruptive behavior of mentally retarded residents of community group homes: the role of self-recording and peer prompted self-recording. Analysis and Intervention in Developmental Disabilities 4: 91–107

Repp A C, Felce D 1990 A micro-computer system used for evaluative and experimental behavioural research in mental handicap. Mental Handicap Research 3: 21–32

Rincover A, Devany J 1982 The application of sensory extinction procedures to self-injury. Analysis and Intervention in Developmental Disabilities 2: 67–81

Rincover A, Cook A, Peoples A, Packard D 1979 Sensory extinction and sensory reinforcement principles for programming multiple adaptive behavior change. Journal of Applied Behavior Analysis 12: 221–233

Schwartz I S, Baer D M 1991 Social validity assessments: is current practice state of the art? Journal of Applied Behaviour Analysis 24: 189–204

Sigafoos J, Dempsey R 1992 Assessing choice making among children with multiple disabilities. Journal of Applied Behaviour Analysis 25: 747–755

Skinner B F 1953 Science and human behaviour. Macmillan, New York

Smith R G, Iwata B A, Vollmer T R, Pace G M 1992 On the relationship between self-injurious behavior and self-restraint. Journal of Applied Behavior Analysis 25: 433–445

Solnick J V, Rincover A, Peterson C R 1977 Some determinants of the reinforcing and punishing effects of time-out. Journal of Applied Behaviour Analysis 10: 415–424

Sprague R I, Horner R H 1992 Covariation within functional response classes: implications for treatment of severe problem behavior. Journal of Applied Behavior Analysis 25: 735–745

Stansfield J, Cheseldine S 1994 Challenging to communicate. Human Communication 3(3): 11–14

Stevens P, Martin N 1999 Supporting individuals with intellectual disability and challenging behaviour in integrated work settings: an overview and a model for service provision. Journal of Intellectual Disability Research 43 (1): 19–29

Stubbings V, Martin G L 1998 Matching training tasks to abilities of people with mental retardation: a learning test versus experienced staff. American Journal on Mental Retardation 102 (5): 473–484

Sturmey P, Carlsen A, Crisp A G, Newton J T 1988 A functional analysis of multiple aberrant responses: a refinement and extension of Iwata et al's methodology. Journal of Mental Deficiency Research 32: 31–46

Sturmey P, Rickets R W, Goza A 1993 A review of the aversives debate: an American perspective. In: Jones R S P, Eayrs C B (eds) Challenging behaviour and intellectual disability: a psychological perspective. BILD Publications, Clevedon, pp 99–120

Thompson T, Hackenberg T, Cerutti D, Baker D, Axtell S 1994 Opioid antagonist effects on self-injury in adults with mental retardation: response form and location as determinants of medication effects. American Jornal on Mental Retardation 99: 85–102

Thorndike E L 1898 Animal intelligence: an experimental study of the associative processes in animals. Psychological Review 2(8)(monograph supplement)

Thurman S 1997 Challenging behaviour through communication. British Journal of Learning Disabilities 25(3): 111–116

Toogood S, Timlin K 1996 The functional assessment of challenging behaviour. Journal of Applied Research in Intellectual Disabilities 9 (3): 206–222

Touchette P E, MacDonald R F, Langer S N 1985 A scatter plot for identifying stimulus control of problem behavior. Journal of Applied Behavior Analysis 18: 343–351

Van Houten R, Rolinder A 1989 An analysis of several variables influencing the efficiency of flash card instruction. Journal of Applied Behaviour Analysis 22: 111–118

Van Houten R, Axelrod S, Bailey J S et al 1988 The right to effective behavioral treatment. Journal of Applied Behavior Analysis 21: 381–384

Vollmer T R 1995 Progressing from brief assessments to extended experimental analyses in the evaluation of aberrant behaviour. Journal of Applied Behaviour Analysis 28: 561–576

Watson J B, Raynor R 1920 Conditioned emotional reactions. Journal of Experimental Psychiatry 3: 1–14

Whitaker S 1996 A review of DRO: the influence of the degree of intellectual disability and the frequency of the target behaviour. Journal of Applied Research in Intellectual Disabilities 9(1): 61–79

Willis T J, LaVigna G W, Donnellan A M 1993 The behavior assessment guide. Institute for Applied Behavior Analysis, Columbia, South Carolina

Wolpe J 1958 Psychotherapy by reciprocal inhibition. Stanford University Press, Stanford, California

Woods P A, Blewitt E 1993 Functional and ecological analysis: a precursor to constructional intervention. In: Jones R S P, Eayrs C B (eds) Challenging behaviour and intellectual disability: a psychological perspective. BILD Publications, Clevedon, pp 34–65

Yoder P J, Davies B, Bishop K 1994 Adult interactional style effects in the language sampling and transcription process with children who have developmental disabilities. American Journal on Mental Retardation 99(3): 270–282

Yule W, Carr J (eds) 1987 Behaviour modification for people with mental handicaps, 2nd edn. Chapman Hall, London

Zarcone J R, Iwata B A, Smith R G, Mazaleski J L, Lerman D C 1994 Re-emergence and extinction of self-injurious escape behavior during stimulus (instructional) fading. Journal of Applied Behavior Analysis 27: 307–316

Zarkowska E, Clements J 1994 Severe problem behaviour: the STAR approach. Chapman Hall, London

Zeigob L, Klukas N, Junginger J 1978 Reactivity of self-monitoring procedures with retarded adolescents. American Journal of Mental Deficiency 83: 156–163

Resources

The following sources of further information concerning the application of behavioural approaches to the assessment and management of behavioural difficulties are especially relevant to people with learning disabilities. However, in a broader sense these resources will be of use to the reader who wishes to acquire further knowledge of both theoretical and practical aspects of the behavioural approach to intervention.

Journals

American Journal on Mental Retardation
http://www.aamr.org

Behavioural and Cognitive Psychotherapy
http://www.cup.cam.ac.uk

British Journal of Learning Disabilities
Frankfurt Lodge
Clevedon Hall
Victoria Road
Clevedon BS21 7HH
Tel: 01275 876519
Fax: 01275 343096

Journal of Applied Behaviour Analysis
http://www.envmed.rochester.edu/wwwrap/behavior/jaba/jabahome.htm

Journal of Behaviour Therapy and Experimental Psychiatry
http://www.elsevier.com/
Journal of Intellectual Disability Research
Blackwell Science
Journal Subscriptions
PO Box 88
Oxford OX2 0NE
Tel: 0 1865 206180/206038
Fax: 0 1865 206219
http://www.blackwell-science.com/products/journals/jidr.htm

Journal of Intellectual and Developmental Disability
http://www.carfax.co.uk/jid-con.htm

Journal of Learning Disabilities
Sage Publications Ltd
6 Bonhill Street
London EC2A 4PU
Tel: 0207 374 0645
Fax: 0207 374 8741
http://www.info@sagepub.co.UK
http://www.churchillmed.com/Journals/LearnDis/jhome.html

Research in Developmental Disabilities
http://www.hbz-nrw.de/

Tizard Learning Disability Review
http://www.speke.ukc.ac.uk/tizard/index/htm/

Academic bodies, associations and organisations
British Institute of Learning Disabilities
Wolverhampton Road
Kidderminster
Worcestershire DY10 3PP
Tel: 01562 850251

American Association on Mental Retardation
444 North Capitol Street
NW, Suite 846
Washington DC 20001–1512
USA
Tel: +1 202 387 1968
Fax: +1 202 387 2193
http://www.aamr.org

Association for the Advancement of Behavior Therapy
305 Seventh Avenue, 16th Floor
New York 10001–6008
USA
Tel: +1 212 647 1890
Fax: +1 212 647 1865
http://server.psyc.vt.edu

Association for Persons with Severe Handicaps (TASH)
29 West Susquehanna Avenue, Suite 210
Baltimore
MD 21204
USA
Tel: +1 410 828 8274
Fax: +1 410 828 6706
hhttp://www.tash.org

European Association of Mental Health in Mental Retardation
c/o Mrs Chris Laming MH-LD
York Clinic
Guy's Hospital
London SE1 3RR
Tel: 0207 955 4792
Fax: 0207 955 4232

Institute for Applied Behaviour Analysis
6169 St. Andrews Road
123 Columbia
SC 29212–3146
USA
Tel: +1 803 731 8597
Fax: +1 803 731 8598
http://www.iaba.net

National Association of Developmental Disabilities Councils
1234 Massachusetts Avenue
NW, Suite 103
Washington DC 20005
USA
Tel: +1 202 347 1234
Fax: +1 202 347 4023
http://www.igc.apc.org/NADDC

Pavilion Publishing and Conference Services
Pavilion Publishing
8 St. George's Place
Brighton
Sussex BN1 4GB
Tel: 01273 623 222
Fax: 01273 625 526
http://www.pavpub.com

The Tizard Centre
Beverley Farm
University of Kent at Canterbury
Canterbury
Kent CT2 7LZ
Tel: 01227 764 000 (Ext.7771)
Fax: 01227 763 674
http://www.speke.ukc.ac.uk/tizard/index.htm/

10 Cognitive behavioural interventions

John Turnbull

Key issues
- Cognitive behavioural approaches have their origins in psychological enquiry and can be used to support people in overcoming specific emotional difficulties
- Cognitive behavioural approaches are based upon the premise that our thoughts, beliefs and expectations (cognitions) have a significant influence over our behaviour
- Cognitive behavioural approaches are used for the treatment of common problems such as depression and anxiety
- Cognitive behavioural approaches have been shown to be as effective as other approaches, although it is uncertain whether it is the behavioural or cognitive elements of the approach that are effective

Overview   Cognitive behavioural interventions constitute some of the most diverse approaches to help people lead more satisfying lives. This chapter shows that the origins of the cognitive behavioural approach can be traced to the beginnings of modern psychological enquiry itself. Since that time, substantial evidence has been amassed to support its use in meeting a range of human needs.

Like other chapters in this section, this chapter opens with an account of the history of cognitive behavioural interventions. This is followed by a discussion of the theoretical and philosophical assumptions underpinning this approach, focusing especially on how emotional and behavioural problems are understood from a cognitive behavioural viewpoint. Next, three case studies will show the versatility of the cognitive behavioural approach and special attention will be paid to its use with people with learning disabilities. Finally, drawing upon research evidence, the strengths and limitations of the cognitive behavioural approach will be examined.

Although the principles of the cognitive behavioural approach are easily explained, anyone applying them should ensure they have received adequate training and supervision in their use. Details of further reading, training and support are given at the end of this chapter.

Introduction

Cognitive behavioural interventions are well researched and increasingly popular approaches that can help people to overcome specific emotional difficulties and to lead more satisfying lives. Cognitive behavioural interventions have their origins in the beginnings of psychological enquiry and they share many of the features of other therapeutic approaches. However, their distinctiveness is based on the premise that our emotions and behaviours are primarily influenced by our thoughts and beliefs. On the basis of our individual experiences, it is supposed that each one of us holds unique assumptions and ways of thinking about the world. Almost without realising, we test out these assumptions in our day-to-day interactions with others and modify them according to our experience. Sometimes, people can hold beliefs or develop ways of thinking that can lead them to experience intense and persistent emotional reactions to events.

Using a cognitive behavioural approach demands a positive and collaborative outlook on the part of the helper. At an early stage, helpers need to enable people to see their problems in normal terms rather than a disorder or mental illness. A major goal is also to develop a shared understanding of people's core beliefs about themselves and others and of how this influences their feelings and actions. Through discussion, role play or simple behavioural experiments, helpers and clients work together to practise different and more flexible ways of construing problems. Gradually, the person being helped learns how to become his or her own 'helper', which includes acquiring strategies to deal with occasions when things do not go according to plan.

Historical overview

As we will see later, cognitive behavioural interventions are based on the assumption that our thoughts, beliefs and expectations (cognitions) have a significant influence over our behaviour. Therefore, helping people overcome emotional problems involves working with them to change the way they view events and to develop a more flexible thinking style.

A number of evaluative studies (Blackburn et al 1981, Hollon et al 1991) have now confirmed cognitive behavioural interventions as the leading psychotherapeutic approach in the last two decades. Cognitive behavioural interventions made their initial impact in the 1950s and 1960s, but the history of the approach can be traced back even further.

The influence of 'non-cognitivists'

The development of cognitive behavioural interventions has been shaped both by people who were fervent proponents of this new approach and by some who would not have described themselves as cognitivists. The origins of the cognitive behavioural approach can be found in the dissatisfaction with two other influential psychological approaches of this century, namely psychoanalysis and behaviourism. In the case of psychoanalysis, criticism was levelled against its introspection and the view that people are driven mainly by instincts and unconscious desires. To many, this explanation did little to distinguish human behaviour from animal behaviour and took little account of people's thoughts and beliefs. Psychoanalysis was also criticised for its portrayal of the therapist as a passive listener and interpreter of what the client said. Du Bois (1909), for example, proposed a more active and persuasive role for the therapist, drawing heavily on logical argument, which later became a key characteristic of the cognitive behavioural approach.

Adler (1927), himself trained in the psychoanalytical tradition, later developed this theme and based his therapy on an exploration of people's personal goals, values and the meanings they attach to events. Again, this became a key principle underpinning the cognitive behavioural approach.

Psychologists and academics also expressed dissatisfaction with the behavioural approach, claiming it forged an unnecessarily strong link between human and animal behaviour. They criticised the behavioural approach for its emphasis on observable, external events. Experimental evidence cast further doubt over behavioural theory. Salter (1949), for instance, reported difficulty in extending the principles of conditioning from animals to humans. Tolman (1925), through his observations of the behaviour of rats in a maze, concluded that the relationship between an external event and a behavioural response was not as straightforward as behaviourists portrayed (Box 10.1). He developed his 'mediational model' of human behaviour which proposed that, between an event and a behavioural response, people develop an internal representation of what is happening to help them make decisions about a course of action.

Box 10.1
A critical experiment

In a famous experiment by Tolman (1932), the authors intended to show that behaviour could be acquired without the direct use of reinforcements. Three groups of rats were required to run through a maze in turn. The rats in the first group were always reinforced with food at the end of the maze. Those in the second group were given no reinforcement. As behaviourists would predict, those in the first group were discovered to make fewer errors during their runs through the maze whilst those in the second group continued to make frequent errors. This would appear to confirm the view that reinforcement brings about learning. The rats in the third group were allowed to run through the maze without reinforcement on 10 occasions and were then given food for their remaining runs. For the first 10 runs, group 3 did as badly as group 1. However, the rats in group 3 were able to catch up with the performance of group 1 once they were reinforced with food. The implication of this is that the rats had been developing a knowledge of the maze even though they were not reinforced for doing so. Although their performance improved with reinforcement, this shows that rewards simply add to motivation: they may not be responsible for learning taking place.

Later, Bandura (1977) extended Tolman's ideas and developed his social learning theory. Through his observations and experiments, Bandura was able to show that someone's behaviour does not have to be directly reinforced but can be learned by observing others. His theory also proposed that people can anticipate events, thereby using cognitions to guide their actions.

The influence of cognitivists

George Kelly (1955) is credited with being the first person to develop a cognitive view of human behaviour, although Kelly himself resisted this label (Neimayer 1986). Kelly's personal construct theory proposes that people develop a set of constructs, or blueprints, about the world through their everyday experiences which helps them understand their own and others' behaviour (see also Box 10.2, below). These constructs can be used to predict events. If something does not match their prediction, the construct can be modified.

In the early 1960s, Albert Ellis (1962) developed rational emotive therapy (RET) which was the first therapeutic approach to be explicitly based on a cognitive model of human behaviour. Ellis proposed that people were not distressed by events but by the way they interpreted them. In other words, emotional problems were influenced primarily by thinking errors and self-defeating beliefs. For example if, on rising to give a speech, someone thinks, 'I'm going to make a mess of this', the chances are that he or she will become anxious and will not make a good presentation. Similarly, someone who believes that 'children should do as they are told' is likely to go through life disappointed and angry. Ellis's approach therefore focused on helping people to recognise and modify irrational thoughts and beliefs. Importantly, Ellis incorporated behavioural components in his therapy, believing that this improved people's motivation during therapy.

Aaron T. Beck (1976) is another central figure in the development of cognitive behavioural interventions. Beck's cognitive therapy was based upon his extensive work with depressed clients. Beck borrowed the term 'schemata', instead of beliefs, to represent the rules or assumptions that people use to guide their actions. Problems occur when the person distorts or misinterprets events (see also Box 10.3, below). For example, a person might exaggerate the significance of a remark made by someone and take it personally. He or she might also interpret events in 'black and white' terms and be unable to cope in situations which are ambiguous. The aim of Beck's therapy was to help the client challenge and modify his or her interpretation of events and develop more flexible thinking styles. He also used behavioural components such as role play to help people rehearse new ways of behaving.

Donald Meichenbaum (1977) is the third influential therapist in the field of cognitive behavioural interventions. Meichenbaum drew attention to the existence and influence of automatic thoughts which can guide our behaviour as well as be symptomatic of our underlying beliefs or cognitive structures. Meichenbaum's work with hyperactive children showed how the use of self-instruction, or thinking out loud (e.g. 'I have to go slowly and carefully . . . remember, go slowly'), enabled them to perform tasks more successfully. Subsequently, Meichenbaum's 'self-instructional training' was used to help people with a range of problems develop greater self-control. He also incorporated inter-personal problem-solving and role play into his work.

This brief history offers you some idea about the basis of cognitive behavioural interventions but we now need to build up a broader picture of the theory underpinning these approaches.

Theoretical development

First principles

Although cognitions lie at the heart of cognitive behavioural interventions, this does not mean that they are the focus of theory. The development of theory has sought to take a holistic view of personality which includes emotions and behaviour, hence the following assumptions which underpin cognitive behavioural interventions:

- Cognitions exist
- External events are processed by cognitions to create personal meaning for an individual

- Almost all behaviour is a product of an interaction between external events, cognitions and emotions
- Cognitions are the primary target for change in therapeutic intervention.

The distinctiveness of the theory underpinning cognitive behavioural approaches is derived from its view of a person as an active seeker, selector and interpreter of experience and information. This is a view first put forward by Kelly (1955), referred to earlier in this chapter. Kelly believed that people developed constructs as a way of making sense of the world. He likened people to scientists, constructing hypotheses about the world and testing them out through everyday experiences. Other people (Wessler 1986) have proposed that the word 'scientist' suggests that people think and act rationally and prefer the term 'manager'. This may be a more appropriate metaphor, since it could be suggested that we rarely act rationally in the face of hard evidence. How many of us, for example, have a fear of flying, despite the fact that it is the safest form of travel? Whatever term we use, Kelly's view is that human beings instinctively want to understand themselves and their world.

How are constructs developed?

Kelly (see Box 10.2) proposed that constructs are the product of recurring themes in our lives. Through our experiences, we develop constructs both to understand what has happened in the past and to anticipate and predict the outcome of future events. This does not mean that constructs are consciously developed. Very often we are only made aware of our beliefs when we either experience problems and crises or are directly asked to explain our behaviour.

There are two key points to remember about constructs. Firstly, they are dynamic phenomena, in that we are constantly revising them in the light of

Box 10.2
Personal construct theory

George Kelly was born in a small farming community in Kansas in the USA in 1905. His first degree was in physics and mathematics though he chose to pursue a career in education, undertaking an educational scholarship to Edinburgh University. He returned to America to study for a doctorate in psychology in 1931. Kelly began his therapeutic work as a Freudian. However, he gradually began to develop his own theories. Kelly came to believe that people live their lives according to their personal contructs of the world which they use to explain and to predict future events (Kelly 1955). In other words, no two people will view events in identical ways. Consider the following example: Imagine you are at the top of a hill looking down over a series of valleys. To what would you pay attention if you were:

1. A property developer?
2. A farmer?
3. An artist?

The activity above is similar to a series of experiments carried out by Kelly and his research students. Kelly hypothesised that personal constructs act in the same way as if people were playing a strictly defined role which guided their behaviour. By using carefully constructed roles for his students to follow over a period of 2 or 3 weeks, Kelly was able to show dramatic changes in their behaviour.

experience. For example, think about how your constructs of education, ageing or parenthood have changed over the years. Secondly, since each person's experience is unique, then so will be their way of looking at the world. For example, one person's construct of the word 'disabled' might contain thoughts of collection boxes, charitable events or someone being pushed in a wheelchair by a relative. Another person's construct might contain images of the paralympic games, a ramp outside a building to promote access for wheelchair users, and a person collecting a certificate at a university graduation ceremony. Neither of these constructs is right or wrong but should be understood and accepted as having a personal meaning for each individual.

How do constructs influence behaviour?

Constructs, then, are at the centre of our cognitive system. Other researchers have referred to them as 'schemata' (Beck 1976), 'beliefs' (Ellis 1962) and 'concepts' (Meichenbaum 1977). Consider the following dialogue:

Father: Come on, you two, it's time we got ready to go shopping.

Elder sister: Yes, Emily, get your shoes on.

Younger sister: Be quiet, Samantha, you're not an adult!

Father: Yes, Samantha, be quiet!

We might conclude several things from this brief extract. First of all, we might suppose that the youngest child has two constructs: firstly, 'sisters should be treated equally, despite their age' and secondly, 'adults are here to tell children what to do'. If we accept this, then we should not be surprised at her reaction when her older sister appears to be behaving like an adult. In other words, the youngest child's expectations have not been met and she appraises, or evaluates, her sister's words as being domineering. Although we would only know by asking her, we might imagine her private thoughts to be 'she's got no right to tell me what to do!'. The combination of the event, her thoughts and beliefs and her feelings of anger result in a sharp retort. However, do all sequences of behaviour follow a similar pattern?

Some of the liveliest discussions of cognitive theory have focused on the issue of whether cognitions actually cause behaviour. Lazarus (1984) proposed that cognitions precede emotional reactions to events whilst Zajonc (1984) took an opposite view and criticised cognitive theorists for playing down the role of emotion in behaviour. Most cognitivists resist the idea that behaviour can only be explained in linear terms, in which a behaviour comes at the end of a chain of events. Instead, they take a more interactionalist viewpoint in which events are seen only as a starting point for behaviour rather than a cause. Blackman (1981) and Hollin (1990), for example, point out that cognitions can both shape and be shaped by events. In his research into the treatment of chronic anger problems, Raymond Novaco (1975) devised a model to explain the relationship between events, cognitions, emotions and behaviour (see Fig. 10.1).

How do cognitivists view problem behaviours?

Like many other theories of behaviour, cognitive theory can be applied to help improve the quality of the lives of many people who would not describe themselves as having emotional or behaviour problems. For example, it can help someone improve their presentation skills, bring them

Fig. 10.1
Interactional model of behaviour (from Novaco 1975, with kind permission from Routledge, London)

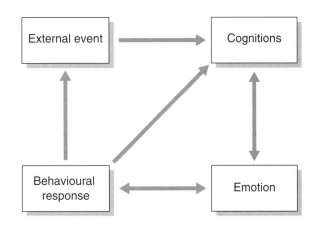

greater success in studying or simply improve their relationships with other people. However, given the focus of this book, we need to ask how cognitive theory explains emotional distress and behavioural problems.

Cognitivists see behavioural problems essentially as exaggerated responses to circumstances. For instance, it is perfectly normal to feel sad when something has not turned out how we would have wanted. Similarly, we would be justified in feeling angry if someone insulted us. The point is that these feelings soon subside. However, according to cognitive theory, problems exist when feelings such as anxiety, sadness or anger become persistent or intense.

At the heart of these problems lie irrational and faulty styles of thinking. Both Ellis (1962) and Beck (1976) have categorised the more common errors of thinking (Box 10.3)

Kendall & Braswell (1985) further proposed that people's problems could be seen to derive from cognitive deficits or cognitive distortions. In the case of cognitive deficits, the person is believed to lack the means to process information appropriately or to choose an appropriate response to a situation. The focus of therapy is therefore to help the person acquire different skills. In the case of cognitive distortions, the emphasis is placed on the specific content of the person's thoughts and beliefs. The approach here is to teach the person how to understand and question their own cognitions in order to think more rationally.

Before moving on, it is important to recognise that we all demonstrate evidence of irrational thinking from time to time. The key issue is that irrational or dysfunctional thinking styles only become problematic when they have a severely negative effect on the person's life, on the life of others, or both.

The philosophical basis of cognitive behavioural approaches

The philosophical underpinnings of cognitive behavioural approaches have been described by many authors as humanistic. In doing this, they have pointed to the characteristics of holism and personal growth:

Holism

As shown in Figure 10.1 (above), cognitive behavioural approaches are based on an interactional model of human behaviour that takes into account thoughts and feelings as well as behaviour. Furthermore, and as we shall see in the case studies, any assessment of an individual should consider external

Box 10.3
Errors of thinking

Aaron T. Beck (1976) was one of the foremost thinkers on the use of cognitive behavioural approaches for people who were depressed. He believed that dysfunctional thinking lay at the heart of people's depressed mood. He categorised these errors as follows:

1. Arbitrary inference – drawing a negative conclusion in the absence of supporting evidence. For example, someone might conclude 'My friend has fallen out with me' because he or she didn't receive a birthday card.

2. Selective abstraction – drawing conclusions about the detail of an issue rather than looking at other evidence. For example, a student might focus on the criticisms of an essay by his or her lecturer of an assignment instead of the good points and conclude 'They think I'm rubbish'.

3. Over-generalisation – drawing a conclusion about a range of issues on the basis of information from a single event. For example, a student who fails one essay will conclude 'I'll never pass any of the other exams'.

4. Magnification and minimisation – evaluating the importance of a negative event and failing to acknowledge more positive factors. For example, one bad day at work could be interpreted by someone to mean 'I'm no good at my job'.

5. Personalisation – relating external events to oneself when this is unjustified. For example, 'If I had warned my friend not to smoke he wouldn't have died of a heart attack'.

6. Absolutist dichotomous thinking – thinking in 'black and white' in which everything is either all good or a total disaster. For example, 'My best friend left the party early so it was a complete failure'.

as well as internal factors such as previous learning history, significant life events, physiological and psychological factors and the influence of family members or friends (Black et al 1997). This approach can be linked to traditional humanistic accounts of health as being an integration of 'mind, body and spirit' (Bermosk & Porter 1979).

Personal growth   Novaco (1997) sees cognitive behavioural approaches as positive and empowering in that people's thoughts and beliefs are held to be valid. In other words, they have a unique meaning for the person and cannot be measured against an objective notion of truth or reality. By acknowledging this, the outlook of the therapist is one of acceptance and one in which the client and therapist work both collaboratively and creatively rather than persuasively and coercively. The aim of therapy is to achieve personal growth through new insights and understanding as well as to acquire different skills. Again, this resembles humanistic concepts in which health is seen as the fulfilment of human potential rather than the absence of disease (Beck et al 1988). It is also in sharp contrast to approaches which have sought to contain or eliminate problems.

Although in this brief account we can see similarities with humanistic traditions, there are also differences. Contrasting the humanistic approach of Carl Rogers (1961) with that of cognitive therapy, Wessler (1986, p.3), for example, believes that cognitive approaches are distinctive because of their emphasis on cognitions whereas humanistic therapies focus on feelings and emotions:

> *the 'self' that so often appears in Rogers' writings is 'experienced' rather than thought about. Cognition and cognitive change seem unnecessary for their [humanists] account of disturbance and prescribed targets for change.*

Other significant differences are noted by Newell & Dryden (1991). Although both humanistic and cognitive behaviour therapists stress the importance of the personal characteristics of the therapist, the authors claim that humanists have emphasised this aspect to the exclusion of any specific techniques of therapy. To summarise, most cognitive behaviour therapists would resist a strict philosophical interpretation of their approach as humanistic though it contains many of its characteristics.

Case illustrations of cognitive behavioural approaches in use

It is only recently that cognitive behavioural approaches have been used with people with learning disabilities. The reasons for this are several, including therapists' own beliefs that people with learning disabilities lack some of the verbal skills that are thought to be a prerequisite for entering therapy. However, a growing number of accounts (cf. Stenfert-Kroese et al 1997) now demonstrate that people with learning disabilities can be helped by cognitive behavioural approaches to overcome a range of difficulties (see the case studies 'Helping a person with learning disabilities to control his anger' (below), 'Helping a young boy with learning disabilities to gain greater self-control' (p. 271) and 'Helping a nurse to overcome a traumatic experience' (p. 272).

Helping a person with learning disabilities to control his anger

This case illustration concerns a 44-year-old man called Bill who, at the time of therapy, was living on a male ward for 12 people in a hospital for people with learning disabilities. Bill was referred for therapy by the ward staff because of frequent episodes of rage which sometimes resulted in him hitting out at other residents and occasionally at staff.

The starting point for any intervention is assessment. In Bill's case, for several weeks, the assessment focused on the following areas:

- Background, including early experiences
- Individual anger pattern, including arousal levels, existing coping strategies, trigger factors
- Cognitions (e.g. thoughts, expectations and appraisals of events)
- Motivation to change
- Capacity to follow therapeutic regime, including completion of 'homework' assignments and self-report measures.

It was important, first of all, to meet with staff to gain background information about Bill and to get their interpretation of factors that angered him. Forming a good relationship with staff was also important to gain their cooperation in recording future incidents and participating in any intervention as 'co-therapists'. However, as we shall see, the bulk of the information must come from the client.

My involvement with Bill followed the pattern of anger management therapy set out in the original work of Raymond Novaco (1975). Novaco describes three essential stages of therapy:

1. Education
2. Skill acquisition and rehearsal
3. Implementation.

Throughout these stages, the goal of the therapist is to work with the client in the following areas:

- To reduce arousal
- To enable the client to recognise and challenge irrational thoughts
- To generate and apply alternative coping strategies.

Although my involvement with Bill followed this pattern, certain aspects of therapy need to be emphasised when working with people with learning disabilities who have anger problems. Firstly, severe anger problems are usually recognised by people who are the object of rage long before the person him or herself seeks out help. Therefore, developing the motivation to change may take time. As Black et al (1997) point out, people with anger problems are usually mistrustful and defensive and they will often attribute responsibility for their behaviour to others. Therefore, Bill was asked to meet with me to discuss his behaviour but care was taken, at this stage, not to imply that he had difficulty in controlling his anger.

The first session with any client is also crucial in clarifying expectations. It is important to establish the therapist's credibility (Stevens 1996) and a relationship that is based on trust and respect. In Bill's case, I had to be mindful of his expectations. People with learning disabilities, especially those who have lived in institutions, may have had specific experiences. For example, in wards or units where people display challenging behaviour, the appearance of staff from outside – such as psychologists or psychiatrists – may be associated by clients with some sort of wrong-doing. Also, it is only recently that services have sought the active participation of people with learning disabilities in planning interventions. Since cognitive behavioural approaches rely heavily on establishing a partnership with clients, it is advisable to go slowly at first.

I first met Bill in his bedroom on the ward. I explained that I was a nurse, like the others on the ward, but that I had received extra training to help people who became very angry. I explained that I had helped other people in the hospital to feel less angry. To establish a good rapport with a client, it is important that the therapist and client share the same expressions and words during therapy. In many institutions for people with learning disabilities, several demeaning adjectives have developed to describe emotional states such 'going high' or 'having a temper tantrum'. In Bill's case, although he used the word 'angry', he commonly used 'getting mad' to describe his feelings.

At this first session with Bill, I continued by telling him that I was interested in the things that made people 'get mad' and asked him to describe some of his experiences. Still a little suspicious, Bill muttered something about staff and 'the others', by whom he meant the other people on the ward. I asked him if he thought he 'got mad' too often and whether he wished it would happen less. Bill said yes. I asked him if he thought this would be difficult. Although Bill believed that things could improve, he was adamant at this point that it was up to other people to change their ways.

Bill agreed to see me again to talk about things that made him angry. He had a job working in the hospital grounds for 4 days a week as well as the self-appointed task of keeping the ward kitchen tidy during the evening. Therefore, we agreed to meet on his day off.

At the second session I took in a flip chart and said that we were going to make a list of some of the good things about getting angry and some of the bad things. To help us, I asked Bill to describe some of his recent experiences of getting angry. Here is an example:

Bill: That Charlie was at it again the other night.

Me: Tell me what he did.

Bill: He got me mad.

Me: What did he do to get you mad?

Bill: The boys were playing cards the other night and he came in to get them crisps and drinks.

Me: What made you get mad with him? Did he say something?

Bill: He just grabbed the stuff and made a mess in the kitchen.

Me: And did you say anything to him?

Bill: I told him alright! I said it wasn't fair 'cos it was me that has to clear up all the time.

Me: What did Charlie do then?

Bill: He swore at me and spat at me.

Me: How did that make you feel?

Bill: I got really mad with him and pushed him against the door. Then he pushed me back and I hit my elbow on the cupboard.

Me: What made you feel like pushing him?

Bill: 'Cos he deserved it! He's always causing trouble and the staff always take his side and they're never bothered about me!

Me: What did the staff do?

Bill: Linda came in to see what was happening but before I had chance to say anything she said I'd better go into my room and calm down.

Me: Was that a good idea?

Bill: I suppose so. My head was thumping by that time and my hands were shaking but it still wasn't fair 'cos Charlie got away scot-free!

Me: What happened later?

Bill: Linda came down half an hour later and asked if I was okay. I said 'Yes'. She asked if I wanted to come and play cards.

Me: Did you?

Bill: Yes, but when I went into the dayroom Charlie and the others said they didn't want to play with me.

Me: How did that make you feel?

Bill: (*pause*) I wasn't bothered. Sometimes it's best to keep yourself to yourself.

Bill and I used this and other examples to make our list of good and bad points about getting angry, as follows:

Good things

■   It lets people know how you feel.
■   It stops people taking advantage of you.

Bad things

■   It gives you a headache.
■   It gets you into trouble.
■   You miss out on good things.

- People don't like you.
- You can get hit.
- It makes you feel bad.

One of the reasons for making a list such as this is simply to give the client more information about anger. Another key reason is to use it as a lever for change. The negative list is nearly always longer than the positive one. This can provide the therapist with the opportunity of getting the person to agree to the need for change. Importantly, however, the therapist must point out that it is not wrong to feel angry. Obviously, being spat at or hit would provoke anyone. However, some of the ways people express anger is wrong. This can be a difficult idea to convey to people with learning disabilities, not least because many people with learning disabilities may have grown up in a culture in which feelings have not been openly discussed and in which violence is a common reaction to provocation. In Bill's case, I used some of my own experiences of getting angry to describe how I reacted to anger: this can often encourage people to disclose their thoughts.

The subsequent two sessions were spent briefly recapping on previous ones and finding out more about Bill's past. This can often give further clues to the way a person sees the world. To do this, I again used a flip chart to draw a 'life-line'. I explained that I wanted Bill to remember as far back as he could and tell me about things that had happened to him. Bill first remembered coming into hospital when he was 7 years old. 'My mam couldn't cope with me,' he said, 'I was wild'. I asked Bill to describe what life was like in the hospital. 'You had to do as you were told,' he replied. I also asked if things had changed. Bill replied that he thought the staff were now 'too soft', by which he meant that they let people get away with too much. He also said that 'This lot aren't real nurses!', referring to the staff on his ward. Bill recalled being on a succession of wards for people who displayed challenging behaviour. He also told me about the day, 20 years earlier, when he got his job working in the hospital grounds. I asked if he'd ever wanted to live outside the hospital. He said that he had. For 2 years he lived with four other people from the hospital in the nearby town. He said he had argued with the staff and been sent back. He said there was no work to do and this is what had got him into trouble. Bill remembered other events such as his sister's wedding, at which he was an usher. He also remembered his mother dying 3 years earlier. He said that this made him feel very lonely but the staff had helped him.

By now, a clearer picture was emerging of Bill. He seemed to be a person whose life had been shaped by clear rules, which could explain his rigid thinking style. Bill's self-esteem had obviously taken several blows during his life and it is not unusual for people in his position to use anger as a way of bolstering their reputation. Certainly, he was very proud of his job which he felt set him apart from his fellow residents.

Bill also showed evidence of unhelpful and irrational thinking styles and beliefs. He had a high and unrealistic expectation of nurses, hence his statement that 'This lot aren't real nurses!' He also showed a feature common to many people with anger problems in which any evidence which contradicts their view of the world is disregarded. For example, Bill didn't acknowledge Linda's attempts to help him to calm down and to include him in the game of cards. His belief about nurses is also unchanged by his statement about how staff had helped him following his mother's death.

The fifth time I saw Bill was a key session in which he needed to take some decisions about my involvement. I began the session by asking him to tell me about some of the things he had learned about anger. I also told him that I thought it must be difficult at times for him to live on a ward like this but that I believed he could have a better time. I explained that it would be hard to make other people do the things he wanted them to and that it might be easier for him to change. Bill said that he could see the sense in this.

In the following sessions I continued to obtain information about Bill's anger patterns and prepared him to take greater responsibility for change. Cognitive behavioural approaches are self-control procedures, in that the person learns to monitor and evaluate his or her own behaviour and set standards for future performance. To achieve this, cognitive behavioural approaches typically encourage clients to keep a diary to record their experiences and thoughts. Many people with learning disabilities cannot read or write. Therefore, Bill was asked to keep a tape-recorded diary. Initially, I trained the staff on Bill's ward to prompt him with a series of questions. It was important that staff did not see themselves in a counselling situation and they were asked not to respond to comments he made. These questions consisted of the following:

- What day is it?
- Did you have a good day or a bad day today?
- What happened to make it good/bad? (If bad, ask Bill to describe the incident)
- What did the person say or do to make you mad?
- Can you remember what were you thinking at the time?
- What happened in the end?

Twice a week, with Bill's permission, I picked up his tapes and listened to them. By the end of 3 weeks, Bill began to use the diary without prompts from staff.

Although clients will continue to learn throughout therapy, it was now time to move on to the next stage of intervention in which Bill needed to acquire the skills to alter his thoughts and behaviour.

In the following 10 sessions we used examples from Bill's diary as a focus for discussion and for role play. It was also important that Bill learned how to reduce his arousal. There were two aspects to this. Firstly, Bill needed to reduce his general arousal levels and feel more relaxed. Secondly, he needed to employ strategies that would help him control his arousal during provocation. Several methods exist to help people feel more relaxed. Imaginal techniques ask people to imagine a relaxing setting, for example lying on a beach, paying attention to the warm sun or the sound of the sea. This can be helped by the use of commercially available tape recordings. In progressive muscle relaxation, the person is asked to tense and relax different muscle groups. Some of these techniques can be difficult for a person with learning disabilities. Therefore, a simpler form has been developed called behavioural relaxation training. This simply involves the person copying the relaxed posture of the therapist and learning to take two or three deep breaths at the beginning of each episode of relaxation. When working with any person who experiences tension, it must be remembered that the person can find the feeling of being relaxed quite aversive at first. In Bill's case, he preferred to copy my own posture which we did at the beginning and end of every session. I also asked him to practise relaxing at the end of each day. Reducing arousal levels during provocation relies on the person monitoring and adjusting their tension levels, for example their breathing, as well as talking themselves through an episode. In Bill's case, he told me he remembered someone once told him to count to 10 and asked if I thought it would work. I suggested he could try it. Later, Bill reported that he did not always get to 10 but he thought it was doing him some good.

Since cognitive behavioural approaches are based on the belief that cognitions influence behaviour, the focus of therapy during this stage was on developing in Bill a more flexible thinking style. Angry people such as Bill have difficulty taking the other person's perspective during interactions. This can often lead to confrontation. Another difficulty can be interpersonal problem-solving skills. The sessions with Bill therefore concentrated on getting him to recognise unhelpful thoughts. In one session, Bill was describing an argument he had with a member of staff called Sandy:

Me: Go back to the beginning and tell me what happened before you started arguing with Sandy.

Bill: The night staff had left the kitchen in a mess and I was cleaning it up. Sandy came in and told me to leave it 'cos I'd be late for work.

Me: Do you always have to tidy the kitchen in the morning?

Bill: No. There was a new man on duty at night.

Me: Do you think he left the kitchen in a mess on purpose?

Bill: I don't know. Some of those night staff are lazy. They leave it for the likes of us to take the blame. They know I'll be the one to tidy up their mess!

Me: But you said he was new on this ward. Do you think he knew that you're the one who tidies up the kitchen?

Bill: No.

Me: So, could there be another reason why the kitchen was in a mess?

Bill: I suppose if he was new, he didn't know what to do.

Me: Yes, you could be right. Anyway, you had the kitchen to tidy. I bet you were feeling mad.

Bill: Too right! I had to tidy it up quick because I had to get to work. Then Sandy came in and started to shout at me. He told me to leave the mess.

Me: What do you think made Sandy get mad?

Bill: I should have been getting ready for work but I was tidying the kitchen.

Me: Do you think he could have been mad that the kitchen was in a mess?

Bill: He could have been.

Me: So, that would mean that he wasn't mad with you but he was mad that it had been left to you to tidy the kitchen?

Bill: Yes, I suppose so.

This is a brief example of how Bill was encouraged to think of alternative explanations for events. Sessions also included role play in which Bill was encouraged to re-enact situations and to apply these new perspectives. Although this could be achieved relatively easily in the calm atmosphere of his room on the ward, Bill needed to learn how to apply these techniques himself during incidents. One approach to helping people has been devised by Castles & Glass (1986) who developed a problem-solving framework for use by people with learning disabilities. Black (1994) later developed this approach and used it as a measure of progress during therapy for people with learning disabilities who have anger problems. Briefly, people are presented with examples of provoking situations and are asked to provide explanations for a person's behaviour and how they would resolve the situation without becoming angry. This worked particularly well for Bill and one of the examples is described below:

Example: You go into the kitchen and find that someone hasn't cleaned their dishes.

Initially, Bill's explanation for the situation was that someone was deliberately trying to get him mad and that he would go into the dayroom and shout at the residents. If we compare this with Bill's response towards the end of therapy, we can see the difference:

Bill: Maybe they forgot to clear away.

Me: Would you feel mad?

Bill: Yes.

Me: So, how could you make things turn out okay?

Bill: I could ask the staff to find out who it was.

Me: What else could you do?

Bill: I could leave the dishes until he cleared away.

Me: But that would mean the kitchen would be in a mess wouldn't it?

Bill: I suppose so. But it wouldn't be my fault, would it?

Twenty-two weeks after I first met Bill, I felt that it was time to reduce my input. I asked him if it was okay to see him once a fortnight and later once a month. The number of incidents Bill had been involved in had reduced considerably over this time. Bill's diary contained fewer incidents of him losing control. Importantly, this did not mean that he never felt provoked. Anger is a necessary emotion and Bill's surroundings provided many sources of annoyance and irritation. However, he learned to think more flexibly about situations and to see alternative courses of action. As Bill told me, he had also learned that being more relaxed 'gave him time to think about things'.

Several years later, Bill now lives in a house in a community setting. The hospital is much smaller and he still has his job on the gardens. Bill never talks about going back to live there.

Helping a young boy with learning disabilities to gain greater self-control

Jaz was a 10-year-old boy attending a special school for children with learning disabilities. Although teachers considered him to be able, they experienced difficulties in helping him to concentrate on his school work. Often, Jaz could be observed rushing his work and quickly becoming frustrated, throwing paper and pens across the room. Sometimes, Jaz would tip over his table and lie on the floor, screaming. Jaz's behaviour improved slightly when teachers sat with him and helped him with his work. However, this was time-consuming. The teachers had also had some success in using tokens for staying on task. The tokens could be exchanged for preferred activities later. However, Jaz obtained so few tokens that this was thought too weak an approach.

Children like Jaz can lack self-control for a variety of reasons. In Jaz's case, he could sometimes be heard muttering 'I have to get it right' when he tried out some new activity during lessons. We can see how quickly Jaz could become caught up in a vicious circle of anxiety and frustration. By demanding high standards of himself and experiencing more failure than success, the pressure to succeed generates further anxiety when presented with unfamiliar tasks. The objective in working with Jaz was therefore to get him to work more slowly on tasks, to have more realistic expectations and to develop his self-control skills.

Vygostky (1962), a Russian psychologist, proposed that a crucial step in the development of self-control in children is learning to use language to direct their behaviour. One view (Luria 1961) is that some people with learning disabilities, as well as people labelled as hyperactive, have not developed this ability. Experimentally, cognitive behavioural researchers such as Meichenbaum & Goodman (1971) have demonstrated that children with learning disabilities and poor self-control skills can be taught to be less impulsive. Their procedures rely primarily upon a trainer modelling a task by talking him or herself through the different steps. Gradually, the child is encouraged to copy the trainer until he or she has internalised the new instructions.

In Jaz's case, I decided to use a shape sorter to develop his self-control skills. In a room on our own, I asked Jaz to watch me and to listen to what I was saying as I matched the shapes:

Me: What am I supposed to do? I have to find which shape fits exactly into these holes. I have to go slowly and remember to look at each shape carefully. Let's begin with this one. This one has lots of points on it like a star. Is there a hole that looks like a star? Yes, there it is. Let me see if it fits. Yes it does. I feel happy. I got it right because I went slowly and carefully.

The use of self-praise here is important, since the long-term objective was to enable Jaz to work independently. In the same way, Jaz needed to know what to do when things did not go well.

In the next extract I deliberately made a mistake:

Me: This shape looks a tricky one. I think I'll try it in this hole. Oops, it's not the right one. I made a mistake. That's okay, but I need to be careful. I should take more time to look at the shape and the holes. Let's try it again. That's better. I got it right because I took my time.

Next, Jaz was asked to copy my actions and words. I carefully corrected him if he missed anything out. At the fourth attempt, Jaz was already showing better performance. When Jaz could complete the task correctly a further four times, I asked Jaz to whisper the instructions instead of talking out loud. Again, after four correct trials, I then asked him to say the words inside his head so that I couldn't hear. Jaz experienced some difficulty, so I asked him to try whispering again until he eventually succeeded in matching the shapes four times using silent self-instruction.

Although Jaz showed a dramatic improvement on this task, we needed to generalise his self-control skills to other situations. It was also important to increase gradually the level of difficulty of these tasks. Over the next 2 weeks, teachers reported an improvement in his behaviour. However, Jaz still became frustrated at times. The teachers and I then thought of combining a self-instructional approach with the use of tokens, as before. However, this time, it was explained to Jaz that he was responsible for deciding if he had showed good behaviour. This was defined as working for 5 minutes on his own without throwing pens or tipping over tables. Jaz was shown how to set a small timer which would 'bleep' when the 5 minutes had passed. If Jaz had concentrated on a task, he took a token from a drawer and placed it on a wooden peg on his table. When the peg was full with 5 tokens, Jaz could leave his task and play for a further 10 minutes.

At the 2 month review, teachers reported excellent progress. We now needed to fade out the use of the tokens which was achieved by doubling the amount of token Jaz needed to fill his peg. At 6 months teachers reported that Jaz worked well on his own with only occasional incidents. The use of tokens could now be phased out completely.

Helping a nurse to overcome a traumatic experience

Cognitive behavioural approaches are successful because they encourage more rational thinking styles and problem solving which lead to more adaptive coping. However, we should not believe that irrational thinking occurs only in people who are depressed, anxious or angry. More recently, cognitive behavioural approaches have been used successfully to help people who are undergoing a major traumatic event in their lives for whom convenient descriptions such as 'depression' or 'stress' seem inadequate. Moorey (1996), for example, describes the feelings of helplessness of a terminally ill person as a perfectly rational response to adverse circumstances. Can cognitive behavioural approaches offer anything to people to whom life has been cruel?

This case study concerns a 28-year-old staff nurse called Rachel. Rachel had a successful career in mental health nursing and frequently deputised on an admission ward in a hospital for people with mental health problems. One evening, a resident became very disturbed and needed to be restrained. The resident showed no sign of calming himself and the staff were becoming exhausted. Rachel decided that he had to be secluded for a short period. In the seclusion room, the resident broke free and began assaulting Rachel. She suffered a broken nose, lost three teeth and had a ruptured spleen.

Rachel spent the following 4 days in a hospital. During this time, the only people from the hospital to visit were her colleagues from the ward and myself. On one occasion, Rachel said to me that she had been thinking why her manager had not been in touch. 'She thinks it was my fault,' said Rachel. 'They're going to blame me. Perhaps I could have handled it better.'

Many victims of violence believe that their own actions could have contributed to their assault (Lanza 1983) and such beliefs can impair future performance. It is therefore important, though sadly unusual (Turnbull 1993), for victims of violence to receive psychological support. Working with Rachel needs to be seen as a process of adjustment. Horowitz (1986) explains how traumatic events can challenge a person's view of the world and the adjustment process is one of enabling a person to reappraise his or her assumptions. In my early contact with Rachel it was clear that her beliefs about managers and her performance in her job had been severely challenged.

Rachel was angry that since her discharge from hospital she had not heard from her managers. She explained their silence as evidence that she was to blame for the incident and asserted that 'managers should support staff in my position'. Her views did not change some days later when the hospital sent her an incident form to complete (a task she had been unable to carry out immediately following her assault). 'Look at this,' she said, 'they're more interested in paper than people. I thought they were different to other managers but they're all the same!'

From a cognitive behavioural viewpoint, Rachel was expressing the sort of dichotomous thinking and over-generalisation that would normally be challenged by the therapist. However, given the circumstances, many people might believe Rachel's apparently irrational thinking to be perfectly rational. Therefore, my intention was not to get Rachel to challenge these thoughts but to recognise them and to regard them as unhelpful. Time spent ruminating on mistakes made by managers could more usefully be applied to planning her return to work and the steps she needed to take to become physically healthy once more.

Although Rachel learned to distract herself, she was also beginning to express anxiety about her return to work. I recognised this from the somewhat flat tone in her voice. When I probed a little further, Rachel admitted she had difficulty with our conversations at times. She felt comfortable with expressing anger, which sometimes can be a positive and energising emotion (Novaco 1975). However, the experience seemed to have not only challenged her views about managers but also her views about her work. She began to claim that her colleagues would not want to work with her again because she had made a bad decision. I tested out the reality of this claim with her by getting her to imagine herself on a 'This is Your Life' programme. I asked Rachel what she really thought people would say about her as they came on stage to talk about her. Rachel admitted that the evidence went against her initial thought. However, by taking the 'This is Your Life' analogy further, Rachel uncovered many beliefs that she had about nursing that could be seen to underpin her anxiety. She told me of two ward sisters she had worked with whom she admired. As she imagined herself on television talking about them, she recalled some of their sayings, for example, 'nurses are always the last resort' and 'surgeons work with their hands, nurses work with their hands, brains and hearts'. This presents a belief system which sees nurses as perfect and invincible. I discussed this with Rachel who recognised that much of her motivation came from her view of herself as strong, indispensable and able to cope with anything. Now that her assumptions had been challenged, her motivation to return to work had diminished.

From a cognitive behavioural viewpoint, Rachel needed to reappraise her beliefs about nursing in order to regain her motivation and return to work. Conversations with her now concentrated on her imagining what she would do on her return. Rachel's thoughts were focused on the risks of injury. Once again, this is natural and is not to be challenged. However, Rachel needed to be assured that a perception of risk is important but that this should lead to active coping instead of avoidance. We also discussed the need to increase the demands on her in a gradual way and to relieve pressure by taking the breaks to which she was entitled.

When the time came for Rachel's return to work, she had negotiated a post on a long-stay ward in the hospital. Six months later, this changed to a position in the hospital's day service. Rachel is currently undertaking a community nursing degree course at the local university. Last time we met, she told me that, in one of her lectures, students had been asked to write down the characteristics of a good nurse. This is what Rachel wrote:

- Good nurses are human beings
- Good nurses aren't reckless
- Good nurses know the risks and take steps to manage them

The strengths and limitations of the cognitive behavioural approach

Considerable evidence exists to demonstrate the usefulness of cognitive behavioural approaches for a range of human problems (Newell & Dryden 1991). Research into cognitive behavioural therapy has gone beyond the 'does it work?' stage to investigate its application to different types of problems or with different groups of people, as well as to compare its effectiveness with other treatments.

Judging the effectiveness of any therapy or treatment is not easy. For example, Wessler (1983) points out that therapists will often differ in their approach. Whereas this demonstrates the flexibility of many of the therapies and is good from the client's perspective, evaluations need to be well controlled. The best evaluations of cognitive behavioural approaches have therefore ensured that the therapy was consistent with the theoretical assumptions that underpin their approach, rather than differences in technique which will inevitably vary between clients.

Using this as the yardstick, a number of controlled studies have shown that cognitive behavioural approaches perform at least as well as other approaches and often lead to more lasting change (Hollon et al 1991, Stark et al 1991). A critical question has concerned the 'active ingredient' of cognitive behavioural approaches: in other words, is it the cognitive or the behavioural aspects of therapy that has the greatest impact? Studies (Hollon & Kriss 1984) are tending to confirm that the cognitive component is the most important. However, this is not the same as saying that it can be as effective on its own. (See also Box 10.4.)

Cognitive behaviour therapy has now established itself as the treatment of choice for more common problems such as depression and anxiety (Hollon et al 1991). Evidence is also emerging for its effectiveness in other areas,

Box 10.4
The Minnesota cognitive-pharmocotherapy project

This study, by Hollon et al (1991), was designed to be a replication and development of an earlier controlled trial by Rush et al (1977) who had demonstrated the superiority of cognitive therapy over drug treatment for depression.

In Hollon et al's study 107 people between the ages of 18 and 65 who requested treatment for depression were randomly allocated to one of four conditions:

1. Cognitive therapy for a 12-week period
2. Drug treatment using imipramine and withdrawal after 12 weeks
3. Drug treatment with continuation after 12 weeks
4. Combined cognitive therapy and drug treatment for 12 weeks.

Outcome measures were administered and evaluated by researchers independent of the therapists. All treatment conditions showed significant change in reported symptoms in the first 6 weeks. At 12 weeks, any gains levelled out and showed no significant difference between conditions. Patients were followed up with a monthly questionnaire and interview every 6 months for 2 years and were asked to refrain from seeking further treatment. People receiving drug treatment for 12 weeks were the most likely to suffer a relapse during the follow-up. The next group most likely to relapse was the drug continuation group. The people least likely to suffer relapse were those who had received cognitive therapy or therapy in combination with drug treatment.

The researchers concluded that cognitive therapy is as good as drug treatment in reducing symptoms but is superior in preventing relapse.

some of which have proved difficult for other approaches. For example, Pretzer & Beck (1996) report on many small-scale studies which point to the efficacy of cognitive behavioural approaches for people with personality disorders. Controlled trials have also been carried out comparing cognitive behaviour therapy with behavioural treatments for people with anorexia nervosa (Vitousek 1996). These studies have shown cognitive behavioural approaches to be more successful but it must be remembered that they have been based on small samples.

Controlled studies have used a variety of outcome measures to compare effectiveness. However, there is a growing need for studies to overcome difficulties in examining clients' own perceptions and preferences. Although many studies have shown the importance of the relationship between therapist and client (Ford 1978, Schaap et al 1993), virtually all therapies stress the need for characteristics such as genuineness, warmth and empathy in the therapist. Therefore, it is difficult to know whether clients' preferences are based on therapist characteristics or styles of therapy. Furthermore, it is rare for people to have had experience of several types of therapy or treatment.

Several authors have pointed to the limitations of the cognitive behavioural approach. Paradoxically, the aspects of cognitive behavioural interventions that some find advantageous are the very ones that cause problems for others. For example, we have seen that the behavioural aspects of this approach are integral to its success. However, this begs the question whether any change in someone's behaviour was brought about by a change in his or her thoughts and beliefs, or whether external contingencies were primarily responsible (Hollin 1990). Linked to this are questions about the nature of self-control procedures such as cognitive behavioural approaches. In their review of self-management approaches for people with learning disabilities, Jackson & Boag (1981) conclude that methodological problems in studies make it difficult to claim categorically that people are exercising self-control as opposed to being controlled by external contingencies.

A key limitation acknowledged by those who use cognitive behavioural approaches concerns the motivation of clients to enter into or complete therapy. Sometimes, the person may show a strong desire to continue but face resistance or scepticism from friends or partners. Others find it difficult to complete homework assignments such as diaries. It is difficult to know precisely what deters some people from entering therapy. However, some research suggests that approaches such as cognitive behaviour therapy work better with people who believe in self-control (Simons et al 1984). This may explain why cognitive behavioural approaches are reported less often for some client groups such as people with learning disabilities or victims of abuse.

Clements (1997) puts forward an interesting view concerning the disadvantages of using cognitive behavioural approaches with people with learning disabilities. He claims that therapists have been too narrow in their interpretation of cognitive behavioural approaches, confining their use to people who communicate through language. Implied in Clements's argument is also the criticism that therapy may have the effect of enforcing compliance with a hypothetical view of the 'normal' world rather than encouraging further exploration of how people with cognitive impairments can be helped to understand their world.

Finally, academic argument persists about the focus of psychological research and enquiry. For some people (cf. Lee 1992), psychology remains the study of human behaviour. It follows that observable behaviour should be the key criterion by which any intervention should be judged. Academics such as Lee therefore regard the attention paid to cognitions as an unhelpful distraction. Although there are many others who would disagree with Lee's analysis of the situation, it is important that any systematic study does not rely solely on self-reported change.

Conclusion

It has only been possible here to provide a brief outline of the theory and philosophy underpinning cognitive behavioural interventions. Knowledge about cognitive behavioural approaches is growing and many professional groups, including nurses, are recognising their usefulness. It is hoped that this will bring greater systematic enquiry into their efficacy. As more people begin to apply a cognitive behavioural approach, the challenge for researchers and practitioners is also to expand the boundaries of practice and remain faithful to its theoretical foundations.

Further reading

The following texts provide a good overview of the application of cognitive behavioural approaches and the range of uses to which it can be put.

Persons J 1989 Cognitive therapy in practice: a case formulation approach. W W Norton, New York

Trower P, Casey A, Dryden W 1988 Cognitive behavioural counselling in action. Sage, London

When using any therapeutic approach, the helper should take into account the particular needs of some groups within society. The following books provide a useful discussion of the key issues.

Ponterotto J G, Pederson P B 1993 Preventing prejudice: a guide for counsellors and educators. Sage, Thousand Oaks, California

Scher M, Stevens M, Good C, Eichenfield G A 1993 Handbook of counselling and psychotherapy with men. Sage, Thousand Oaks, California

Worell J, Remer P 1992 Feminist perspectives in therapy: an empowerment model for women. Wiley, Chichester

All therapeutic approaches demand the application of the highest ethical standards. The following texts are helpful in setting out and helping the reader to deal with the key ethical issues in therapy.

Allison A 1996 A framework for good practice: ethical issues in cognitive behaviour therapy. In: Marshall S, Turnbull J (eds) Cognitive behaviour therapy: an introduction to theory and practice. Baillière-Tindall, London

Beauchamp T L, Childress J F 1994 Principles of biomedical ethics, 4th edn. Oxford University Press, Oxford

Husted G L, Husted J H 1991) Ethical decision making in nursing. Mosby, St Louis

References

Adler A 1927 Understanding human nature. Garden City, New York

Bandura A 1977 Social learning theory. Prentice Hall, Englewood Cliffs, New Jersey

Beck A T 1976 Cognitive therapy and emotional disorders. International University Press, New York

Beck C M, Rawlins R D, Williams S R 1988 Mental health psychiatric nursing: a holistic life cycle approach. C V Mosby, London

Bermosk L S, Porter S E 1979 Women's health and human wholeness. Appleton-Century Crofts, New York

Black L 1994 Helping people with a learning difficulty express anger arousal in socially acceptable ways: the development of a treatment intervention and outcome measures. Unpublished PhD thesis, University of St Andrews, St Andrews

Black L, Cullen C, Novaco R W 1997 Anger assessment for people with mild learning disabilities in secure settings. In: Stenfert-Kroese B, Dagnan D, Loumidis K (eds) Cognitive behaviour therapy for people with learning disabilities. Routledge, London

Blackburn I M, Bishop S, Glen A I M, Whalley L J, Christie J E 1981 The efficacy of cognitive therapy in depression: a treatment trial using cognitive therapy and pharmocatherapy each alone and in combination. British Journal of Psychiatry 139: 181-189

Blackman D E 1981 The experimental analysis of behaviour and its relevance to applied psychology. In: Davey G (ed) Applications of conditioning theory. Methuen, London

Castles E E, Glass C R 1986 Training in social and interpersonal problem solving skills for mildly and moderately mentally retarded adults. American Journal of Mental Deficiency 91(1): 35-42

Clements J 1997 Sustaining a cognitive psychology for people with learning disabilities. In: Stenfert-Kroese B, Dagnan D, Loumidis K (eds) Cognitive behaviour for people with learning disabilities. Routledge, London

Du Bois P 1909 The method of persuasion. In: Parker W B (ed) Psychotherapy: a course of reading in sound psychology sound medicine and sound religion, vol 3. Centre Publishing, New York

Ellis A 1962 Reason and emotion in psychotherapy. Lyle Stuart, New York

Ford J 1978 Therapeutic relationship in behaviour therapy: an empirical analysis. Journal of Consulting and Clinical Psychology 46: 1302-1314

Hollin C 1990 Cognitive behavioural interventions with young offenders. Pergamon, London

Hollon S D, Kriss M 1984 Cognitive factors in clinical research and pratice. Clinical Psychology Review 4: 37-76

Hollon S D, Shelton R C, Loosen P T 1991 Cognitive therapy and pharmocatherapy for depression. Journal of Consulting and Clinical Psychology 59: 88-99

Horowitz M J 1986 Stress response syndromes. Aronson, Northvale, New Jersey

Jackson H, Boag P G 1981 The efficacy of self-control procedures as motivational strategies with mentally retarded persons: a review of the literature and guidelines for future research. Australian Journal of Developmental Disabilities 7(2): 65-79

Kelly G 1955 The psychology of personal construct theory. Norton, New York

Kendall P C, Braswell L 1985 Cognitive behavioural therapy for impulsive children. Guilford Press, New York

Lanza M L 1983 The reactions of nursing staff to physical assault by a patient. Journal of Hospital and Community Psychiatry 34 (1): 44-47

Lazarus R S 1984 On the primacy of cognition. American Psychologist 39: 124-129

Lee C 1992 On cognitive theories and causations in human behaviour. Journal of Behaviour Therapy and Experimental Psychiatry 23: 257-268

Luria A R 1961 The role of speech in the regulation of normal and abnormal behaviour. Liveright, New York

Meichenbaum D 1977 Cognitive behaviour modification: an integrative approach. Plenum, New York

Meichenbaum D, Goodman J 1971 Training impulsive children to talk to themselves: a means of developing self-control. Journal of Abnormal Psychology 77: 115-126

Moorey S 1996 When bad things happen to rational people: cognitive therapy in adverse life circumstances. In: Salkovskis P M (ed) Frontiers of cognitive therapy. Guilford Press, London

Neimayer R A 1986 Personal construct therapy. In: Dryden W, Golden W (eds) Cognitive behavioural approaches to psychotherapy. Harper and Row, London

Newell R, Dryden W 1991 Clinical problems: an introduction to the cognitive behavioural approach. In: Dryden W, Rentoul R (eds) Adult clinical problems: a cognitive behavioural approach. Routledge, London

Novaco R W 1975 Anger control: the development and evaluation of an experimental treatment. Heath, Lexington

Novaco R W 1997 Preface. In: Stenfert-Kroese B, Dagnan D, Loumidis K (eds) Cognitive behaviour therapy for people with learning disabilities. Routledge, London

Pretzer J L, Beck A T 1996 A cognitive theory of personality disorders. In: Clarkin J F, Lenzenweger L W (eds) Major theories of personality disorder. Guilford Press, New York

Rogers C 1961 On becoming a person. Constable, London

Rush A J, Beck A T, Kovacs M, Hollon S D 1977 Comparative efficacy of cognitive therapy versus pharmacotherapy in out-patient depression. Cognitive Therapy and Research 1: 17-37

Salter A 1949 Conditioned reflex therapy. Strauss and Young, New York

Schaap C, Bennun I, Schindler L, Hoogduin K 1993 The therapeutic relationship in behaviour therapy. Wiley, Chichester

Simons A Murphy G Levine J and Wetzel R 1984 Sustained improvement one year after cognitive and/or pharmacotherapy for depression. Paper presented at the meeting of the Society for Psychotherapy Research, June 1984, Lake Loise

Stark K D Rouse L W and Livingstone R 1991 Treatment of depression during childhood and adolescence: cognitive behavioural procedures for the individual and family. In: Kendall P C (ed) Child and adolescent therapy: cognitive behavioural procedures. Guilford Press, New York

Stenfert Kroese B, Dagnan D, Loumidis K (eds) 1997 Cognitive behaviour Therapy for people with learning disabilities Routledge, London.

Stevens A 1996 A framework for intervention. In: Marshall S, Turnbull J (eds) Cognitive behaviour therapy: an introduction to theory and practice. Baillière Tindall, London

Tolman E C 1925 Purpose and cognition: the determinants of animal learning. Psychological Review 32: 285-297

Tolman E C 1932 Purpose behaviour in animals and men. Appleton, New York.

Turnbull J 1993 Victim support. Nursing Times 89 (23): 33-34

Vitousek K B 1996 The current status of cognitive behavioural models of anorexia nervosa and bulimia nervosa. In: Salkovskis P M (ed) Frontiers of cognitive therapy. Guildford Press, London

Vygostky L S 1962 Thought and language. John Wiley, New York

Wessler R L 1983 A critical appraisal of therapeutic outcome studies. British Journal of Cognitive Psychotherapy 1(1): 39-46

Wessler R L 1986 Conceptualising cognitions in the cognitive behavioural therapies. In: Dryden W, Golden W (eds) Cognitive behavioural approaches to psychotherapy. Harper and Row, London

Zajonc R B 1984 On the primacy of affect. American Psychologist 39: 117-123

Resources

Several psychological and nursing journals publish papers on the application of cognitive behavioural approaches. However, two specialist journals are available:

The *Journal of Cognitive Therapy and Research* is published four times a year by:
Plenum Publishing Corporation
233 Spring Street
New York 10013
USA

The *Journal of Behavioural and Cognitive Psychotherapy* is also published four times a year by:
Cambridge University Press
Edinburgh Building
Shaftesbury Road
Cambridge CB2 2RN

Many organisations run conferences and educational events on cognitive behavioural approaches. Further details are available from:

British Association for Behavioural and Cognitive Psychotherapies
P O Box 9
Abingdon
Oxfordshire
http://www.babcp.org.uk

The British Psychological Society
St Andrews House
48 Princess Road East
Leicester LE1 7DR

For nurses, the English National Board (ENB) has approved a number of universities to run a course, number A12, entitled Cognitive Behaviour Therapy for Nurses. Details of the specific universities are available from:

English National Board
Victory House
170 Tottenham Court Road
London W1P OHA
Tel: 0207 388 3131

3 Examining Evidence

11 The problematic nature of evidence   **283**
Jane Wray and Bob Gates

The third section consists of a single chapter, which explores and discusses the problematic nature of evidence. The chapter outlines the relationship between evidence and effectiveness of therapies, and reflects on the potencies and limitations of each of the interventions outlined in Section 2. The final part of the chapter considers how each of these seven therapeutic interventions might be applied within different settings.

11 The problematic nature of evidence

Bob Gates and Jane Wray

Key issues
- Decisions made regarding the effectiveness of an intervention are generally based upon the evidence available to support its claims
- Practitioners in health care are particularly concerned with the promotion and development of evidence-based health care
- The nature of evidence is problematic, and as rationing of resources becomes more commonplace, the issues surrounding the reliability and validity of evidence continue to be debated
- The comparative effectiveness of different approaches needs to be understood in terms of both available evidence and organisational and setting implications

Overview
Any therapeutic intervention designed to support, care for, or treat a person displaying distressing and/or distressed behaviour raises questions such as 'Does this approach work?' and if so, 'How effective is it?' This chapter considers such questions by briefly exploring the problematic nature of evidence. The relationship of evidence to effectiveness and other terms such as evidence-based health care are also discussed. The chapter looks at the strengths and potencies of each of the interventions described earlier in the book and explores potential limitations and boundaries. The final part of this chapter briefly considers the application of the seven approaches to people experiencing different kinds of behavioural distress in different settings.

Introduction
When working with or caring for people who experience behavioural distress, practitioners and carers employ a range of different interventions, seven of which have been outlined in this book. When faced with a person displaying distressed behaviour our wish, usually, is to be as effective as possible in helping and supporting the person and others on whom this distress impacts. A decision is made at this stage about the approach or approaches to be used based on what we know about their 'effectiveness'. The notion of effectiveness is inexorably linked to the nature of evidence, and looking for evidence of effectiveness for a particular intervention requires searching for data to provide some kind of 'proof' that a particular approach or intervention works. This leads us to questions regarding what sort of data might be said to constitute evidence, and from where such evidence might be obtained.

It is likely that people in behavioural distress will come into contact with a large number of specialist services: health, social care, psychology, psychiatry, education and many others. It is the case, particularly within the arena of health, that the practice of many professionals within such services is increasingly governed by a requirement to practice evidence-based health care (Bishop 1996). This is creating a climate where any therapeutic intervention designed to treat or care for someone experiencing behavioural distress requires the support of empirical evidence. This drive to ensure that all treatment and care decisions are evidence-based has many advocates as well as a number of critics (Deigham & Boyd 1996), but it is likely that evidence will continue to play an increasing role in decision making as resources become increasingly scarce and possibly rationed (Sackett et al 1996). The rationing of resources, particularly in the health care arena, has profound implications for those people in behavioural distress. In order to understand the importance of evidence-based decisions, it is important to understand some of the issues that surround the reliability and validity of evidence.

Scientific evidence

This section briefly introduces the reader to what is meant by 'scientific evidence', and how evidence or 'proof' is accumulated. At its simplest, scientists construct knowledge through the processes of induction and deduction. Scientists collect data, generate ideas and theories about those data, experiment to test the validity of theories and generate conclusions. A popular view of science is that scientific knowledge is objectively proven knowledge, and that scientific theories are derived in rigorous ways from the analysis of observation and experiment. Science is based upon observation and experience, and scientists use data gleaned from observation and experience to move from single statements about the world to universal statements and theories that make up scientific knowledge. A theory is essentially an explanation of why certain phenomena happen. Once a universal statement has been generated, a scientist can systematically test that statement under various conditions to see how valid and reliable the statement is. In this way theories about the nature of relationships between the variables of given phenomena are slowly generated and developed.

For most of the 20th century the scientific community has been engaged in investigating and identifying scientific 'truths' that are often superseded by new truths as they are discovered. Scientists researching human behaviour do not search for 'proof' of a particular approach – they look at a behaviour, generalise, develop theories about the phenomena observed and then test the theories. The results of such testing (experiments) leads us to either accept or reject a particular account of the facts.

Although practitioners, academics and researchers alike talk knowledgeably of a particular approach having an established empirical base, the subjective influences inherent in the processes of scientific enquiry raise questions about the value of any intervention. In relation to behavioural distress, this subjectivity can best be illustrated by science's dependence upon the process of observation. Although observation can yield a wealth and depth of data on the behaviour of an individual, it is subject to observational bias (Grey 1998). That is, the emotions, prejudices and values of the person conducting the observing can influence the way in which behaviour and events are observed. Mudford et al (1997) have suggested that, as behavioural states such as 'distress' are not physical phenomena, but are inferred from direct observation of a person's behaviour, they are not directly measurable by observation methods.

Science is neither without bias, nor without a considerable history of accepting theories that have been used to explain some aspects of human behaviour which at some later point have had to be rejected as false. The reasons for this are manifold and range from the emergence of new evidence to different interpretations being placed on existing evidence. Sometimes methodological flaws are discovered in the ways in which that particular evidence has been obtained. An example of this is the work undertaken in the USA by Robert Yerkes (Yoakum & Yerkes 1920) (see Box 11.1).

Box 11.1
The work of Yerkes (Yoakum & Yerkes 1920) and the fallibility of evidence

At the beginning of the 20th century, psychologists were preoccupied with the measurement of intelligence. However, there were at least two problems in undertaking this activity with any reliability or validity. The first was the idiosyncratic ways in which tests were administered, and the second was the fact that different tests yielded different results. Evidently what was needed was a standardised test that could yield a sufficiently large and uniform data source. A psychologist, Robert Yerkes, and his colleagues responded to this by developing two 'mental tests' which they administered to 1.75 million army recruits in the USA. One of the tests (written) sought to measure recruits who were literate, the second (pictorial) tested recruits who were illiterate.

The results of this work were to have a profound impact upon American society. Findings were interpreted by scientists, academics and the general public alike as providing a way of predicting the ability (intelligence) of individuals. For example, recruits who had a low score were unable to apply for officer training. Also, immigration laws were developed to favour certain cultural groups because they were believed to be intellectually superior.

Later, numerous methodological issues were eventually identified that included systematic bias, cultural bias and poor test conditions. However, the consequences of accepting this 'evidence' had already affected people's lives.

The point of recalling this work by Yerkes is to demonstrate the fallibility of scientific evidence, and to show that even when data have been generated in large quantities there may still be fundamental flaws which prevent us from treating that data as 'absolute' evidence. (Readers who wish to explore this further are advised to read *Mismeasures of Man* by J. Gould (1981).)

Scientific understanding of human behaviour and experience is continuously evolving and developing. Consequently, it is likely that our current scientific 'truths' may prove to be incompatible with the evidence obtained from further investigation and experimentation in the future.

Evidence based health care

Interest in 'evidence of effectiveness' can be seen across a number of different disciplines. However, in one particular area, evidence-based health care, interest in the nature of evidence or proof has increased considerably.

People who experience behavioural distress are more likely to come into contact with professional services of some kind (usually health services), particularly if their distress impacts upon others.

The need for evidence of effectiveness in health care has been driven by an increase in the demand for health care resources, and this increase is growing faster than the rate of resource made available. Muir Gray (1997) has identified four main reasons for this: an ageing population, new technology and knowledge, increased patient or client expectations, and professional expectations. As pressure on resources has increased, those who make decisions regarding health care have to do so explicitly and publicly, and they are required to produce and describe the evidence that underpins their decision making.

Evidence-based health care concerns itself with the incorporation of evidence from research, clinical expertise and client preferences into decisions about the health care of individual people. Carefully conducted research should tell us what works and does not work, with whom, and where. Research-based evidence in health care can make a difference to client outcomes: Heater et al (1988) have reported that patients who receive research-based nursing care make sizeable gains in knowledge and in physiological and pyschosocial outcomes compared with those receiving routine nursing care.

Evidence-based health care developed out of the medically led initiative of evidence-based medicine (EBM). EBM was regarded by some as the new paradigm in medical practice (Delisa et al 1999), and by others, including Morgan (1997):

‹the contemporary mantra of many academic physicians ›

Evidence-based medicine, according to Sackett et al (1996), is the integration of individual clinical expertise with the best available external evidence from systematic research. Although there are a considerable number of articles describing what constitutes evidence-based medicine (Rosenberg & Donald 1995, Sackett & Rosenberg 1995, Sackett et al 1996), there appears to be little consensus regarding the definition of evidence based health care (Deigham & Boyd 1996). The term has been broadened to include ‘health care’, and thus acknowledges the contribution made by all members of the health care team.

The kinds of evidence legitimised within evidenced-based health care are: descriptive (cross sectional, longitudinal), analytic (case control study, cohort study) and experimental (randomised controlled trials). Discriminating between knowledge based on opinion and practice, as opposed to scientific evidence, is an important step in understanding evidence-based health care (Kitson 1997). However, the significance and merit of both opinion and practice should not be belittled in terms of understanding the impact of a therapeutic intervention. Tsafrir & Grinberg (1998) undertook a survey and analysed information sources considered most relevant to patient care by a cross section of physicians with varying degrees of experience. They found that physicians considered review articles and meta-analysis extremely reliable for information purposes, but for practical patient care purposes tended to rely upon the opinions of peers and experts.

Evidence-based care, whether it is in the arena of health or not, involves enabling organisations and individuals to assess, appraise and apply information to everyday settings (Anderton 1999). It should be seen as a means of enhancing the role of information in decision making and not as an end in itself (Long & Harrison 1995).

What constitutes evidence and how is it obtained?

The Collins English Dictionary (1995, p. 388) has defined evidence as:

❝ground for belief or disbelief; data on which to base proof or to establish truth or falsehood.❞

Knowledge or evidence on which to base practice originates from a number of different disciplines, and this evidence is generated through the adoption of different research styles and methods. Research methods can potentially provide us with a vast array of evidence sources, and typically reflect questions common to a particular practice setting and seek to give answers in a particular form. Ascertaining the effectiveness of any type of intervention in a practice setting is of prime importance prior to its use with a person in behavioural distress. However, increasingly, the question 'Is this approach effective?' requires a response that takes into account many different factors and opinions. For example, evidence-based health care incorporates not only conclusions about effectiveness, but refers also to aspects of equity, appropriateness and accessibility (Critical Appraisal Skills Programme 1997), all of which are important factors in determining the most appropriate intervention in the care of people whose behaviour distresses themselves or others.

The reliability and validity of evidence

What type of information is considered valid as evidence is open to debate, and is highly dependent on chosen criteria. Morgan (1997, p. 117) has suggested that:

❝the evidence they consider, although superficially convincing, is often slanted, occasionally deliberately, but more often as a result of carelessness and defects in study design.❞

To this end, a combination of research styles and methods may be necessary to generate sufficient and appropriate data about the efficacy of a particular type of therapeutic intervention.

Historically, there has been a continuing dialogue concerning the relative strengths or weaknesses of either qualitative or quantitative research. Parahoo (1997), for example, has delineated the relative strengths and weaknesses of both approaches (see Table 11.1).

Table 11.1

Comparing characteristics of quantitative and qualitative approaches (with kind permission from Parahoo 1997)

Quantitative	Qualitative
Reductionist and/or deterministic	Holistic
Methods are predetermined, structured, standardised and inflexible	Methods are semi-structured and unstructured and flexible
Purpose is to measure	Purpose is to describe and/or theorise

Qualitative and quantitative research approaches have different uses and purposes, and each answers different kinds of questions concerning the effectiveness of a particular therapeutic intervention. Table 11.2 provides a summary of three major research styles and considers a wide range of criteria helpful to choosing methods most likely to yield data useful to answering different kinds of questions.

Table 11.2

A comparison of three research styles (after Sapsford & Evans 1979, with kind permission from the Open University)

	Experiments	Surveys	Ethnography
Emphasis on reliability	A great deal	Generally a great deal	Generally little, observations are acknowledged to differ across observers/settings and to be situation specific
Commitment to generalisation	Generally great	Generally great	Generally less
Emphasis on control of extraneous factors	Generally great	If purely descriptive, none, otherwise generally great	Depends on the stage of the research and progressive focusing
Emphasis on setting	Generally little	Generally little	A great deal
Emphasis on description of 'explanatory variables'	Generally little	Often questionnaire presented in reports but little attention to unwritten and non verbal elements of interaction	Generally a great deal
Data yield	Numerical, easily analysed	Often numerical and easily analysed	Qualitative, often difficult to analyse
Particular strengths leading to generalisability	High internal validity, high construct validity, high reliability	High construct validity, high reliability, high population validity	High ecological validity, high inclusiveness
Potential weaknesses detracting from generalisability	Low ecological validity, usually low population validity, low inclusiveness (content validity)	Low ecological validity, often low inclusiveness (content validity)	Low internal validity, low reliability, low population validity

Table 11.2 continued overleaf

Table 11.2 *cont'd*

A comparison of three research styles (after Sapsford & Evans 1979, with kind permission from the Open University)

	Experiments	Surveys	Ethnography
Types of research for which most appropriate	1. Testing causal hypothesis 2. Establishing statistical association between variables	1. Large scale 2. Establishing statistical association between variables 3. Cross validating, on large representative samples, results obtained from other methods	1. Initial small scale exploratory work to discover areas worth investigating by other methods 2. Cross validating, in a natural setting, results obtained by other methods 3. Investigation of relatively unknown social phenomena in detail and in their natural setting to develop theories which might be further validated by other methods

From Table 11.2 it can be seen that experiments might best be described as scientific investigations in which observations are made and data collected under controlled conditions using randomisation and manipulation of variables, and usually in laboratory conditions. On the other hand, surveys seek to generate responses from a large sample of respondents to fixed questions under comparable conditions. The term ethnography, literally translated, means a story or description of a people or race. Ethnography represents a qualitative research approach to produce cultural theory, it is naturalistic and therefore does not use control, randomisation or manipulation of variables. (To further explore the relative benefits of qualitative and quantitative research methods, see the further reading list at the end of the chapter.)

Within the scientific community, evidence gathered by certain methods are often perceived to be more reliable. For example, the 'well designed randomised controlled trial (RCT)' is seen by many as the gold standard in terms of gathering evidence (Parahoo 1997). Frequently, there are disputes between the proponents of experimental research and the proponents of qualitative research as to which approach is the more valid.

Black (1994) has indicated that qualitative research should be seen as complementary to research trials, and the difference between the two approaches should not be presented as a false dichotomy. Hicks & Hennessey (1997) have suggested that a more eclectic approach to evidence based care is needed, with attention being diverted to qualitative methodologies, particularly at funding and dissemination level. This approach will thus provide a comprehensive and balanced overview of relevant information which has the potential to influence some of the less quantifiable aspects of care delivery. However, despite such arguments for the use of a wider range of methodological approaches, the current emphasis on evidence-based health care has contributed to a continued focus on the use of experimentation and RCTs.

Muir Gray (1997) also outlined the relative strengths of different types of evidence obtained through different types of research method, and these are shown in Table 11.3.

Table 11.3

The strengths of evidence (Muir Gray 1997, with kind permission from Churchill Livingstone)

Type	Strength of evidence
I	Strong evidence from at least one systematic review of multiple, well designed, randomised controlled trials
II	Strong evidence from at least one properly designed randomised controlled trial of appropriate size
III	Evidence from well designed trials without randomisation, single group pre-post, cohort, time series or matched case controlled studies
IV	Evidence from well designed non experimental studies from more than one centre of research group
V	Opinions of respected authorities, based on clinical evidence, descriptive studies or reports of expert committees

This hierarchical approach to the understanding of evidence mirrors that produced by others, such as the Critical Skills Appraisal Programme (CASP) (1997) (see Box 11.2).

Box 11.2

CASP hierarchy of evidence (after Critical Skills Appraisal Programme 1997)

I-1	A well done systematic review of two or more RCTs
I-2	An RCT
II-1	A cohort study
II-2	A case control study
II-3	A dramatic uncontrolled experiment
III	Respected authorities, expert committee
IV	Someone once told me

From these two examples it can be seen that there is a perception that those approaches that are located at the top of such hierarchies are thought to generate evidence that is more reliable and rigorous than other approaches. The more reliable and rigorous the approach to gathering evidence, the more likely that the resultant evidence generated can legitimately determine whether an approach is effective. It would appear therefore that systematic reviews of randomised controlled trials are considered to offer the greatest value. However, although systematic reviews are a powerful and useful way to assemble evidence, just because a review has been undertaken does not guarantee that its results are reliable or valid (Hunt & McKibbon 1997). Increasingly, there is dissatisfaction with this hierarchical approach to evidence and instead the use of multiple methods is generally recommended (Toogood & Timlin 1996).

There are many factors that are significant in deciding the appropriate approaches to obtaining evidence, and these include:

- The type of information to be gathered
- From whom and by whom?
- In what circumstances?
- For what reasons?

Some ways of gathering evidence appear to be more suitable than others in examining human experience and behaviour. In addition to clinically controlled trials and field experiments, qualitative approaches such as case studies, anecdotal evidence, video evidence and carer perspectives (Gates 1996) also make valuable contributions to understanding the client's experience of behavioural distress.

Data that constitutes evidence of effectiveness of therapeutic approaches to helping people in behavioural distress are gathered from many different disciplines and sources. Sources can vary from authoritative journal articles to others such as the Office for National Statistics, and other organisations commissioned by central and local government. In addition, we not only have access to information generated by health authorities such as reports and surveys, but also lobbying organisations, consumer groups, charities, voluntary organisations and service users. The bodies collecting this information may be biased – though how and to what extent it may be difficult to determine – and this bias may influence methods. During analysis, data may also be interpreted in any number of different ways by the various agencies, government departments, pressure groups, scientists, lay people, health care professionals and the media who have access to the research findings. In turn, each of these groups is likely to have an agenda of its own (Katz & Peberby 1997) which may well determine how it chooses to translate its interpretations to others.

Scientists, researchers and others working in the field of behavioural distress might argue against the assumption that their approach is in some way biased by their own professional and personal perspectives. Nevertheless, bias can be present at every stage of an experiment from the admission of subjects to the interpretation and reporting of data (Parahoo 1997). When looking at the relative efficacy of different approaches to gathering evidence, published literature is highly influential. However, Muir Gray (1997) has also identified several types of bias related to the process of publication, including:

- Submission bias – research workers are more strongly motivated to complete and submit for publication positive results
- Publication bias – editors are more likely to publish positive results (Easterbrook et al 1991)
- Methodological bias – methodological errors such as flawed randomisation produce positive biases
- Abstracting bias – abstracts emphasise positive results.

Selection and reviewer bias also occur as decisions to include certain studies are affected by factors such as their results (Centre for Reviews and Dissemination 1996).

In addition, many researchers fail to write up and submit their findings for publication, and pharmaceutical and other private companies are often nervous of publishing or revealing any research results that do not show their products in an advantageous light (Muir Gray 1997). When searching for research evidence in the literature, the first step is generally to consult an electronic database such as MEDLINE, EMBASE, CINAHL and the Cochrane

Library (Cochrane Database of Systematic Reviews (CDSR)). Such databases are known to be limited (Muir Gray 1997): they cover primarily English language journals, they do not cover all available journals world-wide, and, because of inadequacies of indexing systems, relevant papers are not always identified. For example, in a study conducted by McDonald et al (1996), hand searching of the *British Medical Journal* and *The Lancet* added greatly to the number of trails available on MEDLINE – 1100 trials were found before the hand search, and 5200 after. This is a significant difference and shows the scale of material that might be excluded unintentionally.

There is considerable support for evidence-based decision making in health care settings, but many clinicians working in this field lack training and competence in its use (Delisa et al 1999, Moore 1995). In addition, issues such as lack of access to appropriate journals and searching facilities and lack of critical appraisal skills contribute significantly to the theory–practice divide and the slow implementation of research findings into practice (Hicks & Hennessey 1997).

Comparing and contrasting the evidence and research base of interventions

There are many factors involved in making decisions regarding the effectiveness of interventions used in the management of behavioural distress:

"Treatment selection is based upon information obtained during the assessment of behaviour, the risks it poses and its controlling variables; on a careful consideration of the available treatment options including their relative effectiveness, risks, destructiveness and potential side-effects and on examination of the overall context in which treatment is applied."

[Houton et al 1988, p. 382]

As Houton emphasises, the potential limitations of approaches are also important factors to consider. Limitations include the difficulties experienced in the practical application of the intervention in a range of settings, and organisational implications such as resources, time, staff and financial concerns. Establishing 'evidence of effectiveness' for an intervention requires consideration of many complex factors, and this includes the views and wishes of people who are (or who have been) in behavioural distress.

Is evidence of the effectiveness of an intervention merely a reduction in the level of distress experienced by a client or those around him or her? It is suggested that this cannot be so. This is because it is necessary to use holistic and more eclectic criteria for calculating effectiveness. An example of why this is so can be found in the use of 'aversive' behavioural procedures in the care and treatment of behavioural difficulties exhibited by people with learning disabilities. In the past, behavioural approaches used aversive procedures that included contingent electric shock treatment and the use of ammonia and other sprays (Lovaas & Simmons 1969), all of which measures reduced behavioural difficulties exhibited in this group of people. These approaches were 'effective', but only in the very narrowest sense, and the issue became not one of effectiveness as such, but of ethical concerns regarding the use of such procedures. There has been a shift in behaviourism since this time, behaviour modification as a technique per se has diminished, and behaviour analysis has gained prominence. However, ethical concerns continue to have a profound impact on its acceptability. Whoever sets the criteria for 'effectiveness' implicitly also determines ethical criteria.

In Chapter 1 the reader was introduced to a continuum that fell broadly between positivism and anti-positivism, and represented different ways in which we attempt to understand the world. Referring back to Chapter 1 (Fig. 1.1), it can be seen that at one end of this continuum are interventions reflecting views of behaviour described and explained in objective and quantifiable terms, whilst at the other end of the continuum lie explanations more reliant on subjectivity.

It is not difficult to see how hierarchies of evidence emerge when the scientific community uses methods predominately rooted in objectivity such as those identified by Muir Gray (1997) and the Critical Appraisal Skills Programme (1997).

The next part of this chapter briefly reviews the evidence that has been identified in support of the seven intervention described in this book. This evidence is broadly grouped to represent its relative place on the continuum between objectivity and subjectivity.

In Chapter 6, Ibrahim Turkistani explored chemotherapeutic interventions and provided evidence of their effectiveness obtained through experimental studies. For example, Kaplan & Sadock (1995) have reported that the use of medication in the treatment of obsessive compulsive disorder was as effective as response prevention. Klein et al (1980) found that imipramine when compared with a placebo for the treatment of panic disorder was significantly superior. It would be wrong to assume that medicine bases its practice entirely upon scientific evidence, as the contrary is known to be the case (Tsafrir & Grinberg 1998). However, these two examples illustrate the medical focus upon quantitative and outcome based research, and demonstrate one of the fundamental differences between chemotherapy as an intervention when compared with other interventions, in terms of research methods that demonstrate effectiveness.

There is little doubt as to the effectiveness of behavioural interventions in the management of behavioural distress; 'hard' research evidence is abundant and has been comprehensively detailed in Chapter 9. However, the legitimacy, applicability and prospective effectiveness of this approach is questionable in circumstances where the underlying cause of the behavioural distress is due to some kind of internal physiological dysfunction such as mental illness, organic disease or epilepsy. Consequently, the need for a comprehensive assessment of a client's behavioural distress is important in identifying contributing factors and the likely effects of interventions. However, there is evidence to suggest that such assessment, in the form of functional analysis, is rarely undertaken, and when it is, it is carried out inadequately (Murphy 1993). As Mike McCue has pointed out in Chapter 9 (p. 245):

> *The process of assessing and identifying relevant causal factors is often extremely difficult and complex.*

If relevant factors are not identified, or are identified incorrectly, it is likely that behavioural interventions will not be helpful.

In Chapter 8, preliminary evaluation of the effectiveness of TEACCH has indicated that this approach can result in a reduction in the severity and incidence of 'inappropriate' behaviour amongst clients, and simultaneously enhance opportunities for skill development (Sines 1996). It could be tentatively argued overall that service costs might be reduced, as a consequence of the intervention reducing the need for long-term residential care. However, there are high maintenance costs associated with TEACCH, as it is a labour-intensive approach to providing support. It requires highly skilled professional staff and considerable investment of parents' time and money. The extent to which the initial investment actually results in 'value for money' in terms of outcome has yet to be fully researched. Also, TEACCH is an approach developed and used almost exclusively, so far, with people diagnosed as having autistic spectrum disorder, and its lack of applicability to other clients groups is well recognised.

In Chapter 10, John Turnbull has pointed to the considerable evidence that exists to demonstrate the usefulness of cognitive behavioural approaches for a range of human problems (Newell & Dryden 1991). He pointed out a number of controlled studies that have shown cognitive behavioural approaches performing at least as well as other approaches, and often leading to more lasting change (Hollon et al 1991, Stark et al 1991). There is also evidence that cognitive behavioural therapy is a superior treatment for common problems such as depression and anxiety when compared, for example, with chemotherapy (Hollon et al 1991). However, a key limitation, acknowledged by those who use cognitive behavioural therapy, concerns the motivation of clients to enter into and complete therapy. Also, some cognitive behavioural approaches rely exclusively upon the use of verbal and written communication, consequently some client groups such as people with profound learning disabilities who also have complex needs may be excluded and therefore unable to benefit from this approach.

Having briefly reviewed evidence from those interventions most amenable to gathering 'objective' evidence, the remainder of this section briefly reviews evidence for the effectiveness of gentle teaching, Nonviolent Communication (NVC) and the arts therapies. The lack of 'hard' scientific research evidence to date to support claims of effectiveness of approaches such as Gentle Teaching and NVC raises questions, despite their obvious therapeutic potential. Both of these approaches emphasise the significance of relationships and 'connection', and therefore valid measurement is reliant on reports of subjective experiences by participants. When scientific strength lies generally in detachment and impartiality, how would one measure, for example, all of the complex components of a successful marriage or a thriving friendship?

In Gentle Teaching, to establish a relationship between intervention and outcome one might look for indicators such as shared responsibility, taking turns and being supportive. Practitioners of Gentle Teaching have determined outcome measures for shared responsibility and support in terms of eye contact, smiling, accepting, reciprocating and initiating appropriate touch. All of these outcomes may be interpreted as evidence of a shift toward functional participation in a relationship. However, while outcomes such as the radiance of a smile, the strength of a handshake, the peacefulness of a companionable silence can definitely be a shared perception and experience, the interpretation placed on that experience will vary between individuals. Even when two-way mirrors or video recording is used there could still be different interpretations of the relationship. A therapist who knows that he or she is being monitored is also less likely to be focused on the client and this may impact on how they connect with the person or people receiving therapy. This control can be construed as artificial, and distort the relationship between the person with the behavioural distress and those who seek to understand and help.

The outcomes of Gentle Teaching have been outlined in Chapter 7 by Siobhan O'Rourke and Jane Wray. Some research conducted to date questions the claim made by McGee (McGee et al 1987) of the universal successfulness of gentle teaching. McCaughey & Jones (1992) have concluded that any future findings are likely to confirm the findings of Jones et al (1990) that it is effective for some individuals and ineffective for others. The same conclusion could be made regarding many therapeutic interventions, including applied behaviour analysis (Didden et al 1997). Gentle Teaching uses some teaching strategies that are used in behavioural approaches, and these have been proved to be effective (Emerson 1996), therefore it might be argued that Gentle Teaching techniques must also in some sense be effective. Although some of the teaching strategies in Gentle Teaching are shared with the behavioural approach, gentle teaching practitioners have argued that it is not necessarily fruitful to use the same tools for evaluation. Emerging from a psychology of interdependence, Gentle Teaching's effectiveness might best be evaluated using qualitative approaches rather than quantitative ones.

Some qualitative research into the effectiveness of the arts therapies already exists, and has been described by Marian Liebmann in Chapter 5. However, the majority of this research has focused upon process rather than product or outcome. One advantage of art therapy is that it can have very visible and aural outcomes, such as paintings, sculptures, and drama sessions. Case studies are often used to demonstrate evidence of effectiveness, as the experience of a client is a personal and subjective one. An indicator of effectiveness suggested by the author of Chapter 5 is its increasing popularity. Popularity, however, is not a reliable indicator of effectiveness. It is likely to be an indication of arts therapies having captured the imagination of practitioners and a belief in the therapeutic benefits of this approach, which in themselves may make it worthy of further investigation.

In the case of Nonviolent Communication (NVC), major aspects of its utility lie in the simplicity of the concept, and its universal applicability as a fundamental language. Another factor is the potentially profound and deep impact of this approach, and that it can be transformational. NVC can be used at different levels of intervention and in many different ways, and is described as 'useful even with limited skills and practice' (Ch. 4, p. 102). This is a distinct advantage when compared to other approaches that depend upon extensive training. The use of the model has been demonstrated to be effective in very diverse situations (see pp. 91–101) and can support and relieve the experience of behavioural distress in a range of settings. It can also be used in conjunction with, and support, counselling and other therapeutic interventions. However, in common with the learning of any new language, NVC requires regular opportunities for practice and experienced support to achieve fluency.

Technological developments such as video recording have had a profound impact on how we understand the effectiveness of subjective and creative approaches to therapy in that it is possible to accurately record behaviour. For example, client therapist interactions, including responses such as smiling and other indicators of positive engagement can be recorded for subsequent analysis.

Implications for organisations and settings

Evidently there are practical and organisational implications that must be considered before introducing any therapeutic intervention designed to support and care for a person experiencing behavioural distress. On a practical level, organisations need to consider the financial ramifications of training and resource, in addition to the commitment and abilities of individual staff members. Undertaking comprehensive, reliable and valid assessment of distressed and distressing behaviour requires time, experience and expertise. Firstly, there is a dependence upon the reliability of the information gathered and the individual staff member's ability to record it correctly (Toogood & Timlin 1996). Secondly, the ability of the organisation to successfully undertake detailed assessment and evaluation, as in the case of behaviourism, may be limited by time and resource implications.

For practitioners, there is often a significant tension between those methods of assessment that produce the most accurate information and those that are practicable in 'ordinary' settings. Homer (1994) has suggested that while one approach may be excellent under certain conditions, it might be equally disappointing under others. For example, in the case of Gentle Teaching, it is acknowledged that although the approach can be implemented without organisational support, this is likely to be difficult. Gentle Teaching is more likely to be successful when the organisation supports both the philosophy and practice.

The art therapies have a number of organisational and setting implications and these relate primarily to the resources needed to undertake this approach. These include art materials, musical instruments or other specialist equipment and the availability of an appropriately sized (or even soundproofed) room. Such considerations are equally applicable to other approaches such as TEACCH which requires a particularly structured and well-resourced environment and is extremely people intensive.

The cognitive behavioural approach offers the advantage of providing one-to-one support to the person experiencing distress. In addition to the therapist, very little is needed in terms of practical resources other than a quiet, private room in which therapy can take place. However, there are often lengthy waiting lists to see cognitive behavioural therapists, and this is likely to cause difficulties if a person is experiencing acute behavioural distress and requires immediate support.

In relation to chemotherapeutic approaches, the principle consideration in treatment is which medication is the most effective. However, the issue of cost-effectiveness also plays a part. Evidently, there are resource implications in terms of the need to properly assess, monitor and evaluate the effect of any medication upon an individual. Nevertheless, medication can provide a relatively quick and cost-effective way of managing behavioural distress. As Ibrahim Turkistani has pointed out (p. 132), this is perhaps a reason why this approach is widely used, although sometimes inappropriately, resulting in adverse side-effects. The prescription of medication to manage the behavioural distress of people with learning disabilities has been called into question (Schaal & Hackenbury 1994), particularly as pharmacological control of behaviour often reflects the poor availability of other support services (Hogg 1992).

Clearly, each approach is subject to many different organisational factors, some of which have been outlined in this chapter. For more detailed explanation of organisational and settings factors readers are referred back to the relevant chapters. Look also at the activity below.

Choosing an approach

This activity can be undertaken within a small discussion group, or individually. Consider someone you know who was in distress and required the support of specialist services. What type of approach was chosen to help them and why? Reflect upon the following factors:

- The nature of the difficulty
- The situation or settings in which it occurred
- The individual's experience of distress
- The skills needed by the individual to 'cope'
- The carer/supportive environment
- Access to training and support
- The availability of expertise in a particular approach
- Research evidence
- Preferences of the individual experiencing the distress
- Preferences of the practitioner or carer.

Which of these factors do you believe were important in making the decision regarding the approach used? If possible, rank these factors in order of 1 to 10 in terms of their priority in making your decision (1 = most important, 10 = least important).

Conclusion

At the outset readers were informed that the intentions of this book were to explore how we view behaviour, to present seven different kinds of therapeutic intervention used by professionals, and then, finally, briefly to examine, as problematic, the nature of evidence that is available to support the use of each of the interventions.

This chapter commenced with two questions: 'Does this approach work?' and if so, 'How effective is it?' For a synopsis of the specific evidence available for each of the approaches, readers are referred, once again, back to the chapters in question. Each of the therapeutic interventions outlined is currently used in practice settings and is supporting people who are in behavioural distress. However, given that there are many different possible kinds of evidence, the issue of whether these approaches provide sufficient evidence of their effectiveness remains open to debate.

The issue of evidence-based practice must also be considered along with other contemporary issues such as 'empowerment' and 'service user involvement'. The use of evidence is not only an issue for professionals; carers, families and service users also have to make informed decisions about their own needs. It follows that some of the 'best' evidence may not come from professionals, scientists or academics, but from the people who actually experience, or have experienced, behavioural distress. For the concept of 'effectiveness' to hold meaning, the individual and that individual's experience must be at the centre of decisions made regarding the selection of any intervention.

Further reading

Bradford Hill A 1984 A short textbook of medical statistics, 11th edn. Hodder and Stoughton, London
This excellent textbook provides a most straightforward account of the statistical method of research applied to medicine. The contents include sampling, correlation, clinical trials, evidence and inference. Although some highly technical terms are used, the text is supported with some definitions of these terms.

Muir Gray J A 1997 Evidence-based health care: how to make health policy and management decisions. Churchill Livingstone, Edinburgh
This book explains how evidence can be applied to health policy and management decisions for populations rather than for individual patients. The book concentrates on the facts, figures, skills and knowledge that are needed when making evidence based health care decisions.

Parahoo K 1997 Nursing research: principles, process and issues. Macmillan, London
This excellent textbook is essential reading for pre-registration students and qualified practitioners of nursing who have little or no prior knowledge of research. The text provides a clear and comprehensive outline of the concepts and principles of nursing research.

Mark R 1996 Research made simple: a handbook for social workers. Sage, London
This very useful book provides a non-technical guide to understanding research. The contents include research and the scientific methods, ethics, sampling, measurement, analysis and hypothesis testing.

Breakwell G M, Hammond S, Fife Schaw C 1998 Research methods in psychology. Sage, London
This is a comprehensive textbook in four parts. The first provides a useful overview of issues relevant to research in the field of psychology. The second part explores measurement and issues of research design and the third methodological issues. The final part provides a useful summary concerning bivariate, mulivariate and meta analysis.

References

Anderton P 1999 Evidence based practice: what is evidence based practice and what are the skills practitioners will need? Link Up: The Newsletter for Nurses working in Learning Disabilities. Royal College of Nursing RCN Learning Disabilities Nursing Forum, Summer 1999, RCN, London

Bishop V 1996 Editorial. Focus: evidence based health care. Nursing Times Research 1(5): 328–329

Black N 1994 Experimental and observational methods of evaluation. British Medical Journal 309: 540

Centre for Reviews and Dissemination 1996 Undertaking systematic reviews of research on effectiveness. Centre for Reviews and Dissemination (CRD), York

Collins English Dictionary and Thesaurus 1995 HarperCollins, Glasgow

Critical Appraisal Skills Programme 1997 Critical Skills Programme, Institute of Health Studies, Oxford

Deigham M, Boyd K 1996 Focus: defining evidence based health care in a health care learning strategy. Nursing Times Research 1(5): 332–339

Delisa J A, Jain S S, Kirschblum S, Christodoulou C 1999 Evidence based medicine in psychiatry: the experience of one department's faculty and trainees. American Journal of Physical Medicine and Rehabilitation 78(3): 228–232

Didden, Duker P C, Korzilius H 1997 Meta analytic study on treatment effectiveness for problem behaviours with individuals who have mental retardation. American Journal on Mental Retardation 101(4): 387–399

Easterbrook P J, Berlin J A, Gopalan R, Matthews D R 1991 Publication bias in clinical research. Lancet 337: 867–872

Emerson E 1996 Early interventions, autism and challenging behaviour. Tizard Learning Disability Review 1(1): 36–38

Gates R 1996 Issues of reliability and validity in the measurement of challenging behaviour behavioural difficulties: a discussion of implications for nursing research and practice. Journal of Clinical Nursing 5(1): 7–12

Gould S J 1981 Mismeasures of man. W W Norton & Co, New York

Grey M 1998 Data collection methods. In: LoBiondo-Wood G, Haber J (eds) Nursing research, methods, critical appraisal and utilisation, 4th edn. Mosby Year Book, Missouri

Heater B S, Becker A M, Olson R K 1988 Nursing interventions and patient outcomes: a meta-analysis of studies. Nursing Research 37: 303–307

Hicks C, Hennessey D 1997 Mixed messages in nursing research: their contribution to the persisting hiatus between evidence and practice. Journal of Advanced Nursing 25(3): 595–601

Hogg J 1992 The administration of psychotropic and anticonvulsant drugs to children with profound intellectual disability and multiple impairments. Journal of Intellectual Disability Research 36: 473–488

Hollon S D Shelton R C, Loosen P T 1991 Cognitive behaviour therapy and pharmacotherapy for depression. Journal of Consulting and Clinical Psychology 59: 88–89

Homer R H 1994 Functional analysis: contributions and future directions. Journal of Applied Behaviour Analysis 27: 401-404

Houton R V, Axelrod S, Bailey J S et al 1988 The right to effective behavioural treatment. Journal of Applied Behaviour Analysis 21: 381-384

Hunt D L, McKibbon K A 1997 Locating and appraising systematic reviews. Annals of Internal Medicine 126: 532-538

Jones L J, Singh N N, Kendall K A 1990 Effects of gentle teaching and alternative treatments on self-injury. In: Repp A, Singh N (N eds) Perspectives on the use of non-aversive and aversive interventions for persons with developmental disabilities. Sycamore Publishing, Sycamore, Illinois

Kaplan H I, Sadock B J 1995 Comprehensive textbook of psychiatry, 6th edn. Williams and Wilkins, Baltimore

Katz J, Peberby A (eds) 1997 Promoting health: knowledge and practice. Open University Press, Buckinghamshire

Kitson A 1997 Using evidence to demonstrate the value of nursing. Nursing Standard 11(28): 34-39

Klein D F, Gittelman R, Quitkin F H, Rifkin A 1980 Diagnosis and drug treatment of psychiatric disorders: adults and children. Williams and Wilkins, Baltimore

Long A, Harrison S 1995 The balance of evidence. Health Services Journal Management Guide, Supplement 6: 1

Lovaas I O, Simmons J Q 1969 Manipulation of self destructive behaviour in three retarded children. Journal of Applied Behaviour Analysis 2: 143-157

McCaughey R E, Jones R S P 1992 The effectiveness of gentle teaching. Mental Handicap 20: 7-14

McDonald S J, Lefebvre C, Clarke M J 1996 Identifying reports of controlled trials in the BMJ and Lancet. British Medical Journal 313: 1116-1117

McGee J J Menolascino F J, Hobbs D C, Menousek P E 1987 Gentle teaching: a non-aversive approach to helping people with mental retardation. Human Sciences Press, New York

Moore P 1995 The utilisation of research in practice. Professional Nurse 10 (8): 536-537

Morgan W K 1997 On evidence, embellishment and efficacy review. Journal of Evaluation in Clinical Practice 3 (2): 117-122

Mudford O C, Hogg J, Roberts J 1997 Interobserver agreement and disagreement in continuous recording exemplified by measurement of behaviour rate. American Journal on Mental Retardation 102(1): 54-66

Muir Gray J A 1997 Evidence-based health care: how to make health policy and management decisions. Churchill Livingstone, Edinburgh

Murphy G 1993 Understanding challenging behaviour. In: Emerson E, McGill P, Mansell J Severe learning disabilities and challenging behaviour: designing high quality services. Chapman and Hall, London

Newell R, Dryden W 1991 Clinical problems: an introduction to the cognitive behavioural approach. In: Dryden W, Golden W (eds) Cognitive behavioural approaches to psychotherapy. Harper and Row, London

Parahoo K 1997 Nursing research: principles, process and issues. Macmillan, London

Rosenberg W, Donald A 1995 Evidence based medicine: an approach to clinical problem solving. British Medical Journal 310: 1122-1126

Sackett D, Rosenberg W 1995 On the need for evidence based medicine. Journal of Public Health Medicine 17(3): 330-334

Sackett D L Rosenberg W M C, Gray J A M, Hayes R B, Richardson W S 1996 Evidenced based medicine: what it is and what it isn't. British Medical Journal 312: 71-72

Sapsford R, Evans J 1979 Evaluation of research. Open University Press, Milton Keynes, block 8, part 1: 14

Schaal D W, Hackenbury T 1994 Toward a functional analysis of drug treatment for behavioural problems of people with developmental disabilities. American Journal on Mental Retardation 99 (2): 123-140

Sines D T 1996 A study to evaluate the effectiveness of the TEACCH project. University of Ulster, Jordanstown

Stark K D, Rouse L W, Livingstone R 1991 Treatment of depression during childhood and adolescence: cognitive behavioural interventions for the individual and family. In: Kendall P C (ed) 1991 Child and adolescent therapy: cognitive behavioural procedures. Guildford Press, New York

Toogood S, Timlin K 1996 The fundamental assessment of challenging behaviour: a comparison of information based experimental and descriptive methods. Journal of Applied Research in Intellectual Disability 9 (3): 206-222

Tsafrir J, Grinberg M 1998 Who needs evidence based health care? Bulletin of the Medical Library Association 86 (1): 40–45

Yoakum C, Yerkes R 1920 Mental tests in the American army. Sidgwick and Jackson, London

Index

A

Absolutist dichotomous thinking, 264

Accountability, 72

Acheulian axe, 19–20

Acting in good faith, 52

Activities
  Gentle Teaching, 165–168
  scheduling/rescheduling, 236–237

Adaptive Behaviour Scale, 38

Adaptive style, 22, 23–27

Addiction, 12
  alcohol *see* Alcohol dependency

Adolescent and Adult Educational Profile (AAPEP), 195, 198, 206

Adrenaline, 17–18, 22–23, 25

Akathisia, 142
  beta-blockers, 151
  trifluoperazine, 155–156

Akinesia, 142

Alcohol dependency, 12, 137–138
  aversion therapy, 137–138, 152
  benzodiazepines, 137, 147
  dance movement therapy case illustration, 120–121
  detoxification, 147
  drug treatment, 137–138, 147, 152
  withdrawal, 137

Alienation, 10

Alprazolam, 146, 147

American Association for Mental Retardation (AAMR), 255
  learning disability model, 45–46

American Nurses Association
  Code of Ethics, 50

American Psychiatric Association
  code of ethics for psychologists, 50, 55
  Diagnostic and Statistical Manual, 132, 135–136

Amisulpride, 140

Amitriptyline, 135, 144, 145

Amoxapine, 145

Anger, 17, 23, 25–26, 81–82, 87, 263
  case illustration, 265–271

Anorexia nervosa, 135
  cognitive behaviour therapy, 275
  drug treatment, 135

Antecedent-based interventions, 236–237

Antecedent-behaviour-consequence triad, 217, 218, 235–245
  record format, 225

Anthropology, 12–13

Anticholinergic drugs, 152

Anticonvulsants
  affective disorders, 151
  psychogenic pain, 138

Antidepressants, 132, 144–146
  bulimia nervosa, 135
  classes, 145
  depression, 134, 144
  drug interactions, 146
  generalised anxiety disorders, 144
  indications, 144
  obsessive-compulsive disorders, 144
  panic disorder, 135, 144
  pharmacokinetics, 145
  phobias, 144

post-traumatic stress disorder, 137
  psychogenic pain, 138
  side-effects, 145–146

Antimuscarinic (antiparkinsonian; anticholinergic) drugs, 152

Antiparkinsonian drugs, 152

Anti-positivism, 3, 293

Antipsychotics, 132, 140–144
  antiadrenergic effects, 143
  antimuscarinic effects, 143
  behavioural difficulties, 155
  classification, 140–141
  dosage, 141
  drug interactions, 143, 144
  ECG, 143
  extrapyramidal side-effects, 140–141, 142–143
  indications, 140
  learning disability, 139
  long-acting depot, 143, 144
  mania, 134
  mechanism of action, 141
  neuroleptic malignant syndrome, 143
  personality disorders, 136
  pharmacokinetics, 141
  schizophrenia, 133
  side-effects, 140–141, 142–144
  weight gain, 143

Anti-Semitism, 80, 81

Anxiety
  APM-A theory (orientation), 22–27
  benzodiazepines, 146
  beta-blockers, 151
  case illustration, 155–156
  cognitive behaviour therapy, 274, 294

Anxiety, *cont'd*
  generalised anxiety disorders, 144
  trifluoperazine, 155–156
Anxiolytics, 146–149
  panic disorder, 135
  post-traumatic stress disorder, 137
  psychogenic pain, 138
APM-A (orientation) theory, 13, 14–27, 42
  and Nonviolent Communication, 27, 79, 85–86, 101–102, 103–104
Applied behaviour analysis, 217, 295
Arbitrary inference, 264
Aristotle, 4–5
Arousal
  and anger, 25
  APM-A (orientation) theory, 14–27
  and expression, 18–26
  and impulsivity, 15, 24
  conscious and unconscious, 20
  limbic, 17, 19, 22
Art, 19–20, 28
Art therapy
  behavioural difficulties, 115–116
  case illustrations, 115–117
  drawings as metaphors, 116–117
  history, 109
  learning disability, 115–116
  and personality, 23–24
  theoretical basis, 111–112
  outcome research, 114
Arts therapies, 107–127
  see also Art therapy; Dance movement therapy; Dramatherapy; Music therapy
  case illustrations, 113, 115–125
  child-centred approach, 108
  effectiveness, 294, 295
  emotional safety, 127
  evidence base, 108, 113–115
  history, 108–111
  limitations, 125–127
  outcome research, 113–114
  philosophical basis, 112
  physical requirements, 126, 296
  process research, 114–115
  state registration, 108–109
  supervision, 126

  theoretical basis, 111–112
  training, 126, 130
Assault, 62–63, 66
Association for the Advancement of Behaviour Therapy, 255
Association for Dance Movement Therapy, 111, 130
Association for Persons with Severe Handicaps (TASH), 255
Association of Professional Music Therapists, 110, 130
Attention, 14–27
Attention deficit-hyperactivity disorder *see* Hyperkinetic disorder
Attention-seeking, 218
Authoritarianism, 160–161
Autism *see* Autistic spectrum disorder
Autism Europe (AE), 213
Autism Research Unit, 213
Autism Resources (website), 213
Autistic spectrum disorder (ASD)
  aetiology, 186
  assessment, 194–195
  behavioural approach, 190
  case illustrations, 202–204
  characteristics, 186–187
  cognitive strategies, 190
  communication deficit, 187–188, 190, 191, 194
  continuum, 186–187
  developmental profile, 195–196
  family stress, 206–207
  goals for intervention, 187
  inclusion, 193
  individuality, 193, 195
  music therapy case illustration, 122–124
  prevalence, 186
  rating scales, 195, 206
  social skills, 187–188, 190
  structured teaching, 185, 188–209
  time concept, 197
  visual processing, 190
Autonomic nervous system, 17–20, 22
Autonomy, 20, 52–53
Aversion therapy, 138, 152
Aversive control, 54, 162–163, 292
  and Gentle Teaching, 177–178
Awareness *see* Arousal

B
Bandura, A., 10, 82, 217, 259
Barbiturates, 132, 149
Battery, 63–64, 66–67
Bayley Scales of Infant Development, 195
Beck, Aaron T., 260, 264
Behaviour
  applied behavioural analysis, 217, 295
  functional alternatives, 237–240
  interactional model, 263
  mediational model, 259
  psychological theories, 5–10, 33–34
  socially acceptable/ unacceptable, 25
  theories, 4–13
  understanding, 3–28
Behaviour modification, 6–7
  ethics, 54–55
Behavioural difficulties (challenging behaviour)
  analogue studies, 230–233
  art therapy case illustration, 115–116
  assessment, 222–233
  behavioural interventions, 215–249
  benzodiazepines, 155
  bio-physiological factors, 229–233
  drug treatment, 156
  drug treatment case illustration, 154–155
  environmental factors, 229–233
  functional hypotheses, 229–233
  Gentle Teaching *see* Gentle Teaching
  learning disability, 139
  legal issues, 61–68
  skill deficits, 234
  terminology, 32, 35–36
Behavioural interventions, 215–249
  antecedent based approaches, 236–237
  approaches to behaviour change, 235–245
  assessment, 222–233, 246, 247–249
  autism, 190
  behaviour based approaches, 237–240

Behavioural interventions, *cont'd*
  behavioural difficulties,
      215–249
  cognitive *see* Cognitive
      behavioural
      interventions
  consent, 247, 248
  consequence based
      approaches, 243–245
  costs/benefits, 248
  displacement model, 237–240
  early intervention, 248
  effectiveness, 293
  ethics, 246, 247
  evaluation, 248–249
  extinction, 243–244
  functional alternatives,
      237–240
  versus Gentle Teaching,
      175–177, 179–180
  history, 216–217
  interviews, 223–225
  limitations, 245–247
  observational assessment,
      225–229
  outcomes analysis, 235
  planning, 233–235, 248
  practical applications,
      222–233
  prevention, 248
  punishment, 217, 219,
      243–245
  rating scales, 224–225
  reinforcement *see*
      Reinforcement
  response consistency,
      239–240
  response cost, 245
  response interruption, 237,
      243
  risk analysis, 235
  self-management approaches,
      240–241
  structured teaching, 190, 191,
      205
  theoretical basis, 218–221
  time-out, 54, 55, 244
  topographically compatible
      behaviours, 240
  visual/facial screening, 245
Behaviourism, 5–7, 33–34
  cognitive behavioural
      interventions, 258–259
  Gentle Teaching, 179–181,
      295
Beliefs, 260–262
Beneficence, 52–53

Benzhexol, 152
Benzodiazepines, 132, 146–148
  absorption, 147
  alcohol dependency, 137, 147
  anxiety, 146
  behaviour difficulties, 155
  dosages, 147
  drug interactions, 148
  elimination half-life, 147
  epilepsy, 146
  indications, 146–148
  overdose, 148
  panic disorder, 135
  personality disorders, 136
  pharmacokinetics, 148
  potency, 147
  psychogenic pain, 138
  psychosis, 147
  receptors, 147
  side-effects, 148
  status epilepticus, 147
  withdrawal, 148
Benztropine, 152
Beta-blockers, 151
Biological alternatives, 25
Biperiden, 152
Blindness
  autistic spectrum disorder,
      186
  socialisation of clients, 43–44
Bolam test, 58
Boyle, Jimmy, 25–26
British Association of Art
      Therapists (BAAT), 109,
      130
British Association for
      Behavioural and
      Cognitive
      Psychotherapies, 279
British Association of
      Dramatherapists, 110,
      130
British Institute of Learning
      Disabilities, 255
British Psychological Society,
      279
British Society for Music
      Therapy, 110, 130
Bromide, 149
Bulimia nervosa, 135, 144
Buspirone, 149
Butylpiperidines, 140
Butyrophenones, 140

C
Camphor, 152
Carbamazepine, 151

drug interactions, 151
  mania, 151
  manic-depressive illness, 151
  personality disorder, 136
  psychogenic pain, 138
  side-effects, 151
Caregiver Interactional
      Observation System
      (CIOS), 178
Caring for People (Department
      of Health), 71, 73
Categories of behavioural
      distress, 38–39
Challenging behaviour *see*
      Behavioural difficulties
Change
  behavioural, 235–245
  mutual, 162
  setting events, 237
Chemotherapy *see* Drugs
Child-centred approaches, 40
  arts therapies, 108
Child development model of
      intervention, 40–41
Childhood Autism Rating Scale
      (CARS), 195, 206
Childhood sexual abuse case
      illustration, 119–120
Children and Young Person's Act
      (1933), 62, 71
Children's Act (1989), 60, 67
Chloral hydrate, 132, 149
Chlordiazepoxide, 146, 147
Chlormethiazole, 149
Chlorpromazine, 140
  anorexia nervosa, 135
  dosage, 141
  metabolism, 141
  potency, 141
  side-effects, 140, 143
  weight gain, 143
CINAHL, 291
Citalopram, 145
Citizen's Charter, 54
Citizenship, 28, 192
Citrated calcium carbimide, 152
Civil law, 60–61, 64–68
Classical conditioning, 5–7,
      216–217
Clobazam, 146, 147
Clomipramine, 134
Clonazepam, 146
Clozapine, 140
  dosage, 141
  side-effects, 141
  tardive dyskinesia, 143
Cochrane Library, 291

Cognitive approaches, 7–9
Cognitive behavioural
        interventions, 257–276
    anger case illustration,
        265–271
    anorexia nervosa, 275
    anxiety, 274, 294
    autism, 190
    and behaviourism, 258–259
    case illustrations, 265–274
    cognitivists, 259–260,
        262–263
    constructs (schemata; beliefs;
        concepts), 260–262
    depression, 294
    effectiveness, 294
    evaluation, 274–275
    history, 258–260
    holism, 263–264
    humanistic, 263–265
    learning disability, 265–272
    limitations, 275–276
    motivation, 276, 294
    non-cognitivists, 258–259
    overcoming traumatic
        experiences case
        illustration, 272–274
    personal growth, 264–265
    personality disorders, 275
    philosophy, 263–265
    practical requirements, 296
    and psychoanalysis, 258–259
    self-control, 271–272, 276
    strengths, 274–275
    structured teaching, 191
    theoretical development,
        260–263
Cognitive deficits/distortions,
        263
Cognitive needs, 19
Common law, 60
Communication
    autism, 187–188, 190, 194
    compassionate see Nonviolent
        Communication
    father/son, 93–95
    interpersonal skills, 28
    nonviolent see Nonviolent
        Communication
    skills, developmental
        approach, 191
    structured teaching, 205
Community psychology, 83–84
Compassion, 81–82
Compassionate communication
    see Nonviolent
        Communication

Compliance
    behavioural interventions,
        218
    drug treatment, 153–154
Conditioning, 5–6, 216–217
Connectionism, 5
Consciousness, 20
Consent, 68–70
    behavioural interventions,
        247, 248
Consequence-based
        interventions, 243–245
Constructional orientation, 221
Constructs, 260–262
Costs of treatment
    behavioural interventions, 248
    drug treatment, 296
    structured teaching, 207,
        293–294
Council for Professions
        Supplementary to
        Medicine, 108
Creativity, 19–20
    and adaptive style, 23–27
Crime
    reformed criminals, 25–26
    sociological theories, 12
Criminal law, 60, 62–64
Critical Appraisal Skills
        Programme (CASP),
        290, 293
Crown Prosecution Service, 60,
        61
Culture, 12–13
Cyproheptadine, 135

D
Dance movement therapy,
        110–111
    outcome research, 114
    case illustrations, 120–121
    depression, 120–121
    learning disability, 121
    theoretical basis, 111–112
Dangerousness, 70–71
Dantrolene, 143
Deafness, 186
Deduction, 5
Defence mechanisms, 7
Defusion, 172
Delirium tremens, 137
Denial, 7
Deontology, 52
Depression, 133–134
    see also Antidepressants
    cognitive behaviour therapy,
        274

dance movement therapy case
        illustration, 120–121
drug treatment, 133–134, 144
ECT, 134, 152
lithium, 150
noradrenaline, 145
Descriptions of behavioural
        distress, 38–39
Destruction, 19–20
Developmentally Delayed
        Children's Behaviour
        Checklist, 59
Deviants, 11, 12, 27
Diagnosis, 41
Diagnostic and Statistical Manual
        (DSM), 132
Diazepam, 134, 146
    absorption, 148
    elimination half-life, 147
    overdose, 148
    status epilepticus, 147
Differential diagnosis, 41
Differential reinforcement of
        alternative behaviours
        (DRA), 242
Differential reinforcement of
        incompatible
        behaviours (DRI),
        242–243
Differential reinforcement of
        other behaviour (DRO),
        241–243
Disability
    medical model, 32
    perceptions of, 34–35
    terminology, 31–47
Disintegrative disorder, 186
Disorientation, 15–17
Displacement model of
        behavioural change,
        237–240
Distance, 160–161
Distress, definitions, 36–37
Distributed practice, 240
Disulfiram, 138, 152
Division TEACCH see TEACCH
Domestic violence, 95–101
Dopamine receptors, 141
Doxepin, 145
Dramatherapy
    case illustrations, 118–120
    childhood sexual abuse,
        119–120
    history, 110
    learning disability, 118–119
    theoretical basis, 111–112
    outcome research, 114

Drives, 7
Droperidol, 140, 142
Drug addiction, 12
Drug treatment, 131–156
  alcohol dependency, 137–138, 152
  anorexia nervosa, 135
  behavioural difficulties, 156
  bulimia nervosa, 135, 144
  case illustrations, 154–156
  compliance, 153–154
  cost-effectiveness, 296
  depression, 133–134, 144
  effectiveness, 59, 293, 296
  evidence, 293
  history, 131–132
  hyperkinetic disorder, 136
  inappropriate use, 296
  insomnia, 138
  learning disability, 139, 154–155
  legal issues, 57–60
  mania, 134
  negligence, 58–59
  non-psychotropic, 151–152
  obsessive-compulsive disorder, 134, 144, 293
  overuse, 132
  panic disorder, 135, 144, 293
  personality disorders, 136
  pharmacotherapy, 139–152
  psychogenic pain, 138
  psychotropic, 140–151
  record-keeping, 60
  schizophrenia, 133
  sensory extinction, 244
  side-effects, 132
  withdrawing treatment, 60
Durkheim, Émile, 10
Duty, 52
Duty of care, 67–68
Dysarthria, 142
Dystonias, 142

E
Education (schools), 28
  expectations and child's self-concept, 43
  Nonviolent Communication case illustrations, 91–101
  Nonviolent Communication programmes, 84–85
Edwards, S., 50, 53
Effectiveness
  arts therapies, 294, 295
  behavioural interventions, 293

cognitive behavioural interventions, 294
  drug treatment, 59, 293, 296
  ethics, 292
  evidence, 283–284, 286, 291, 292–295
  Gentle Teaching, 175–177, 294–295
  Nonviolent Communication, 294, 295
  structured teaching, 206–207, 293–294
  TEACCH, 293–294
Ego, 7
Elective mutism, 186
Electroconvulsive therapy (ECT), 134, 152–153
Electronic databases, 291–292
Elementalism, 3
Ellis, Albert, 260
EMBASE, 291
Emerson, E., 35–36, 39, 217, 229
Emotion, 14–18, 23, 25–27, 88–89, 101, 103, 127, 258, 260, 262–263
Emotional deprivation, 186
Emotional literacy, 28
Emotional safety, 127
Empathy, 80, 86–87
Enculturation, 12–13
English National Board, 279
Epilepsy
  benzodiazepines, 146
  phenobarbitone, 149
  status epilepticus, 147, 149
Equity, 162
Errors of thinking, 264
Ethics, 49–51
  behaviour modification, 54–55
  behavioural interventions, 246, 247
  codes, 50, 55
  and effectiveness, 292
  Gentle Teaching, 161
  group, 50
  personal, 50
  philosophical, 50
  professional behaviour/practice, 50, 52–53
  reinforcement, 246
Ethnography, 288–289
Eugenics movement, 34
European Association of Mental Health in Mental Retardation, 255
European Union, 84–85

Evidence, 283–297
  critical appraisal skills hierarchy, 290
  definition, 287
  drug treatment, 293
  of effectiveness, 283–284, 286, 291, 292–295
  fallibility, 285
  gathering, 290–292
  recording, 294–295
  reliability, 287–292
  research see Research
  scientific, 284–287
  validity, 287–292
Evidence-based health care, 284, 285–287
Evidence-based medicine (EBM), 286
Evidence-based practice, 32, 41, 42
  arts therapies, 108, 113–115
  Nonviolent Communication, 84–86
Evolution, 13, 14, 15, 21
Expression, 14, 15, 20–28
  and arousal, 17–19, 25–26
  of behavioural distress, 37–39
Externalisers, 22–23, 24
Extinction, 243
  sensory, 244
Extroverts, 23
Eysenck, H.J., 23

F
False imprisonment, 62, 65–66
Family stress, 206–207
Family therapy, 83
Fear, 17, 19, 23, 24, 26, 261
Feelings see Emotion
Fight-flight response, 17
Flumazenil, 148
Fluoxetine, 134, 144, 145
Flupenthixol, 140, 143
Fluphenazine, 143
Flurazepam, 146
Fluvoxamine, 134, 144, 145
Freud, Sigmund, 7
Fulcher, G., 45
Functional analysis, 41, 247–249, 293
Functional Analysis Interview Form, 223
Funkenstein, D.H., 17

G
Gamma-aminobutyric acid (GABA), 147

Gates, B., 33, 34
Gear, J., 13, 14, 18, 20, 23, 28, 79
Generalised anxiety disorders, 144
Geneva Convention on Human Rights, 51
Gentle Teaching, 41, 159–181
    activities, 165–168
    aversive properties, 177–178
    versus behaviour therapy, 175–177, 179–180
    behavioural techniques, 179–181, 295
    criticisms of, 175–180
    development, 162–163
    effectiveness, 175–177, 294–295
    entry points, 168–169
    equity, 162
    ethics, 161
    history, 162–163
    information gathering, 164–165
    mini-breaks, 167–168
    mutual change, 162
    objective evaluations, 178–179
    organisational principles, 173–175, 296
    outcomes, 178–179, 294–295
    philosophy, 160–161
    practical application, 163–173
    respect, 162
    response to behavioural distress, 169–170
    self-injurious behaviour, 175
    training, 173–175, 182–183
    value system, 161–162
Gestalt psychology, 7–9
Global mediation, 84

H
Hakeem, Michael, 82
Haloperidol, 140
    dosage, 141
    metabolism, 141
    schizophrenia, 133
    side-effects, 140, 142
Hazards, 70
Health and Safety at Work Act (1974), 72
High intensity, low frequency behaviour, 171–173
Holism, 3, 263–264
Human rights, 51–52
Humanistic psychology, 9–10, 163

cognitive behavioural interventions, 263–265
Husserl, Edmund, 9
Hyperkinetic disorder (attention deficit-hyperactivity disorder; ADHD), 135–136
    drug treatment, 136
    stimulants, 151
Hyperparathyroidism, 150
Hyperthyroidism, 150
Hypnotics, 146–149
    insomnia, 138
Hypothyroidism, 150

I
Id, 7
Imagination, 19–20
Imipramine, 135, 145
    depression, 144
    panic disorder, 293
Impulsivity, 7, 15, 24
Inclusion, 193
Inclusiveness, 192
Individual differences, 22–23, 24, 27
Individual educational programmes (IEPs), 195, 196
Individuality, 193, 195
Induction, 5
Information processing, 20
Informed consent *see* Consent
Insight, 20
Insomnia, 138
Institute for Applied Behaviour Analysis, 255
Intelligence, 25
Interaction, 220, 221
Interactional model of behaviour, 263
Interactional styles, 236
Internal world, 7
Internalisers, 22–24
International Classification of Mental and Behavioural Disorders version, 10 (ICD-10), 132–133
    alcohol dependency, 137
    depression, 133
    hyperkinetic disorder, 135–136
    learning disability, 139
    personality disorders, 136
International League for Societies for the Mentally Handicapped, 53–54

Interpersonal communication skills, 28
Interpersonal styles, 236
Interventions, 4
    antecedent-based, 236–237
    assessment, 296
    behavioural *see* Behavioural interventions
    child development model, 40–41
    client's rights, 54–55
    cognitive behavioural *see* Cognitive behavioural interventions
    consequence-based, 243–245
    early, 248
    Gentle Teaching *see* Gentle Teaching
    language of, 39–42
    limitations, 292
    medical model, 41
    models of service delivery, 39–42
    organisational factors, 296
    personal approach, 42
    psychotherapeutic, 41
    research evidence, 292–296
    settings, 296
    socio-ecological models, 42
    technical model, 41–42
Interviews, 223–225
Introverts, 23
Irish Society for Autism (ISA), 213

J
Johnson, Bob, 26
Justice, 52–53

K
Kelly, George, 259–260, 261
Koffka, Kurt, 7–9
Köhler, Wolfgang, 7–9

L
Laban movement analysis, 111, 114
Labelling, 10–11, 37, 43, 44–45
Language, 31–47
    of behavioural distress, 35–37
    impact of message, 43–45
    of intervention, 39–42
    psycholinguistics, 190, 191, 205
    sociological approaches, 45
    of special services, 45

Learning disability, 139
    AAMR model, 45–46
    art therapy case illustration,
        115–116
    aversive practices see Aversive
        control
    behavioural difficulties, 139
    client's rights, 53–55, 162–163
    cognitive behavoural
        intervention case
        illustrations, 265–272
    dance movement therapy
        case illustration, 121
    definition, 45–46
    dramatherapy case
        illustration, 118–119
    drug treatment, 139
    drug treatment case
        illustration, 154–155
    Gentle Teaching see Gentle
        Teaching
    high intensity, low frequency
        behaviour, 171–173
    idiopathic, 186
    labelling, 44
    legal issues, 57–68
    low intensity, high frequency
        behaviour, 170–171
    music therapy case
        illustration, 124–125
    participation, 164–165
    prevalence of behavioural
        distress, 37
    psychiatric disorders, 139
    self-concept, 44
    terminology, 31–47
Learning theories, 5–6, 216–217
Legal issues, 57–68
    behavioural difficulties, 61–68
    client's rights, 54–55, 162–163
    common law, 60
    criminal law, 60, 62–64
    definitions, 60–61
    drug treatment, 57–60
    learning disability, 57–68
Leiter International Performance
    Scale, 195
Levy, A. & Kahan, B., 49, 55–56
Liberty, restriction of, 62, 65–66
Literature searches, 291–292
Lithium, 149–150
    personality disorder, 136
Loprazolam, 146, 147
Lorazepam, 146, 147
Lormetazepam, 146, 147
Low intensity, high frequency
    behaviour, 170–171

Loxapine, 141
Luria, A.R., 18

M
Magnification, 264
Makaton, 197
Maladaptive postures, 160–161
Mania, 134
    carbamazepine, 151
    drug treatment, 134
    ECT, 152
    lithium, 150
Manic-depressive illness, 150,
    151
Maprotiline, 145
Maslow, Abraham, 10, 163
Mediation, global, 84
Mediational model of behaviour,
    259
Medical models
    of disability, 32
    of intervention, 41
Medication see Drugs
MEDLINE, 291–292
Meichenbaum, Donald, 260
Memory, 14–27
Mental Deficiency Acts (1913,
    1927), 33
Mental Health Act (1959), 71
Mental Health Act (1983), 33, 34,
    62, 153
Mental Health Foundation, 36
Mental retardation see Learning
    disability
Meprobamate, 149
Merrill-Palmer scale, 195
Metaphysics, 49–50
Methohexitone, 149
Methylphenidate, 136
Metrazol, 152
Minimisation, 264
Minnesota cognitive-
    pharmacotherapy
    project, 275
Mirtazapine, 145
Moclobemide, 145
Monoamine oxidase inhibitors
    (MAOIs), 145, 146
Mood stabilisers, 149–151
Moral philosophy, 50–51
Morphine, 132
Motivation, 276, 294
Motivational Assessment Scale,
    224
Multimodal Diagnostic and
    Intervention Model,
    224

Music therapy
    autism, 122–124
    case illustrations, 122–125
    history, 109–110
    learning disability, 124–125
    outcome research, 113
    theoretical basis, 111–112
Mutism, elective, 186

N
Naltrexone, 244
Narcolepsy, 151
National Arts Therapies Research
    Committee, 115, 130
National Association of
    Developmental
    Disabilities Councils,
    255
National Autistic Society (NAS),
    213
National Health Service and
    Community Care Act
    (1990), 54
Needs
    cognitive, 19
    first- and second-order, 20
    Maslow's hierarchy, 10
    Nonviolent Communication,
        89–90
    orientation needs, 14–20
    sensory, 19
    spiritual, 19
    universal human needs, 90
Nefazodone, 145
Negligence, 67–68
    long-term medication, 58–59
Neuroleptic drugs see
    Antipsychotics
Neuroleptic malignant
    syndrome, 143
Neuroticism, 23
Neurotransmitters, 141, 145
Nitrazepam, 146, 147
Nocturnal enuresis, 144
Non-compliance see Compliance
Non-maleficence, 52–53
Nonviolent Communication
    (NVC), 79–104
    and APM-A theory, 27, 79,
        85–86, 100–102,
        103–104
    case illustrations, 91–100
    classroom case illustration,
        91–92
    and community psychology,
        83–84
    definition, 80

Nonviolent Communication
    (NVC), *cont'd*
  domestic violence counselling
    case illustration, 95–100
  effectiveness, 294, 295
  empathy, 80, 86–87
  evidence base, 84–86
  and family therapy, 83
  father-son communication
    case illustration, 93–95
  feelings *versus*
    interpretations, 88–89
  global mediation, 84
  identifying needs, 89–90
  and labelling, 11
  limitations, 102
  misconceptions about,
    102–103
  model, 87–91
  needs, 89–90
  observations *versus*
    evaluations, 87–89
  and personal growth, 80–84
  process, 86–87
  programmes, 84–85
  and psychological theories,
    82–83
  qualities, 102–103
  requests *versus* demands, 90
  training, 84, 103
  usefulness, 102
  uses, 102–104
Noradrenaline, 17–18, 22–23, 25,
    145
Noradrenaline re-uptake
    inhibitors, 145
Normalisation, 162, 192
Nortriptyline, 145

O
Object relations theory, 7
Objectivity, 3
Observational assessment,
    225–229
Observational bias, 284–285
Obsessive-compulsive disorder,
    134
  drug treatment, 134, 144, 293
Oculogyric crisis, 142
Olanzapine, 140, 143
Operant conditioning, 6–7,
    216–217
Orientation, 15–17
  constructional, 221
  needs, 14–20
  theory *see* APM-A theory
Orphenadrine, 152

Outcome research
  arts therapies, 113–114
  behavioural interventions,
    235
  Gentle Teaching, 178–179,
    294–295
  structured teaching, 205–
    206
Over-generalisation, 264
Over-protectiveness, 160–161
Oxazepam, 146
  absorption, 148
  dosage, 147
  elimination half-life, 147

P
Pain
  chronic, 144
  psychogenic, 138
Panic disorder, 134–135
  drug treatment, 135, 144, 293
Paraldehyde, 149
Parasympathetic nervous system,
    17–22, 24
Parents and Professionals and
    Autism (PAPA), 213
Parkinsonism, 142
Paroxetine, 134, 145
Participation, 164–165
Patient's Charter, 54
Pavlov, I.P., 5, 17, 216
Perception, 8, 9, 15–22, 27
  of disability, 34–35
  orientation theory, 14–27
Perceptual disorders, 23
Person-centred approaches, 192
Person Interactional
    Observation System
    (PIOS), 178
Personal construct theory,
    261–262
Personal growth, 80–84, 264–
    265
Personalisation, 264
Personality, 15
  individual differences, 22–23,
    24, 27
Personality disorders, 11, 15, 23,
    136
  cognitive behaviour therapy,
    275
  drug treatment, 136
Personality traits, 25
Phenobarbitone, 149
Phenomenological approaches,
    9–10
Phenothiazines, 140

Phenytoin, 138
Philosophy, 4, 49–51
Phobias, 144
Physical restraint, 55
Pimozide, 140
  arrhythmias, 143
  dosage, 141
  side-effects, 140, 142
Pindown, 55–57
Plato, 4
Political correctness, 31–32
Positive behaviour support, 221
Positivism, 3, 293
Post-traumatic stress disorder,
    136–137
Prevalence of behavioural
    distress, 37
Prevention, 248
Proactivity, 3
Problem-solving capacities, 20
Procyclidine, 152
Projection, 7
Protriptyline, 145
Psychiatric disorders, 139
Psycho Educational Profile (PEP),
    194–195, 206
  revised (PEP-R), 194–195,
    198–200
Psychoanalysis, 7
  and cognitive behavioural
    interventions, 258–259
Psychodynamic approaches, 7
Psychogenic pain, 138
Psycholinguistics, 190, 191, 205
Psychological survival, 14–27, 42
Psychological theories, 4, 5–10
  and arts therapies, 112
  behaviourism *see*
    Behaviourism
  and Nonviolent
    Communication, 82–83
Psychopathology, 24–25
Psychosis, 147
Psychosurgery, 153
Psychotherapeutic interventions,
    41
Psychoticism, 23
Punishment, 217, 219, 243–245

Q
Quality of life, 219
Quetiapine, 140

R
Rabbit syndrome, 142
Randomised controlled trials,
    289–290

Rating scales
    autism, 195, 206
    behavioural interventions,
        224-225
Rational emotive therapy (RET),
    260
Rationalisation, 7
Rationing, 284
Reactivity, 3
Reboxetine, 145
Recklessness, 63, 64
Regression, 26-27
Reinforcement, 6, 217, 219-220,
        229-230, 234-235,
        239-240
    differential reinforcement,
        241-243
    ethics, 246
    intervals, 243
    limitations, 246
    punishment, 217, 219,
        243-245
    response cost, 245
    visual screening, 175, 245
Relationships, 7, 31, 32, 40, 45-46
    and communication, 28, 42,
        83-87, 92-95, 170,
        186-188
    Gentle Teaching, 159-161, 169
    skills, 28
Repression, 7
Research, 287-295
    arts therapies, 113-115
    bias, 291
    ethnography, 288-289
    experiments, 288-289
    interventions, 292-296
    literature searches, 291-292
    outcomes see Outcome
        research
    quantitative versus qualitative,
        287-288
    randomised controlled trials,
        289-290
    surveys, 288-289
Respect, 162
Response consistency, 239-240
Response cost, 245
Response interruption, 237, 243
Restriction of liberty, 62
Retreatism, 12
Rett's syndrome, 186
Reversible monoamine oxidase
        inhibitors (RMAOIs),
        145
Rights of client, 53-55, 162-163
Risk assessment, 70-72, 235

Risk management, 70-72
Risperidone, 140
    antiadrenergic effects, 143
    dosage, 141
Rogers, Carl, 9-10, 79, 81, 82,
        163, 264-265
Rosenberg, Marshall, 79-104

S
Scatter plot analysis, 225-226,
        227-228
Schemata, 260-262
Schizophrenia, 133
    catatonic, 152-153
    creativity, 23
    drug treatment, 133
    ECT, 152-153
Schools see Education
Scientific method, 4-5
Scottish Society for Autistic
        Children (SSAC), 214
Seclusion, 55, 62
Seedhouse, D., 50, 51, 52
Selective abstraction, 264
Self-actualisation, 9-10, 162-163
Self-concept, 43, 44
Self-consequation, 241
Self-control
    case illustration, 271-272
    cognitive behavioural
        interventions, 271-272,
        276
Self-destruction, 19-20
Self-empathy, 86-87
Self-esteem, 10, 44
Self-evaluation, 241
Self-hatred, 80-81
Self-injurious behaviour (SIB)
    Gentle Teaching, 175
    lithium, 150
    naltrexone, 244
    restraint, 66-67
    visual screening, 175
Self-instruction, 241
Self-instructional training, 260
Self-management training,
        240-241
Self-monitoring, 241
Semantic pragmatic disorder, 186
Sensory extinction, 244
Sensory needs, 19
Serotonin, 145
Serotonin reuptake inhibitors
        (SSRIs), 134, 145
Sertindole, 140
Sertraline, 145
Setting events, 237

Sexuality, 71
Skills
    behaviour difficulties, 234
    communication, 187-188,
        190, 191, 194
    deficits discrepancy analysis,
        225
    relationships, 28
    social, 187-188, 190
Skinner, B.F., 6-7, 217, 225
Slee, R., 32, 45
Smilekeepers programme, 84-85
Social exclusion, 10
Social learning theory, 10, 217,
        259
Social role valorisation, 162
Social skills, 187-188, 190
Socio-ecological model of
        intervention, 42
Sociological theories, 4, 10-12
Sodium valproate, 151
Special needs children, 24
Spiritual needs, 19
Status epilepticus, 147, 149
Stimulants, 151
Stress response, 17
Structured teaching, 185,
        188-209
    assessment, 194-195
    autism, 185, 188-209
    behavioural techniques, 190,
        191, 205
    building on strengths, 193
    case illustrations, 202-204
    cognitive techniques, 191
    communication, 205
    costs, 207, 293-294
    dimensions, 191-192
    effectiveness, 206-207,
        293-294
    empirical basis, 204-207
    environment, 196-197
    evaluation, 193, 198-201
    history, 188-190
    implementation, 195-198
    individual educational
        programme (IEP),195,
        196
    integrated approach, 190-192
    introducing, 209
    key concepts, 188, 194
    limitations, 207
    objectives, 189
    outcome measures, 205-206
    parental involvement, 193,
        204, 207-208
    philosophical basis, 192-193

Structured teaching, *cont'd*
  planning, 195-198
  practical application, 194-204
  psycho-educational model, 190-191
  psycholinguistic approach, 190, 191, 205
  quality enhancement, 201
  resources, 212-214
  structured classrooms, 196-197
  TEACCH programmes *see* TEACCH
  teaching environment, 196-197
  teaching goals, 196
  theoretical basis, 190-192
  time structure, 197
  timetables, 197, 198
  training, 192
  visual instruction, 198
  work system, 198
Styles, 22-23
  adaptive, 22, 23-27
  artistic, 23-24
  dynamic model, 22-23
  external, 22-23, 24
  individual, 14, 15, 22-28, 236
  interactional, 236
  internal, 22-24
  interpersonal, 236
Subjectivity, 3
Sublimation, 7
Suicide, 10
Sulpiride, 141
Sumarah, J., 40, 42
Superego, 7
Surrogate actions, 51
Suxamethonium chloride, 54
Sympathetic nervous system, 17-22, 24
Symptoms, 41
Szasz, Thomas, 10-11, 82

T
Tardive dyskinesia, 142-143

TEACCH, 185, 188-190, 193-194, 204-209, 213
  effectiveness, 293-294
  environment, 296
Technical model of intervention, 41-42
Temazepam, 146, 147
Terminology, 31-47
Therapeutic holding, 55
Therapeutic interventions *see* Interventions
Thiamine deficiency, 137
Thinking errors, 264
Thioridazine, 140
  dosage, 141
  side-effects, 140, 143
Thioxanthenes, 140
Thorndike, E.L., 5, 217
Threats, responses to, 18
Time, concept of, 197
Time-based lag sequential analysis, 229
Time-out, 54, 55, 244
Tolman, E.C., 5, 7, 259
Torticollis, 142
Torts, 61, 64-68
Touching, unlawful, 63-64
Training
  arts therapies, 126, 130
  Gentle Teaching, 173-175, 182-183
  Nonviolent Communication, 84, 104
  structured teaching, 192
Tranquillisers, major *see* Antipsychotics
Traumatic experiences, 272-274
Trazodone, 145
Trespass to the person, 64
Trifluoperazine, 140
  akathisia, 155-156
  anxiety case illustration, 155-156
  dosage, 141
  side-effects, 140, 142, 155-156

Trimipramine, 145
Trust, 26

U
Unconsciousness, 20
UNICEF, 84
United Kingdom Central Council for Nursing, Midwifery and Health Visiting (UKCC)
  Code of Conduct, 50, 52-53, 72
  Exercising Accountability, 72
United Nations Declaration of Human Rights, 52
Universal human needs, 90
Utilitarianism, 52

V
Validity, 287-292
Venlafaxine, 145
Violence
  domestic, 95-101
  non-physical, 80-81
  personal, 64, 66-67
  roots of, 81-82
Visual instruction, 198
Visual processing, 190
Visual screening, 175, 245
Vitamin E, 143
Vulnerability, 20-23, 27
  risk assessment, 70-71

W
Watson, J.B., 5, 6, 216
Wechsler intelligence tests, 195
Weight gain, 143
Wernicke-Korsakoff syndrome, 137
Wertheimer, Max, 7-9
Wessler, R.L., 261, 264-265
Wolfensberger, W., 34, 53, 162

Z
Zolpidem, 149
Zopiclone, 149
Zotepine, 140